Clinical Skills for Nursing Practice

Employing an evidence-based approach, this comprehensive textbook introduces the core clinical skills and competencies a newly qualified nurse is required to have for professional practice. It is divided into five broad sections looking at:

- **Care and compassion and communication**, including personal care and pain assessment
- **Essential skills**, including observations, monitoring and emergency management
- **Organisational aspects of care**, including moving and handling, and wound care
- **Safety and protection**, including medicine management and infection control
- **Nutrition and fluid balance**, including hydration and nutrition.

Designed to allow readers to develop and enhance their clinical skills with one key textbook, each chapter contains learning outcomes, recommendations for practice, case studies, activities, 'clinical significance' highlights and step-by-step guides to important procedures.

This invaluable clinical skills textbook is an essential reference for pre-registration nursing students of all fields of nursing.

Tina Moore is a Senior Lecturer in Adult Nursing at Middlesex University, UK. She teaches nursing assessment, clinical skills and care interventions for both pre-qualifying and post-qualifying nurses. She is also a Middlesex University Teaching Fellow.

Sheila Cunningham is an Associate Professor in Adult Nursing at Middlesex University, UK. She has a breadth of experience teaching nurses both pre- and post-registration and she supports mentors supporting students in practice. She is also a Middlesex University Teaching Fellow and holds a Principal Fellowship at the Higher Education Academy. She is currently programme leader for the BSc European nursing and is passionate about the future of nursing and nurse education.

Clinical Skills for Nursing Practice

Edited by Tina Moore and Sheila Cunningham

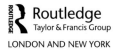

Routledge
Taylor & Francis Group

LONDON AND NEW YORK

First published 2017
by Routledge
2 Park Square, Milton Park, Abingdon, Oxon OX14 4RN

and by Routledge
711 Third Avenue, New York, NY 10017

Routledge is an imprint of the Taylor & Francis Group, an informa business

British Library Cataloguing-in-Publication Data
A catalogue record for this book is available from the British Library

Library of Congress Cataloging in Publication Data
Names: Moore, Tina, 1962- , editor. | Cunningham, Sheila, 1962- , editor.
Title: Clinical skills for nursing practice / edited by Tina Moore and Sheila Cunningham.
Description: Abingdon, Oxon ; New York, NY : Routledge, 2017. | Includes bibliographical references and index.
Identifiers: LCCN 2016014016| ISBN 9781138791190 (hardback) | ISBN 9780273767947 (pbk.) | ISBN 9781315528779 (ebook)
Subjects: | MESH: Nursing Care--methods | Clinical Competence
Classification: LCC RT51 | NLM WY 100.1 | DDC 610.73--dc23
LC record available at http://lccn.loc.gov/2016014016

ISBN: 978-1-138-79119-0 (hbk)
ISBN: 978-0-273-76794-7 (pbk)
ISBN: 978-1-315-52877-9 (ebk)

Typeset in Times
by Typeset by Fakenham Prepress Solutions, Fakenham, Norfolk NR21 8NN
Printed by Ashford Colour Press Ltd.

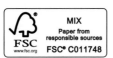

Contents

PART II: Essential and Advanced Skills

PART III: Organisational aspects of care

PART IV: Safety and protection

PART V: Nutrition and fluid balance

Figures

Colour plates

The colour plate section appears between pages 72 and 73 of the text.

Tables

Contributors

Dee Anderson (RN, RNT, MA, BSc (Hons), PGCHE)
Lecturer in Child Nursing, Middlesex University

Nora Cooper (RN, BA (Hons) PGCEA, MA (Higher Education))
Senior Lecturer, Practice Based Learning, Middlesex University

Sheila Cunningham (DProf, MSc, PGDipEd (Adult), BSc (Hons), RN, RNT, OncNCert, PFHEA) Associate Professor in Adult Nursing at Middlesex University

Kirstie Dye (RN, BSc(Hons) Nursing, MPhil, PGCHE)
Senior Lecturer in Adult Nursing, Middlesex University

Margaret Herlihy (RN, RM, MSc, PGCHE)
Senior Lecturer in Adult Nursing, Middlesex University

José Manuel Hernandez-Padilla (RN, PhD, MSc Nursing Science, BSc Nursing, PGCHE)
Lecturer in Emergency Life Support, Middlesex University

Marion Hinds (RN, DN, RNT, Diploma in Nursing Studies, MSc, PGCHE)
Senior Lecturer in Adult Nursing, Middlesex University

Susan Kaur Lawrence (RN, MA Ethics and Law in Healthcare Practice, BSc (Hons) Child Health Studies, PGDip Practice Education, NMC Registered Teacher)
Paediatric Practice Education Lead, North Middlesex University Hospital NHS Trust

Tina Moore (RN, Diploma in Nursing, BSc (Hons) Nursing, MSc Nursing, PGCEA)
Senior Lecturer in Adult Nursing at Middlesex University

Carolyn Perriman (BSc (Hons) Child Nursing, PGCE)
Lecturer in Child Health, Middlesex University

Jenny Phillips (Dip HE Child Nursing, BSc (Hons) Neonatal Nursing Science, PGCE)
Lecturer Practitioner in Child Nursing, Middlesex University

Jane Preece (RN, BA (Hons))
Tissue Viability Nurse Specialist, Whittington Health NHS, Whittington Hospital

Sinna Ramonaledi (RN, RNT, BA Nursing, PGCHE, MA Ed Curr, MSc Health Education and Promotion)
Senior Lecturer in Adult Nursing and Moving and Handling, Middlesex University

Brian Richardson (RMN, RN, RSCN MA, BSc (Hons), PGCHE, LP)
Senior Lecturer in Child Nursing, Middlesex University

Mariama Seray-Wurie (RN, MA)
Senior Lecturer in Practice Adult Nursing, Middlesex University

Fiona Suthers (RN, BEd (Hons) MA Teaching and Learning in Higher and Professional Education)
Senior Lecturer in Resuscitation, Enterprise Fellow, Middlesex University

Kathy Wilson (RN, MSc, BSc (Hons), PGCHE)
Head of Practice-based Learning, Middlesex University

Foreword

Alina Garofil

It is an honour to write the foreword of *Clinical Skills for Nursing Practice.* In many places you may find other books with a similar topic, but nowhere will you find a book like this – that does not only educate but also create a defining moment on how students and nurses will from now on look at their clinical skills. The authors have brought to light the grim truth that without some important clinical skills in nursing practice there is no future for nursing development. The authors show us how everyday clinical skills such as communication or pain assessment are not to be taken for granted and can result in serious immoral decisions, that are not tolerated in the healthcare environment.

Moore and Cunningham show that professionals need to be skilled and knowledgeable people. The reality is that we need to provide the best nursing care possible. These should be learnt and practiced in authentic ways so the reality is you can succeed in the nursing profession! These clinical skills are not from the future, but the authors will walk you through how you too can use these core and advanced "magical skills" displayed in this book with little time to spare and an open mind.

The *Clinical Skills for Nursing Practice* is a very useful instrument for nursing assistants, student nurses or RNs and is not a book for those who are afraid to look into the void and not blink! This is a book for those who dare to ask, "Why? How?" and who are never afraid to answer a question such as, "What should I do to make my job more effective?".

Go forth, reader, and learn of the wonders of skilled patient care, protection and safety and how your job is appreciated more than you think!

Enjoy,
Alina Garofil (Adult student nurse)

Foreword

Lisa Smith

It's been thirty years since I started my nurse training at University of Surrey. Most of the university based time was spent studying the sciences such as anatomy, physiology and pathology, but apart from the contact with patients or clients, the parts that I loved the most were the opportunities to practice clinical skills on each other. When I was in my second year, along with some friends, I was lucky enough to be chosen to teach the first year students how to "do a bed bath" before they went out onto the wards for the first time. We proceeded to teach the class under the watchful eye of our clinical tutor, who had a wry smile on her face for the whole session. The water that we used was cold – a fundamental mistake, and by the end of the session, my friend was blue. Surprisingly we are still close friends.

When I look back, nursing is almost unrecognisable today, and so it is fitting that this new book has been published, that takes students through the steps required to carry out their skills effectively in practise. What I feel sets this book apart from others is that it gives the reader guidance on how to carry out the skills effectively, not just technically, but also interpersonally. Compassionate care is covered in the first section of the book and is a key theme running through. For patients and their families, this is often the thing that they remember the most about their care in hospital or care that they receive in the community. At Whittington Health, we rarely receive compliments on how technically brilliant our nursing staff are, but we do receive compliments on how kind they are. Each chapter is thorough, but concise and extremely well laid out with clear illustrations. There are a number of activities in each section which encourage the reader to reflect on a situation or a case study, which I feel make this book invaluable to qualified nurses who are undergoing revalidation as well as student nurses. Top tips are highlighted and many are the sorts of points that bring the patient experience to another level, for example in the chapter on personal care, the author suggests that the nurse should check if the patient would like to have moisturiser applied after they have washed. Simple but to some patients vitally important to maintaining a sense of comfort and normality. The watch out sections are also useful at pointing out areas of concern for the reader for example, in chapter four, the author warns the reader that drainage of large volumes of urine on catheterisation can lead to hypotension. In addition to this, where techniques differ in a community setting compared to an acute setting, this is also addressed, making the book particularly relevant for nursing care today. All in all, this book is a must have for all student nurses, all newly qualified nurses and all health libraries.

It is of no surprise to me that this book is of such high quality. I have known the editors for over twelve years now and they have made a massive contribution to nursing locally, nationally and internationally. Tina Moore is a senior lecturer in Acute Care Nursing and work based learning at Middlesex University and has a number of previous publications in both fields . Her role in spearheading the work based learning agenda locally has enabled many of our staff to become motivated to study at masters level and through work based projects, make a real difference to nursing care. Dr Sheila Cunningham is an Associate Professor and a prolific author. She has presented at numerous conferences nationally and internationally. Her doctoral thesis was on widening participation in higher education and she leads on the Erasmus international nursing exchange programme at Middlesex University.

It is a great privilege and honour to recommend this essential text book to you. It is the book that I wished I had when I was training. I know that Maureen would have approved.

Lisa Smith
Assistant Director of Nurse Education and Workforce – Whittington Health
Honorary Clinical Fellow – Middlesex University
Lead Nurse – Nurse Training Superhub, North Central London Community Education Provider Network
Florence Nightingale Scholar

Preface

Over the years approaches to nursing practice have become increasingly more complex, with the delivery of care being influenced by advances in technology, disease prevention and management. All of which require the nurse to develop a wider repertoire of skills to enable the provision of optimal, effective nursing care. The consequence of this is greater accountability.

In order for nurses to meet these expectations and provide efficient and effective care, there is now an anticipation that they engage in a high-level critical thinking and analysis as an essential component of clinical decision-making. Clinical nursing skills when performed with confidence, care, compassion and competence are highly valued by patients, their families and the nursing profession.

Skills serve to assess, plan and deliver care, be it promoting health, recovery, comfort, dignity or daily functioning and ensure patients have a positive healthcare experience. The content of this book is derived from a number of sources, including practice and education which have influenced the development of skills in clinical practice.

This book has been written especially for nursing students who are embarking on and developing their clinical skills (theory and practice) in their journey towards the provision of excellent nursing care. It aims to provide rationale on how and why certain skills are performed. We believe that this book is relevant to student nurses in the main three fields of nursing (child, mental health and adult), although much of the presenting material will also be relevant to the field of learning disability. Nursing skills discussed within this book include those that are fundamental within nursing and are relevant to first year students (although second and third year students can access these areas to serve as revision) to more complex approaches in order to particularly prepare the third year students for some of the clinical demands of being a registered nurse.

All the authors come from a variety of nursing backgrounds within clinical practice and education. They have developed a high level of knowledge, experience and expertise within their respective fields.

Structure of the book

The format of this book is based on the core domains of the NMC (2010) Essential Skills Clusters, however, the categorisation reflects our interpretation while keeping their distinctiveness yet structured to support student nurse development. Chapter 1, 'The professional role of the nurse' is a theme threaded through all the chapters and thus we consider it a distinct domain on its own. The book is set out in chapters which clearly outline the topic. Each chapter starts with simple skills suitable for year one students of any field of nursing. As the chapter progresses, the skills become more complex. Certain chapters have some quite complex skills and may need revisiting to absorb and develop those skills. Case studies reflect the variety of nursing fields and enable students to apply learning to their own developing clinical practice.

The book is divided into five parts to reflect the Essential Clusters. The core foundations of nursing practice are: Care and Compassion and these are explored in chapters addressing skills such as Communication and Personal care. The remaining themes are: Essential skills, Organisational aspects of care, Safety and protection, Nutrition and fluid balance. Each chapter contains a range of activities to assist a student's learning and points of clinical significance or concern in clinical areas ('Watch out', 'Don't forget!' or 'Top tip'). Overall it is designed to enable the students to think about skills in action and critically appraise the effectiveness of those skills.

Throughout this book it is recognised that terminology and descriptors (including patient, family) will vary. This means that while the term 'patient' is used mostly, there are times when 'client' or 'service user' may appear – these terms are synonyms and should be considered in light of the particular environment the skill is to be practised. Similarly the term 'relatives' may also be used and mean 'family' or 'significant other', again depending on the context.

This textbook provides a comprehensive approach to nursing skills which will support nursing students and any other healthcare student who works with patients and has to engage with the monitoring and care management of patients.

Acknowledgements

We would like to recognise our nursing students and professional colleagues (past and present) for the contributions that they have made throughout the years in helping to shape and develop our delivery of nursing education. We would also like to acknowledge their engagement, perceptiveness, receptiveness and challenge to the ever-changing world of nursing.

Finally, we are appreciative of the team at Routledge for commissioning this book and of the support provided.

For Vincent, Charlene, Calvin and Kiara – Tina Moore

For Andrew, Katherine, Lizzie and Mark – Sheila Cunningham

Chapter 1

The professional role of the nurse

Kathy Wilson and Nora Cooper

My aunt's basic human rights as a person, never mind her special needs and rights as a person with severe disabilities, were totally disregarded and neglected. I am certain that she was in great distress and felt totally alone and abandoned (Mrs H's niece).
(Health Service Ombudsman, 2011, p. 23)

Key concepts

Care, compassion
Professional role
Beliefs and values
Culture

Leadership
Raising concerns
Duty of candour
Fitness to practice

Learning outcomes

By the end of this chapter you will be able to:

- Discuss some of the key historical influences that have shaped nursing over the years
- Explore the underpinning beliefs and values of the nurse
- Identify relevant professional standards and regulations
- Debate key policy drivers that influence the professional role of the nurse
- Reflect on the knowledge and skills required by the nurse in contributing effectively to the transformation of services and care delivery models.

Introduction

The statement that opened this chapter may cause emotions of shock and outrage but this is unfortunately one of many similar statements that have been reported by the media over the past few years, reflecting serious incidences of poor practice. While care delivery involves a large number of multi-professional staff across a range of levels, often it is nurses who have been singled out as culprits in many of these cases.

Discussions about professionalism and why compassion appears to have disappeared from nursing values have been widely and thoroughly debated with a number of key policies published just prior to and following the investigation and publication of the final Francis Report in January 2013 (Francis, 2013; Keogh, 2013). This report detailed the serious failings at the Mid Staffordshire NHS Foundation Trust, highlighting poor leadership, in particular, as one of the main reasons for these organisational failures. The Francis Report details 290 recommendations for improvements in care, culture and education. Twenty-nine of these recommendations specifically focused on nursing. This report and the subsequent dissection and analysis by the media, professionals and policy-makers are considered a watershed moment for nursing.

This negates the fact that over the past 15 years, nursing has gained increasing recognition as a profession, with the inception of an all-graduate education and the development of advanced practice, together with an increase in the autonomous roles of the nurse.

Ensuring pride in our profession and giving patients the very best care with compassion are key aims for the nursing workforce and this was specifically expressed by the Chief Nursing Office for England in 2012. The publication *Compassion in Practice* outlined a vision and strategy for nursing, midwifery and care staff (Commissioning Board Chief Nursing Officer and DH Chief Nursing Advisor, 2012).

To be a professional is to be engaged in activities that are guided by a body of knowledge and evidence. The registered nurse must understand what it means to deliver professional practice within this constantly changing environment (Murphy *et al.*, 2009). Nurses need to feel confident and proud of their profession and strive further to make positive contributions to multi-disciplinary care in an ever-changing and politically-driven healthcare arena. In this chapter a number of views of nursing will be represented and the public perception of professionals, i.e. the social and historical context of professional practice will also be discussed.

It is important that student nurses aiming to be admitted to the register have an understanding of why all nurses are bound by a professional code of conduct and what constitutes the hallmarks of professional behaviour as dictated by the Nursing and Midwifery Council (NMC, 2015a). In addition to practising in accordance with the Code and as a reflective practitioner, nurses also need to consider their own values, beliefs and actions in terms of how these translate into 'professionalism'.

The aim of this chapter is to explore the professional role of the nurse. Being able to articulate the essential duties of the nurse will aid critical reflection which is crucial to the delivery of safe, competent and compassionate care, which should lead to an enhanced patient/service user experience, promote the uniqueness of nursing within an inter-professional team and support a strong professional identity for nurses. The remaining chapters in this book will help facilitate the integration of theory and practice and enable the student nurse to develop a thorough understanding of the evidence base that supports practice and builds on the knowledge and skills required by all nurses in the delivery of high quality care.

The nurse of today

The role of the nurse is constantly changing in every field of practice as services evolve and patient/service user needs alter as a result of the changing sociocultural environments we live in: developments in science and technology; new models of service delivery; flexible pathways to registration; health inequalities and an ageing population with co-morbidities are some of the factors that impact on the role of the registered nurse practitioner.

Activity 1.1

It is useful to reflect on your reasons for becoming a nurse and if your values have remained the same. Consider the following questions fully and seek opportunities to discuss your thoughts with colleagues.

- Why did you decide to become a nurse?
- What did you think you would do as a nurse? If you are already qualified, try to remember how it felt to be starting out in your nursing career.
- What is it that you value most about being a nurse?

One of the most common reasons cited at interview by prospective nursing students for wanting to be a nurse is helping people, perhaps as a result of having witnessed sick relatives being cared for in a hospital or community setting. It is noted that those who enter the profession later in life, sometimes after a number of years in other jobs, voice concerns about wanting to do something worthwhile. Anecdotally, it would appear that few candidates have stated that they want to be part of a distinct professional group (perhaps like medicine) or indeed fully recognise the autonomous role undertaken by many practising nurses. With the introduction of an all-graduate profession, it will be interesting to note if these views change with more candidates considering the excellent opportunities to combine an academic and clinical career with the increase in availability of Post-Graduate programmes, with initial registration as well as post-registration pathways to Masters and Doctorate programmes.

When one considers why nurses remain in the profession, it is more complicated as there are many reasons why people continue in an occupation that is often stressful and demanding. Some may see nursing as a job which pays the bills and provides job security but many remain highly committed and enjoy their roles, and, despite very negative and sometimes shocking reports, they remain proud of their profession and continue to strive to deliver a high standard of care. *Nurses in Society*, a report commissioned by the Chief Nursing Officer on behalf of the Department of Health (DoH, 2008), interviewed a number of senior practising nurses and identified five aspects they valued most about nursing:

1   Making a difference to patients' lives
2   Close contact with people

3   Delivering excellent care
4   Working in a team and being a role model
5   Continuous development.

The increased number of career opportunities that nursing offers nowadays (nurse consultant, advanced nurse practitioner, nurse researcher, nurse educator) together with a high level of respect for nursing within the multi-disciplinary team appeals to many who are keen to progress in their careers. An occupation that brings relative security, job satisfaction and career progression is an attractive career option. This needs to be promoted more fully to ensure that this essential workforce is maintained. While the professionalisation of nursing has developed over the years, the image of the nurse has not always been portrayed in this light. It seems that the role of the nurse remains largely misunderstood by the wider public.

A professional image is influenced by the views of the society it serves and nursing is no exception. The social context has shaped nurses' attitudes, public attitudes and in many ways, the direction of nursing practice. Hoeve *et al.* (2013) refer to the work of Bridges in 1990 which identified 34 different nursing stereotypes, many of which are unflattering and inaccurate and unfortunately still seem to influence public perception today. They advocate that nurses should stand up for themselves more, increase their visibility and use their professionalism to enhance understanding about what nurses actually do. Much of the negativity still stems from the fact that nursing has always been a largely female occupation. However, a Nursing and Midwifery Council (NMC) report states that there are now 65,755 male nurses, representing over 10 per cent of the nursing workforce (NMC, 2010). An understanding of the history of nursing will enable a better understanding of the development of the profession and how the past has shaped the present.

Historical perspective

Throughout history, nursing has existed formally or informally in the form of caring for the sick. Historically care has been seen as a feminine practice, almost exclusively performed by women and often viewed as low-level and low-profit work.

Charles Dickens, in his 1843 novel, *Martin Chuzzlewit*, depicts the poor state of nursing care in his representation of the drunken character Sairy Gamp, whom he claimed was based on a nurse he knew. At the other extreme, nurses were often also described as members of religious orders in the Middle Ages.

In the mid-1800s in Europe, changes in the way nurses were trained were evident with the establishment of the Deaconess Institute at Kaiserswerth in Germany. A training programme for deaconesses had been set up in Kaiserswerth, and Florence Nightingale, who is widely viewed as the 'pioneer nurse' and founder of modern-day nursing, undertook her nurse training there in 1850 over a period of three years. In the mid-nineteenth century, the attitude remained that training was not required for nursing or for any other profession undertaken by women. Florence Nightingale challenged those who supported this sexist view of nursing and proposed that the 'new nurse' was to be trained and to have thoroughly mastered her subject just as a man masters his: 'an uneducated man who practices physics is justly called a quack, perhaps an imposter but why are uneducated nurses not called quacks and imposters?' (Seymour, 1932, p. 92), The general opinion at the time was that anyone could be a nurse, all that was required was instinct. Some of these beliefs have been perpetuated over many years and have had a significant impact on the development of nursing as a profession.

The most famous images and stories of the nursing practices of Florence Nightingale stem from her involvement in the Crimean War (1853–1856). After hearing of the terrible conditions there suffered by British soldiers, Florence volunteered to go to Turkey. Despite an initial reluctance by the British Government she was eventually granted permission to go, along with a group of other nurses.

Nightingale's work during the war earned her national recognition and several medals for bravery. Her legacy remains through the Florence Nightingale Foundation. This foundation was established following a proposal at the International Council of Nurses Congress by Ethel Bedford Fenwick to pay tribute to Florence Nightingale's life and work. The foundation continues today and provides scholarships to support professional development and a voice for nursing. Florence later set up a training school for nursing at St Thomas' Hospital in London with the first recruits joining in 1860.

Some of the history of Florence Nightingale and the foundation can be found on the foundation's website which is written by Dame Sheila Quinn (see below). An annual commemoration service is held each year at Westminster Abbey, tickets are open to all nurses and can be applied for online through the foundation's website: www.florence-nightingale foundation.org.uk/uploads/Short_History_by_Dame_Sheila_Quinn_PDF_Version.pdf.

Mary Seacole, a Jamaican-born nurse, also sought permission to travel to Turkey at that time but her appeals were rejected on several occasions, largely, as she believed, to be due to racial discrimination. Others believe it might have been related to her age; she was 50 at the time. In addition, the medical establishment were also wary of the treatments that she offered. Nevertheless she persisted with her plan and travelled to Turkey at her own expense. On arrival, Mary Seacole set up a hotel and there are numerous stories of how she treated and cared for wounded soldiers.

Mary Seacole's story was largely overlooked for many decades after her death, but for the past 15–20 years, her caring and courage have been widely acknowledged. As well as appearing in nursing texts, these characteristics have formed the basis of discussion in many primary school curricula. Some question her elevated role. While Mary Seacole never did claim to be a nurse, there is no doubt about her kindness, commitment and dedication and the number of men she helped during the Crimean War.

Mrs Ethel Bedford Fenwick, a matron at St Bartholomew's Hospital (1881–1887), is recognised because of her work with the International Council of Nursing and as chairwoman of the Florence Nightingale Foundation. She also founded the British Nursing Association in 1887 and over many years argued fiercely for the regulation and professional status of nursing.

Achieving regulation was, however, a lengthy and challenging process. Despite the British Nursing Association being formed in 1887, the first Bill for registration was not put forward until 1904. It took a further five attempts between 1906, and 1918 until a Bill was finally passed in 1919. The Nurses Act (1919) established a regulatory system and the introduction of the General Nursing Council responsible for the maintenance of the register for nurses.

Despite the tireless work of some very dominant and influential nurses, it took many years for nursing to move forward. It was not until 1970 that the Briggs Committee was established to explore the nature of nursing within the NHS and the quality of professional nurse training. Briggs recommended a number of changes to the education system and proposed a change in structure which became evident in the Nurses, Midwives and Health Visitors Act of 1979 coming into force in 1983. The United Kingdom Central Council (UKCC) was established in 1983, with the main function of maintaining a register of UK Nurses, Midwives and Health Visitors.

Throughout history there have been many powerful influences on the development of nursing as a profession. Three influential women have been highlighted here though many others have played a significant part in the building of hospitals, creating schools of nurse training and in the development of nursing knowledge. One such person was Edith Cavell who was sentenced to death by firing squad for helping British and French troops to escape from occupied Belgium in the First World War. Her bravery is recognised by a commemorative coin to mark the centenary of her death, which was in 1915. There are many other inspiring historical figures represented in books and films who do not accurately reflect nursing as it is today but they do nevertheless often demonstrate the journey that nursing has travelled.

Defining nursing

There has been a lot of debate about the definition of nursing's remit. Many nurse theorists have proposed definitions and one of the most quoted for many years was by Virginia Henderson (1966) who stated the role of the nurse is 'to assist individuals to gain independence in relation to the performance of activities that contribute to health or its recovery (or a peaceful death), that he/she would perform unaided, if he/she had the necessary strength or knowledge'.

Henderson's definition (1966) focuses on tasks that nursing seeks to accomplish. This definition with an emphasis on caring and helping patients move towards wellness remains relevant but lacks the emphasis on the complexities of practice, education and professionalism that is more in tune with modern nursing. Older definitions of nursing, such as Henderson's, have been seen as echoing the female perspective of caring, close to mothering, and say little to dispel ideas of nursing as a handmaiden to the medical profession. Nurses would hope that ideas such as these are long outdated, though there is a wealth of evidence suggesting that the development of the profession as previously discussed has been greatly influenced by them, and unfortunately some may still resonate in areas of practice.

The NMC provides an alternative definition in their *Standards for Pre-Registration Nursing Education* (2010), produced by the European Tuning project (2009):

> The nurse is a safe, caring, and competent decision maker willing to accept personal and professional accountability for his/her actions and continuous learning. The nurse practises within a statutory framework and code of ethics delivering nursing practice (care) that is appropriately based on research, evidence and critical thinking that effectively responds to the needs of individual clients (patients) and diverse populations.

This definition acknowledges the importance of education in developing the range of knowledge and skills needed to deliver evidence-based care supported by an ethical framework. It could be argued it does not sufficiently address the knowledge and skills needed for complex care management and the co-ordination of patient-led pathways across professional boundaries (Willis Commission, 2015).

Activity 1.2

Reflect on your 'personal' definition of nursing. Do you think that these are the essential skills that nurses need to fulfil the requirements of being a professional nurse?

■ From your experiences in practice, what are the images that you think nurses portray today?
■ Think of a nurse whom you consider to be a positive role model. What is it about them that gives positive messages about nursing?

Numerous definitions and descriptions of what constitutes high quality nursing care have been reflected in the literature over the years. In 2011, the Royal College of Nursing (RCN) produced *The Principles of Nursing Practice: A Set of Statements Reflecting What Constitutes Safe and Effective Nursing Care* (RCN, 2011). Eight principles were developed by the RCN in partnership with the Department of Health and the Nursing and Midwifery Council.

It is unfortunate that one of the main drivers for the development of these principles has been the numerous reports of poor care practices that have been reflected in both government-led reports and the media. While these instances involve a small minority of the nursing profession, it is essential that these are not ignored. A significant amount of learning can take place by exploring and analysing such reports.

As highlighted in the Francis Report (2013), poor practice is often evident across the organisation and many different members of the team may be implicated in this care. However, the importance of team working and the role of the nurse in leading by example, influencing high standards of care and being conscientious in reporting concerns are reflected in the principles of nursing practice (RCN, 2011). This is also clearly reflected in the revised *Code: Professional Standards of Practice and Behavior for Nurses and Midwives* (NMC, 2015a).

Lord Willis, in the *Shape of Caring* review, an independent review undertaken on behalf of Health Education England in 2013, celebrated many excellent examples of nursing and models of nurse education. Registered nurses were acknowledged as expert clinicians, change agents, champions and leaders of multi-disciplinary teams (Willis Commission, 2015).

Lord Willis did, however, levy some criticism at the current preparation of nurses and felt that new models needed to be developed to prepare students for contemporary nursing with more advanced skills. The report also emphasised the need for changes in education to enhance the role of the registered nurse in supporting the transformation of services based on population needs as outlined in the *Five Year Forward Review* (NHS, 2014).

The role of healthcare assistants and the need to develop this workforce to better support the registered nurse practitioner were also recommended. In response to these recommendations, in 2016, Health Education England (HEE) launched a consultation in relation to a new 'associate nurse' role. The role is designed to bridge the gap between healthcare assistant roles and that of the registered nurse. This initiative has been supported by many nurse leaders. There is a strong call for career pathways into nurse registration, however, a number of concerns have been raised, particularly from those already familiar with what was known as the enrolled nurse, a role that was phased out in the early 1990s. The inception of this new role has again raised the question about whether nurses really do need a degree to care. It is also a reminder of the insulting 'too posh to wash' headlines, depicting the continued widespread misunderstanding about the role of the registered nurse and the complexities of care.

Nursing is guided and influenced by many professional, statutory and policy factors that can have a direct and immediate impact on the outcomes for clients and their families or carers. The nurse needs to understand what it means to deliver professional practice within this constantly changing environment and the aspects of behaviour, attitude and approach that underpin good nursing care (RCN, 2011).

Beliefs and values

Activity 1.3

Identify the values and beliefs that are important to you:

- Are the beliefs and values that you held before entering into nursing the same as those you hold now? If not, identify what has changed and why this might be so.
- What would you consider to be the values and performance expectations to which all nurses subscribe?

Whether aware of it or not, every individual has a core set of personal values that shape their thinking. Values help define what is right and what is wrong and are the basis for judgements and behaviour. The identity of a nurse is defined by the values held, both personally and in relation to how nurses view their role. This identity shapes actions and interactions with patients and others and translates into the way in which nurses practise (Fagermoen, 1997).

The nurse working within a mental health setting may attach most value to the importance of interpersonal skills that allow them to demonstrate therapeutic use of self. On the other hand, a nurse working in a critical care setting, while still valuing interpersonal skills, may place greater value on observation and the knowledge of altered physiology in order to anticipate or alleviate life-threatening situations for patients.

Activity 1.4

Consider the following scenario:

■ A girl aged 14 comes into the sexual health clinic seeking 'the morning-after pill' (emergency contraception). She informs you that she has had unprotected sex at the weekend while under the influence of alcohol. What is your reaction? (Think about your PERSONAL feelings about this situation and the PROFESSIONAL REACTION that you might be expected to hold.) Are there any differences?

Analysing the above situation, it can be surmised that personal beliefs and values are affected by the socialisation that occurs within families/background. Cultural values will emerge and influence perceptions in relation to under-age sex and alcohol consumption. There are of course legal aspects also to be considered in this scenario. The main questions here are, how much influence do personal values have in the way nurses interact with patients, and how much should they be allowed (if at all) to do so?

In an under-age sex scenario, parents reading this might want to immediately inform the girl's parents (arguing that if other parents were in a similar situation, they would want to know). However, in healthcare, sexual health practice is characterised by a commitment to confidentiality and the nurse cannot (unless the client is deemed to be at risk of harm) inform others of the patient's health-related information. One's personal values may potentially conflict with the organisational and one's professional values. In terms of good practice guidelines, the sexual health nurse should seek to encourage the girl to inform her parents or guardian of the situation, but cannot insist on this.

The Fraser Guidelines (named after Lord Fraser) are used to guide professionals in the care of under 16-year-olds in decisions about contraception. Balancing children's rights and wishes and keeping them safe from harm do raise challenges for professionals working with children. An understanding of policy, legislation and statutory guidance related to child protection is paramount in guiding practice.

As reflected in the above discussion, personal values might not always be shared by others. Nurses should try and find out from patients/clients/carers what their values are and what is meaningful to them. It is only by eliciting from them their notion of what their health/illness means to them and explaining the choices being offered, that nurses can truly care for patients in a professional manner.

Personal values may also conflict with organisational values, possibly causing tension. For example, a nurse may hold a personal value that medical and nursing care should be given to all those in need of such care and that nurses should not be involved in determining who is eligible for that care. This may conflict with the government's agenda of collecting fees from those who are not eligible for NHS care, e.g. foreign visitors.

The terms beliefs and values are often used interchangeably. However, it is useful to look at the difference between the two. A *belief* is essentially an opinion that is generally held to be true. Many beliefs develop from upbringing and family influences. *Values* are ideas that are held to be important and can influence the development of our beliefs. They are personal beliefs and attitudes about a person, object, idea or action which can influence both decisions and actions as nurses.

Professional values are acquired through socialisation into nursing from codes of ethics, nursing experience, teachers and peers. In 2011, the Department of Health published the NHS Constitution, which set out rights to which patients, public and staff are entitled, in addition to responsibilities that they each owe to one another to ensure that the NHS operates fairly and effectively (DoH, 2011). The core values of respect, dignity, compassion, improving lives, working together for patients and that everyone counts are an integral part of the NHS Constitution (DoH, 2015).

In focusing on professionalism and nursing values, one of the most widely promoted resources post the Francis Report has been the national strategy 'Compassion in Practice', a vision and strategy for nursing, midwifery and care staff which was launched at the Chief Nursing Officer's Conference in 2012. Much of the emphasis in the promotion of this policy has been on the exploration of six specific values, i.e. Care, Compassion, Competence, Communication, Courage and Commitment (Box 1.1), known as the six Cs. While there has been some debate and discussion about the value of defining nursing and midwifery practice in this way, they have nevertheless become an integral part of many developments in nursing strategies and educational curricula.

The underpinning principles required to deliver the vision of the six Cs are:

- Helping people to stay independent, maximising well-being and improving health outcomes
- Working with people to provide a positive experience of care
- Delivering high quality care and measuring the impact of care
- Building and strengthening leadership
- Ensuring we have the right staff, with the right skills, in the right place
- Supporting positive staff experiences.

These six values are obviously not new to nursing and have always been embedded in good nursing practice, with the aim of delivering high quality care. It has been difficult for nurses to accept the implicit and sometimes very explicit criticism of the way in which their practice has been viewed. However, discussions involving staff delivering frontline care as well as Members of Parliament and senior nurse leaders have created a better understanding of the impact of negative culture, poor staffing levels and weak leadership on the patient experience and the environments in which care is delivered.

Two years on from the launch of the national strategy, Jane Cummings, the Chief Nursing Officer, England, stated: 'The Compassion in Practice Strategy is changing the culture of how we care, the culture of how we work and the culture in which we work' (Cummings, 2014) and in 2015, NHS England launched a Culture of Care barometer, which again emphasises the importance of developing a positive work culture.

There are a significant number of strategies and policies that have been released post Francis and other reports about poor and neglectful practice. It is important that nurses keep abreast of these and contribute to the debates and developments that will inevitably impact on the delivery of care.

Box 1.1 Compassion in Practice (2012)

Care

Care is our core business and that of our organisations, and the care we deliver helps the individual person and improves the health of the whole community.

Compassion

Compassion is how care is given through relationships based on empathy, respect and dignity. It can also be described as intelligent kindness, and is central to how people perceive their care.

Competence

Competence means all those in caring roles must have the ability to understand an individual's health and social needs and the expertise, clinical and technical knowledge to deliver effective care and treatments based on research and evidence.

Communication

Communication is central to successful caring relationships and to effective team working. Communication is the key to a good workplace with benefits for those in our care and staff alike.

Courage

Courage enables us to do the right thing for the people we care for, to speak up when we have concerns and to have the personal strength and vision to innovate and to embrace new ways of working.

Commitment

A commitment to our patients and populations is a cornerstone of what nurses do.

(Commissioning Board Chief Nursing Officer and
DH Chief Nursing Advisor, 2012)

The Nursing and Midwifery Council (NMC)

The principal role of the Nursing and Midwifery Council (Nursing and Midwifery Order, 2001) is to safeguard the health and well-being of the public and they do this by:

■ Keeping a register of all nurses and midwives in the UK and ensuring that they are appropriately qualified to work

■ Setting standards of education and training and providing guidance to both qualified nurses and midwives as well as students

■ Ensuring the Code is upheld and investigating any allegations made that nurses or midwives have breached the Code.

The NMC registers almost 685,000 nurses and midwives, who are eligible to work in the UK. They describe fitness to practice as a person's suitability to be on the register without restrictions. Suitability to be on the register without restrictions includes:

■ Achieving the standards required for entry to and maintenance on the register

■ Maintenance of good health and good character to enable safe and effective practice

■ Adherence to the principles of good practice set out in the Code and other guidance by the Code (NMC, 2015a).

The Standards of Competence for pre-registration nursing (NMC, 2010) set out the standards for competency for entry onto the register. Every pre-registration nursing programme validated from September 2011 must be underpinned by these standards. These standards are due to be reviewed in 2017.

The Standards of Competence identify the knowledge, skills and attitudes the student must acquire by the end of the programme. This framework comprises four sets of competencies, one for each field of practice: adult, mental health, learning disabilities, and children's nursing. Each set comprises both generic competencies and field-specific competencies. The competencies are organised into four domains:

■ Professional values

■ Communication and interpersonal skills

■ Nursing practice and decision-making

■ Leadership, management and team working.

The NMC (2010) also recommend a number of skills that they define as the Essential Skills Clusters (ESCs) to be used as guidance and to support the achievement of the standards outlined above. There are five ESCs:

■ Care, compassion and communication

■ Organisational aspects of care

■ Infection prevention and control

■ Nutrition and fluid management

■ Medicines management.

In each cluster there are a number of nursing skills that student nurses need to demonstrate at specific points in their programme. The NMC introduced the ESCs in response to feedback on a number of practice-related issues around fitness to practice at the point of registration in the belief that achievement of the ESCs will ultimately improve patient care.

Throughout the three-year programme students will be facilitated to learn and practise these skills. These skills are reflected in many practice assessment documents and require assessment at various points throughout the curriculum. The remaining chapters in this book will present the underpinning theory and evidence for many of the ESCs and support the development of knowledge and skills for practice. The standards for nurse education are currently under review and are due to be published in 2017.

Adherence to the principles of good practice set out in *The Code: Professional Standards of Practice and Behaviour for Nurses and Midwives* (NMC, 2015a) is not negotiable, and by being on the register nurses are committed to upholding these standards and other guidance by the NMC. It is essential therefore that student nurses become familiar with the Code. The four key principles of the code are set out in Box 1.2.

Activity 1.5

- What do you understand by the Code?
- How is the Code relevant to you as a student?
- How can you improve your practice by adhering to the Code?

It would be good to have access to the Code as you work through this section.

Box 1.2 The Code

1   *Prioritise people* – incorporates the need to act in the best interest of people at all times, respecting people's right to privacy and confidentiality and treating people as individuals and with dignity.
2   *Practise effectively* – incorporates evidence-based care, effective communication, cooperative working, record-keeping and accountability.
3   *Preserve safety* – incorporates working within limits of your own competence, being open and candid, raising concerns and reducing harm.
4   *Promote professionalism and trust* – incorporates upholding the reputation of the profession, being a model of integrity and leadership for others to aspire to and cooperating with all investigations and audits.

(NMC, 2015a)

Not all sections of the Code will be discussed here but students are encouraged to become familiar with all aspects of it and consider how the Code can be applied in practice. It is the NMC's aim that this revised Code will remain a 'live' document and encourage nurses to use it in their daily practice for reflection and development, and hence this is why the Code is an integral part of revalidation, which will be discussed later in the chapter.

Case study 1.1

When facilitating a seminar with a group of year 1 students recently, they were asked to consider what dignity meant to them. The students had just returned to the university after a period of six weeks clinical practice, which was for many of the students their first experience of hospital care. The following questions were posed and the students were given time to consider these initially on their own and then discuss with colleagues in groups of three.

▪ What do you understand by dignity?
▪ Give examples from practice where you or others had positively maintained a patient's dignity.
▪ Give examples from practice where you felt that a patient's dignity had not been maintained.

The four most popular answers to the first question are shown in Figure 1.1.

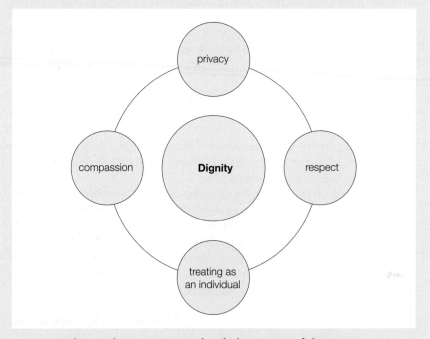

Figure 1.1 **The words most associated with the concept of dignity**

Many positive incidents reflecting excellent patient care were shared. However, some negative ones were also shared and these related mainly to patient privacy. These examples were explored in depth and the NMC guidance on 'Raising Concerns' was revisited.

The key themes in the Code include: Dignity, Health and Good Character, Raising Concerns, Duty of Candour and Revalidation.

Dignity is a concept that has formed the basis of many of the government reports which have focused on improving the quality of care and the patient experience. Many reports have been instigated because of patient accounts of poor care practices in which patient dignity was not maintained and indeed completely neglected at times.

The RCN's 'Dignity: at the heart of everything we do' campaign was launched in 2008 to support the delivery of care in every environment amidst concerns that patient dignity was being lost, particularly in caring for older people. Respect, compassion and sensitivity are viewed as being integral to the provision of dignity, which is viewed as the essence of care. Janet Davies, Executive Director of Nursing and Service Delivery at the RCN at that time, said:

> Some of this goes beyond nursing, and is related to the overall attitude of society towards older people and their needs and dignity. Nurses can and should be leaders in developing the right attitudes and ensuring that all older people are treated with respect and kindness both in healthcare and in the rest of their lives.
>
> (RCN, 2008)

Good health and good character are viewed as fundamental to fitness to practice as a nurse or midwife, and so all approved education institutions (AEIs) have a responsibility to ensure that all applicants meet the NMC requirements for entry to the programme and the subsequent entry to the register.

Student nurses must have a clear understanding of what is meant by good health and good character so that they honestly and accurately disclose this information. Certain health issues or disabilities might not preclude a student from entering the profession as reasonable adjustments can be made. However, failure to disclose key information could raise concerns about an individual's honesty and hence their fitness to practice.

In 2005, the Disability Discrimination Act was updated and required organisations to have a 'positive duty' to 'promote equality of opportunity and positive attitudes; eliminate unlawful discrimination and encourage disabled people's participation' (HMSO, 2005). Under the terms of disability legislation, individuals are entitled to receive 'reasonable adjustments' to help them overcome their difficulties. Students are encouraged to disclose their disabilities and seek appropriate levels of support, though they are not required to do so.

The Raising Concerns policy

The Raising Concerns policy was first published in 2010, entitled *Raising and Escalating Concerns* but reviewed and reprinted in 2015 and entitled *Raising Concerns: Guidance for Nurses and Midwives* (NMC, 2015b). The NMC advises that essential guidance for nurse and midwives, including students, should be read in conjunction with the institution's whistleblowing policy and clinical governance procedures. This guidance is underpinned by the Code and sets out principles that will support nurses in taking appropriate action in the interest of patients. This guidance advises the nurse to either raise their concerns with the individual involved or their line manager.

If a staff member raising concerns still feels that these are not being addressed appropriately, the guidance advises that the concern be escalated to a more senior member of staff. If they remain dissatisfied, then they should escalate the situation to an external regulatory body, i.e. in this instance, the Nursing and Midwifery Council.

Activity 1.6

■ Was there ever an occasion that you observed care that made you feel uncomfortable and was not at the standard that you expected care to be delivered but felt unsure about what to do?

■ What do you think are the factors that influence students in their decisions to report poor practice?

A number of references have been made to the Francis inquiry and the failures in Mid Staffordshire, but another high profile systems failure was aired in a *Panorama* programme on BBC1, looking at the care received by learning disability service users at Winterbourne Nursing Home. This sent shockwaves throughout the country and created a great deal of discussion and debate around raising concerns. The essential message outlined in the Department of Health strategy 'Valuing People' (DoH, 2009) and by the Royal College of Nursing Learning Disability Forum (RCN, 2010) is that all people with a learning disability have the right to lead their lives like any others, and to be treated with the same dignity and respect. The RCN provides guidance on how to improve practice and also provides examples of good practice and practical ideas on what nurses can do to improve the experiences of people with learning disabilities.

In response to the Winterbourne scandal, in October 2015, NHS England pledged £45 million to fund a policy called 'Homes Not Hospitals'. This policy is aimed at ensuring people with learning difficulties can live as independently as possible and has led to what many view as a very positive outcome.

As well as an emphasis on raising concerns, there have been renewed calls for openness and honesty and the introduction to a 'duty of candour' to the Code. Guidance on the 'duty of candour' has been published in collaboration with the General Medical Council and highlights the necessity for nurses and midwives to be honest when things go wrong, not only regarding patients but also within organisations in reporting adverse incidents or near misses that might have led to harm.

In 2016, the Care Quality Commission (CQC) appointed its first National Guardian for speaking up safely within the NHS. The purpose of this role is to support healthcare organisations in developing a culture of openness to raise concerns about any issues that might affect patient safety. This post is viewed as a very positive move in changing the culture within the NHS.

Revalidation

In addition to maintaining appropriate professional values as reflected in the six Cs, nurses are required to continually reflect on their professional development and performance to enhance their practice. One of the key frameworks implemented by the NMC to support the nurse in achieving these standards is 'revalidation'.

As required by current legislation, nurses and midwives renew their registration every three years and declare their fitness to practice. As part of the 'Prep' requirements published in 2008, all registrants had to confirm that they have practised for 450 hours during those three years and have demonstrated a commitment to continuing professional development.

In 2013, the NMC announced its intention to introduce a process of revalidation from April 2016 at the point of renewal as part of its commitment to the enhancement of public protection. Revalidation requires registered nurses and midwives to demonstrate that they remain fit to practice. Nurses and midwives will also need to reflect on feedback from patients, service users, carers and colleagues to enhance their practice. The model agreed will require a third party (such as an employer or manager) to confirm that the nurse or midwife who is revalidating is complying with the Code. It is essential that student nurses become familiar with this process though they are likely to be comfortable with reflecting on practice and on patient/service user feedback as it is integral to the pre-registration programme.

The Fitness to Practice directorate

Fitness to Practice is the largest directorate in the NMC and the largest area of expenditure. According to the NMC, nurses are personally accountable for their actions and omissions in their practice. Nurses are required to work within the law and are accountable to their patients, the public, their employer and the profession.

Fitness to practice is defined by the NMC as a person's suitability to be on the register without restrictions. Registered nurses maintain appropriate standards, ensure good health and character and adhere to the principles of good practice that are set out in the various standards, guidance and advice.

If someone has concerns about the fitness to practice of a nurse or midwife, they can raise these with the NMC, which will investigate all allegations, and following this, a decision will be made by an independent panel about whether or not the individual nurse's or midwife's fitness to practice has been impaired. The panel will be provided with evidence and can hear from witnesses and from the nurse or midwife against whom the allegations have been made. In some cases the panel may decide that no action is necessary, given all the circumstances of the case. If the panel decides that action is necessary, they can direct one of the following orders:

- Caution order
- Conditions of practice order
- Suspension order
- Striking-off order.

The NMC emphasises that the overwhelming majority of nurses and midwives on the register do practise safely and effectively, and currently it is approximately only 0.7 per cent of the 686,782 on the register, about whom concerns have been raised. In the 2014–2015 report, there was an increase of 10 per cent in referrals from the previous year and employers remain the biggest source of referrals. However, there was a notable increase in the total number of referrals made by members of the public, a 47 per cent increase from 2013–2014. This is an important issue to reflect on and the NMC must explore some of the reasons why this might be occurring and the impact on a number of the issues highlighted in this chapter. It might be related to enhanced processes at the NMC, as they have been heavily criticised in the past for the delay in responding to referrals and during the investigation process, but also related to the extensive debates, discussion and policy changes related to raising concern.

Top tip

Fitness to practice hearings are held in public venues. Practitioners or members of the public can attend a hearing to observe. This can be a very useful learning experience for both student nurses and qualified practitioners, and attendance can be booked via the NMC website.

Summary

While it is clear that the role of the nurse has changed throughout the decades, some of the negative stereotypes persist alongside doubts about whether nurses really do need to be educated to care. These uninformed opinions appear to be based on an assumption that care is merely a series of tasks and ignore the fact that nursing is multifaceted and at times challenging, and that we need better-educated professionals to manage this demanding but rewarding and privileged role.

Reports of appalling poor and neglectful practices, attributed to some nurses and the wider healthcare team, have led to a plethora of reports, policies, strategies and debates about how we can improve healthcare for people across all fields of nursing, and nurses need to engage positively with these to ensure their voices and those of the people in their care are heard.

The NMC highlights the importance of nurses reinforcing their professionalism, and presents the underpinning values and principles for nursing and midwifery practice within a revised Code, which the majority of registrants already uphold. Revalidation is intended to encourage nurses to reflect more regularly on their practice and the principles in the Code, and many expert practitioners are positively embracing this, so that it is meaningful and integral, rather than being a duty to be undertaken every three years.

Nurses are working in an ever-changing socio-political environment where care needs to be better coordinated with greater integration between healthcare and social care to manage the complex and diverse population needs. Effective leadership is vital and nurses need to continue to be at forefront of developing innovative approaches to empower people, promote independence and work effectively in multi-disciplinary teams and across professional boundaries. In-depth knowledge and advanced practical skills are needed to undertake increasingly complex care management as the transformation of services continues to require intelligent ways of working.

References

Commissioning Board Chief Nursing Officer and DH Chief Nursing Advisor (2012) *Compassion in Practice: Nursing and Midwifery and Care Staff: Our Vision and Strategy*. London: Department of Health NHS Commissioning Board.

Cummings, J. (2014) *Compassion in Practice, Two Years On: Experience Matters*. Available at: www.england.nhs.uk/wp-content/uploads/2014/12/nhs-cip-2yo.pdf (accessed 10 February 2016).

DoH (Department of Health) (2008) *Nurses in Society*. London: HMSO.

DoH (Department of Health) (2009) *Valuing People Now: A New Three-Year Strategy for People with Learning Disabilities*. London: HMSO.

DoH (Department of Health) (2015) *NHS Constitution: The NHS Belongs to Us All*. London: HMSO.

Fagermoen, M. (1997) Professional identity: values embedded in meaningful nursing practice. *Journal of Advanced Nursing Practice*, 25: 431–441.

Francis, R. (2013) *Report of the Mid Staffordshire NHS Foundation Trust Public Inquiry*, vol. 3, *Present and Future Annexes*. London: The Stationery Office.

Health Service Ombudsman (2011) *Care and Compassion? Report of the Health Service Ombudsman: Investigations into NHS Care of Older People*. London: Department of Health.

Henderson, V. (1966) *The Nature of Nursing: A Definition and Its Implications for Practice and Education*. New York: Macmillan.

HMSO (2005) *Disability Discrimination Act*. London: The Stationery Office.

Hoeve, Y., Jansen, G. and Roodbol, P. (2013) The nursing profession: public image, self-concept and professional identity: a discussion paper, *Journal of Advanced Nursing*, 70(2): 295–300.

Keogh, B. (2013) *Review into the Quality of Care and Treatment Provided by 14 Hospital Trusts in England: Overview Report*. London: NHS.

Murphy, J., Quillinan, B. and Carolan, M. (2009) Role of clinical nurse leadership in improving patient care. *Nursing Management*, 16(8): 26–28.

NHS (2014) *Five Year Forward Review*. Available at: www.england.nhs.uk/ (accessed 19 February 2016).

NMC (Nursing and Midwifery Council) (2010) *Standards for Pre-Registration Nursing Education*. London: NMC.

NMC (Nursing and Midwifery Council) (2015a) *The Code: Professional Standards of Practice and Behaviour for Nurses and Midwives*. London: NMC.

NMC (Nursing and Midwifery Council) (2015b) *Raising Concerns: Guidance for Nurses and Midwives*. London. NMC.

Nursing and Midwifery Order (2001) Article 253, HMO.

RCN (Royal College of Nursing) (2008) Definition of dignity in Dignity resource. Available at: www.rcn.org.uk/development/practice/dignity/rcns_definition_of_dignity

RCN (Royal College of Nursing) (2010) *Mental Health Nursing of Adults with Learning Disabilities*. London: RCN.

RCN (Royal College of Nursing) (2011) *The Principles of Nursing Practice: A Set of Statements Reflecting What Constitutes Safe and Effective Nursing Care.* London: RCN.

Seymour, L.R. (1932) *A General History of Nursing.* London: Faber and Faber.

Willis commission report (2012) *Quality with Compassion: the future of nursing education,* Royal College of Nursing.

Willis Commission (2015) *Shape of Caring: A Review of the Future Education and Training of Registered Nurses and Care Assistants.* London: Health Education England. Available at: http://hee.nhs.uk/wp-content/blogs.dir/321/files/2015/03/2348-Shape-of-caring-review-FINAL.pdf (accessed 4 September 2015).

Part I

Care and compassion and communication

Chapter 2

Communication

Brian Richardson

Being able to communicate effectively is perhaps the most important skill a nurse can have. Without it, achieving competence in the other skills described in this book will be difficult.

Key concepts

The humanistic approach to communication
Skills for effective communication

Empathy
Professional communication

Learning outcomes

By the end of this chapter you will be able to:

- Reflect on the humanistic approach to communication and apply it to practice
- Decide how to enhance communication by using the appropriate skills
- Understand the importance of empathy when caring for patients across the fields and their families and carers
- Use communication skills to enhance professional communication.

Introduction

Most people would say that they were excellent at communicating and that their communication skills were good and perhaps in some situations that may be true. However, the way in which the nurse communicates with their families and friends is different from the way in which they will need to communicate within the healthcare setting. As nurses, their communication skills will be tested in ways that the average person may never have imagined. This is due to the fact that nursing involves working with a wide range of people across the life span, within a multicultural society when they are at their most vulnerable. Feeling vulnerable can lead people to behave in ways that may be challenging and difficult. These challenges, if dealt with appropriately, can also be some of the most rewarding experiences for the nurse and patient within nursing.

A simple tool, called PER (Propose, Engage and Reflect) (Box 2.1) is provided to help support reflection and to help improve communication. In order to help identify with the case studies, the responses will be directly addressed to the reader. It is anticipated that these opportunities to reflect on the case studies will raise awareness of the ways that communication with service users, families, carers and the other members of the healthcare team can be developed so as to be more effective and professional.

Box 2.1 Propose, Engage and Reflect: the PER tool

The PER tool is designed to help explore and examine communication in all aspects of practice in order to develop skills and promote effective communication. It involves three simple steps:

- *Prepare* – before any communication ensure that all aspects are taken into consideration and that preparation is carried out, e.g. who will be involved? What does the communication concern? Are you informed? Is the environment appropriate?
- *Engage/Communicate* – introduce yourself, gain the person's attention, check that their responses are appropriate, clarify those that you may not be sure of, make sure that each aspect of communication, both verbal and non-verbal, is complementary.
- *Reflect* – Did you achieve what you planned? Was there any aspect you felt could have been done better? Were you prepared? Was the communication clear?

The rationale for communicating clearly and effectively is to achieve a particular purpose, e.g., exploring feelings or passing on information. It is important to adopt an approach that is recognised and understood so to provide a reference point for reflection and development. This requires meeting people at different stages in their own development and all are individual, as in philosophical approaches such as rationalism or humanism: valuing the person. This may be slightly different for different fields of nursing (adults, child and young person, or mental health) but the principles remain similar.

The humanistic approach to communication

There are many different methods and means of communication discussed in the literature. However, for the purposes of this chapter, the main focus will be on the 'humanistic' approach. The reason for this is that it relates very closely to the principles underlying the guidelines and standards set by the Nursing and Midwifery Council (NMC) that guide all nurses on the register and students in training. Communicating with patients and service users will require nurses to use their basic humanity, to ensure delivery of care that is safe, effective and compassionate. Nurses will be called on to help resolve difficulties in communication between those in their care, their families and other healthcare professionals. The most important aspect of the humanistic approach is that it empowers the patients and their families and encourages professionals to work in partnership with those they are caring for.

One of main proponents of the humanistic approach to communication was Carl Rogers. His philosophy was that all people are deserving of respect and that they are all equal. He believed that professionals should not set themselves up as experts when helping people solve problems, as everyone is capable of finding their own solutions. However, at times they may need help in clarifying what steps to take to make the best choices and reach their full potential and this is where professionals can help (Rogers, 1980). Carl Rogers explored what he considered to be the basic requirements for effective therapeutic communication; that is to say in the simplest terms: *being congruent, being empathic and being non-judgemental*. Nurses need to develop these qualities as they will be required to help those in their care to make important decisions in relation to their health needs. These situations entail a great deal of responsibility, necessitating the use of communication skills safely and effectively.

What is meant by 'being congruent, being empathic and being non-judgemental'?

Carl Rogers describes being congruent as being real. He states that when communicating it is important to be genuine within the relationship, to acknowledge to yourself how you are feeling in response to the other person; it is important to recognise and acknowledge these feelings as they can cloud communication (ibid.). Recognising where the emotions originate will help the nurse communicate more effectively because they will be responding directly to the emotional needs of the other person and not their own.

Second in the Rogerian approach to communication is the use of empathy and the development of an empathic relationship. According to Rogers, empathy is developed through a process of putting oneself in the other person's world and seeing it from their point of view. It requires sensitivity to the feelings of the other person and sensitivity to their lived experiences. However, it is important to check that these perceptions are correct, and this can be achieved through a series of questions to elicit if the perceptions as to what the person is feeling are correct (ibid.). The skills of being congruent and being empathic need to be used in conjunction with the third skill described by Rogers, being non-judgemental. It is important to remember that these therapeutic communication skills were developed to be used within counselling relationships and therefore need to be adapted to the way in which the nurse communicates with those in their care and the multi-disciplinary team. While the skills have been described separately, they are in fact closely interwoven and need to be used in conjunction to achieve effective communication.

Being real in practice

When following these three basic principles proposed by Carl Rogers, the nurse would need to be real (congruent) with the people they were caring for. But how real can a nurse be? It is important to remember that these are professional relationships and not personal ones. While there are things that a nurse might say in response to their own family and friends, it would not be acceptable for them to respond in the same way to someone in their care or to a colleague. For example, showing certain emotions, such as anger. While a display of anger may be acceptable and healthy in a personal relationship, it would not be so in a professional relationship. They need to recognise and acknowledge their own feelings of anger or distress but know that it is not necessary to act on them.

So, what can be done in situations like these? First, it is important that the nurse does not take it personally but is able to stand back and think before responding. The patient or service user, who is expressing their anger, may have a valid reason for doing so. It is important to find out why, without causing more distress. It is at this point that the skill of being empathic needs to be used. Perhaps there are valid reasons for the patient or service user to be angry? Unless one asks, the nurse might never know the reason for the aggression and make judgements that may be unfounded.

Being empathic

Nurses need to understand the importance of being empathic and displaying empathy. However, in its purest form, this may be difficult because if the nurse has empathy for all the people in their care, the emotions may soon become overwhelming, making it difficult to practise effectively. The Rogerian approach that the professional 'enter' the world of the other person needs to be adapted for nursing. As mentioned above, if empathy is used in the psychotherapeutic sense, it would soon become overwhelming (Williams and Stickley, 2010). The most important aspect of empathy is again that the nurse responds to the patient's experiences, not their own. The student nurse with experience will learn how to withdraw after the interaction and separate their own feelings from those in their care. It is important that all nurses recognise that boundaries can become blurred and that they need to seek support in addressing the situation if this happens.

Activity 2.1

Find an empathy questionnaire on the internet to assess your level of empathy.

- How empathetic are you?
- What does empathy mean to you now?

There are many empathy questionnaires but completing one will give you points to reflect on. You may find this useful: www.midss.org/content/toronto-empathy-questionnaire

Being non-judgemental

There may be occasions when the nurse starts to form opinions and judge those in their care and their colleagues according to their own beliefs. As Carl Rogers describes it, when this happens, the other person, in this case, the patient, service user or colleague is no longer being heard (Rogers, 1980). The nurse is not hearing the other person, instead they are 'listening' to their own reactions to what they are hearing. Once this happens, objectivity is lost and it does not matter if the judgements are critical or sympathetic, communication will be compromised. Rather than help the other person reach their own conclusions as to how they feel and why, the nurse may influence them because of their own judgements and therefore they are no longer effective in their communication.

Don't forget!

The basic humanistic principles underlying communication (Rogers 1980) are:

- Be real
- Be empathic
- Be non-judgemental.

Case study 2.1

Staff Nurse Smith has spent the last hour caring for Mr Basset, aged 55 years, who has been on the ward for four weeks. He was admitted after having being involved in a car accident and is confined to bed. He sustained multiple fractures and relies on others to meet all of his needs. Mr Basset has been quiet throughout the hour and had kept his head down and avoided eye contact with the nurse, despite the fact that Nurse Smith did his best to chat and keep the conversation going by talking about his own planned trip to Spain. Nurse Smith was pleased with the care he had given and decided that he would go for his break. As he turned to go, he says cheerfully: 'I'll be back later.' However, as he walked away Mr Basset became angry because he was not offered a drink. Nurse Smith was surprised and a little irritated but he went back and assisted Mr Basset with drinking a glass of water, after which Mr Basset became very apologetic. Nurse Smith responded by saying he did not need to apologise and went on his break.

Now look at the answers in Box 2.2.

It is important in situations like that shown in Case study 2.1 that the nurse reflects on and uses the skills described by Carl Rogers and put the needs of the patient or service user first (NMC, 2010a). Was the nurse communicating from the three humanistic principles? Was he being real? Did he show empathy? Was he non-judgemental?

Box 2.2 Answers using the PER tool

Prepare

- Was Nurse Smith prepared to care for Mr Basset?
- While he felt excited about his trip to Spain, he needed to focus on the care he was about to give Mr Basset
- He should have taken time to read through Mr Basset's medical notes so as to be aware of his needs and focus on Mr Basset's reality, that he was immobile and unable to care for himself
- Nurse Smith needed to think about how this might have affected Mr Basset.

Engage/Communicate

- When Nurse Smith first introduced himself to Mr Basset, he should have noted his response as this would have influenced the way communication developed
- He did not act sensitively and talked about his forthcoming trip without thinking about how Mr Basset might feel about it
- Nurse Smith did not demonstrate empathy; he was carrying out nursing care routinely without thinking about the impact of his conversation.

Reflect

- Nurse Smith could have responded sooner to Mr Basset's behaviour and turned the focus of the conversation away from himself to Mr Basset
- Perhaps this was not the time to 'chat' but was a time to be empathic
- He could have asked if there was anything Mr Basset needed before he went on his break
- He also could have asked himself if it was appropriate to feel irritated by Mr Basset's request for a drink
- Was he judging Mr Basset for becoming angry?
- Perhaps it would have been more appropriate for Nurse Smith to have delayed his break and to have spent more time with Mr Basset to find out if there was anything worrying him.

Remember that being real in this situation is not in relation to the nurse but the patient. Focus on the reality of the patient's or service user's situation, reality is not a trip to Spain but that of being restricted to bed. This is when it is important to use the skill of empathy and to think what it feels like to be in that position. Imagining the situation will help develop empathy and maintain focus on the patient. At times, aspects of a patient's or service user's behaviour such as anger may be difficult to accept. But it is important not to make judgements. There could be many reasons why patients become angry and it is important to elicit the cause, rather than making assumptions and forming judgements. Being real, showing empathy and accepting patients and service users as they are when they are at their most vulnerable ask a great deal of the nurse's emotions. Communication can become clouded, especially if the situation is similar to one the nurse may have experienced previously. This may confuse their reality with that of the patient and it can at times be difficult to realise what is appropriate and what is not. The nurse always needs to ensure that the patient is at the centre of the communication.

Don't forget!

- Know your patient
- Focus on the patient and their reality
- Use the necessary communication skills to meet their needs
- Communication skills can be developed with thought and practice.

What are communication skills?

The humanistic approach discussed previously will support and underpin the more practical and cultural aspects of communication that are now to be explored. The rationale for nurses adopting a philosophy is to guide their overall interactions with patients and colleagues, and to combine this with the practical aspects of communication in order to communicate effectively. Communication skills can be said to fall into three main categories, each of which involves a complex set of skills. These three categories are: (1) verbal skills; (2) non-verbal skills; and (3) perceptions and judgements.

Verbal communication skills include far more than merely the words used: the language; they also involve the way they are said: the paralanguage. Non-verbal communication skills include the use of facial expressions and the body, from head nods to hand gestures, to the way someone stands or sits. Finally, there is the category described as perceptions and judgements, which is a more subtle but important aspect of communication that may not always be obvious. The way that people perceive each other has a profound impact on communication and this type of communication occurs constantly throughout the day or night, whenever someone is being observed. As an example, the nurse on the ward may not be aware of the fact that they are 'communicating' whether they are actively interacting with another person or not. They are communicating by just being there.

Vocabulary

Language or words are what most people would consider to be the most important way in which they communicate. In some respects this is true. One of the first aspects consciously noted by the listener when someone speaks is the type of vocabulary or words used and the way in which they construct their sentences. Nurses need to see beyond the words the patients use, e.g. if the patient is swearing, they need to see the emotions behind the language and respond to those rather than judge them because of their language and use of words.

Another example of the influence of vocabulary on communication is when the speaker uses terms and expressions that are considered to belong to particular social groups. Perceptions and judgements depend on the person who is listening and their own social background or command of English, and these perceptions can have an impact on the development of communication. Nurses also need to be aware of words that are *not* being used in conversations. When working with young people and adults who may not be comfortable in disclosing their sexuality, they may omit the gender of their partner when discussing their relationships. The fact that patients or colleagues feel that they cannot mention the gender of their partner indicates they feel that they will not be treated with equal respect. Patients or service users who are depressed may heighten concern about their welfare if they do not talk about their future, as it may indicate they are having suicidal thoughts because they do not feel that they have a future.

As professionals, it is important that nurses think about and reflect on the vocabulary they use, and this is particularly relevant for student nurses. There is a whole new vocabulary related to the nursing profession and health care that needs to be learned. Initially this can seem daunting, it can feel as if another language is being spoken, and to some extent it is. However, it is the responsibility of all nurses to learn and understand it. By listening to other nurses and healthcare professionals, the nurse will learn to use the relevant terminology and understand it. Competence in using this new language will develop with experience. However, nurses will often be in a position when they have to 'translate' medical and nursing terms into a language that the patient can understand, so that the patient can be fully involved in decisions relating to their care.

Paralanguage

The second and possibly more important aspect of verbal communication is the way in which the words are said. This is referred to as paralanguage, that is to say, pitch, volume, rate, tone and intonation. While people may consciously think about the words someone is using, it is usually their intuition that is used to interpret the way in which the words are being said. It is paralanguage that makes clear what the meaning is and it is this 'meaning' that people are trying to understand when listening to what someone is saying. They are attempting to understand the mood or emotional state of the person. The patient or service user may be consciously communicating their emotional state by using the appropriate tone and volume that complements the words. However, at times they may not be conscious of the fact that the paralanguage does not match the language which can cause confusion for the nurse. For example, a patient or service user may say that they are not worried about going for surgery or being admitted to a psychiatric unit. The fact that their voice is low and shaky should lead the nurse to think that perhaps they are anxious.

Before exploring the different components of paralanguage, it is necessary to think of another less obvious aspect of verbal communication but one which is potentially important and influential in respect to perceptions and judgements. In a multicultural country such as Britain, with a wide variety of accents and dialects, it is important that nurses are aware of this subtle but essential aspect of verbal communication and be aware how it may influence the perception of others.

Nurses need also to be aware of the pitch, volume, rate, tone and intonation. Each aspect is important in its own right; however, in order to be understood, they need to be related to each other to get the most accurate interpretation of the message being conveyed. When thinking about paralanguage, it is also important to remember that while the aspects such as tone and intonation can be similar, they can vary between cultures, ranging from the culture within the family to the different cultures found in the UK. This can mean it might be normal for some people to speak loudly and appear to be shouting at each other. If questioned, the person may say that it is the way they speak with their family and it is natural for them.

Clinical significance

When communicating with patients, it can also be difficult to interpret what the emotion is if the language being spoken is not understood, as it can be difficult to match the words and the paralanguage. If unsure how to interpret what the patient is trying to say, check understanding by asking if they really feel that or are they 'putting on a brave front'?

Case study 2.2

Tom is 16 years old and a keen rugby player. He has been in hospital for a week following an operation. However, he has been seen by the surgical team and has been told he can be discharged and go home. His mother has arrived to collect him and he is very keen to leave the ward. Nurse Ramsay has spent 45 minutes going through the discharge plan which is almost completed, however, they have spent some of the time chatting about Tom's school and Mrs Nolan's journey to the hospital. Nurse Ramsay notices that when giving him advice about when he can begin to play rugby or participate in contact sports, he and his mother do not appear to be paying attention, as they are packing his bag and looking around his locker to make sure they have not forgotten anything. Before saying goodbye she asks if they have understood what she has said, he just says 'Yeah, yeah' and Mrs Nolan nods.

Look at the answers in Box 2.3.

When communicating important information to patients, keep it simple and to the point, do not include information that is irrelevant. Ensure that the patient is 'listening'. It will be difficult for them to concentrate if the ward is busy and noisy. It is the responsibility of the nurse communicating the information to make it clear. Give information that relates directly to safety first, such as how to store and use medication. Use terms the patient understands and check their understanding by asking them to explain what has been said. Paralanguage, such as intonation and volume, can be used to emphasise important information and to maintain attention.

Box 2.3 Answers using the PER tool

Prepare

▪ When Nurse Ramsay was told that Tom could be discharged home, she would have begun to prepare by ensuring that everything was ready for him to leave the ward on time

▪ One essential aspect of discharge is the information that he will require to ensure a safe post-operative recovery at home

▪ It is Nurse Ramsay's responsibility to make sure the patient and their family understand the discharge information.

Engage/Communication

▪ Nurse Ramsay had initially engaged Tom and his mother. However, during the discharge she spent time talking to them about things not directly related to the discharge

▪ She lost their attention while giving them key information, i.e. returning to sport post-operatively

▪ Their actions of packing should have alerted her to the fact that they were not listening.

Reflect

▪ Nurse Ramsay could have started the discharge by giving the most important information first

▪ She could have made use of paralanguage to emphasise the most important information

▪ This could have included using Tom's name to regain attention when it wandered

▪ She could have had the general conversation after the essential information.

Watch out

When giving patients or service users important information, choose the most appropriate time and place.

▪ Gain their attention
▪ Give the information related to safety first
▪ Repeat important information
▪ Use paralanguage to emphasise the most important information and keep their attention
▪ Check understanding and give written information as required.

Non-verbal communication

It has been stated that non-verbal communication is the aspect of communication that is the most influential (Knapp *et al.*, 2014). Yet, at times it can be the one that nurses are the least aware of. Therefore, it is essential that nurses develop their non-verbal skills in the same way that they develop their verbal skills. They need to be constantly aware what they are communicating through the use of their facial expressions and the use of their body. More often than not, people do not consciously think about their facial expressions or the bodily movements they are making when interacting and communicating with someone, unlike their choice of words. This can lead to communications being mixed. On the whole, non-verbal communications are almost automatic, however, it is important that nurses develop awareness and be sensitive to the non-verbal messages they are giving and receiving, so as to communicate professionally and effectively. For example, even the way nurses walk will communicate a message to the observer, i.e. they are in a hurry? Bored? Confident?

In order to develop awareness of the impact of non-verbal communication, such as facial expressions, head movements, the use of hands and touch and the body itself will be explored and discussed. The main discussion will be from a Western perspective, although cultural differences need to be considered when developing skills for non-verbal communication.

Head movements

Before thinking about the specific aspects of facial expressions, it is worth looking at how head movements are used to enhance communication. In Western cultures people nod their head to show understanding and agreement; they shake their head to disagree or to 'say' no. The head is inclined to show that someone is listening but it can also indicate that the person is thinking. People look down or drop their head when feeling shame or sadness. Nurses need to think about the way they are using their head movements to strengthen their communication, particularly when listening to someone, one of the most important communication skills in nursing. They can do this by nodding at times to show understanding, affirming what is being said. Head inclinations towards the speaker indicate that the nurse is focusing on what is being said. Head movements aid communication but they need to be used in conjunction with the appropriate facial expressions.

Facial expressions

When listening to patients and colleagues, nurses can use their head to show that they are actively listening. However, these movements of the head will also need to be complemented by the appropriate facial expression. Basic facial expressions, such as smiling, sadness, anger, disgust, fear and joy, are said to be universal throughout the world, from Western Europe to the forests of Borneo! A smile will be recognised as a smile wherever you are, as would an expression of sadness (Ekman, 1999). The reason for this is that they are some of the oldest ways in which people have communicated over the centuries from the Stone Age to the present. But that does not always make them simple to use or understand. People can smile with genuine happiness or to be polite, the way to tell which is through the subtle use of the eyes. Are they being used to enhance the smile or is it only the mouth that is being used? If the smile is related to happiness, the eyes will be involved in the expression. Nurses will find that a person's face will tell them many things that perhaps they are unable to say or express. This is especially relevant when working with children or those who are unable to communicate through speech. Nurses will also need to use their facial expressions to express emotions that perhaps they do not have the words for, to show compassion and empathy when patients are at their most vulnerable.

Eye contact

Eyes are very important ways in which people communicate, not only as part of the overall facial expressions but in the way they express thoughts and emotions to others; eyes can be used to indicate interest, attraction or hostility. They are also one of the best ways to express more subtle emotions, such as compassion, empathy, and sadness and perhaps that is why they have been described as 'the windows to the soul'. The emotions and thoughts expressed through eye contact are complicated and complex and can often depend on things such as the duration that the gaze is held between the people involved. If the gaze is held for too long, it can indicate hostility or attraction. When eye contact does become uncomfortable, one of the participants breaks the gaze. For nurses working with children and young people, it is important to remember that babies have difficulty in focusing their eyes at birth and initially can only see up to 30 cms by the age of 6 weeks. As they develop, they can see up to 60 cms, and by 6 months they will be able to see the same distance as that of an adult. As children grow older, they will learn the skills needed to use eye contact to communicate effectively, 'Don't stare' is something that most people would be told as they grew up.

However, if asked, few people could identify where they learned these skills. It is often from the people around them and the culture that they live in. In some cultures, maintaining eye contact is not considered polite, in others, such as West African cultures it is considered rude for younger people to look directly at their elders as it shows a lack of respect, but in Western cultures not to make eye contact is thought to be devious. It is important to appreciate cultural differences so as not to cause or take offence (McCarthy et al., 2006). For nurses caring for patients and service users from other cultures, it is important to ensure that they pay attention to how they use and interpret eye contact. When interpreting eye contact, the nurse needs to take into consideration aspects such as culture, gender and the mental and emotional state of the other person, as each of these will have an impact on the type of eye contact.

Clinical significance

It is the nurse's responsibility to ensure their non-verbal communications do not add to the patient's discomfort or anxiety.

Proximity, orientation and touch

Other forms of non-verbal communication that are culturally specific, hence may not be regulated consciously, include how close someone stands to another person (proximity) or the way people face each other (orientation). Facing someone shows interest and facing away can show disinterest. The way in which hands are used when making gestures and when touching someone is also important. Hand gestures can be used to beckon someone, or to stop them to emphasise what is being said. Hands are also very important in the use of touch. This is a key aspect of communication in nursing and one that requires close monitoring. The use of the body is related to personal culture, from one's own family culture to the wider society in which one lives. In order not to give offence, it is very important that nurses think about proximity, orientation and touch because they will often be in situations where the normal social rules in relation to these will not apply.

The distance people keep between themselves and others depends on the environment and their relationship. People in a lift or on public transport may have little control over how close they stand next to someone or how close someone stands next to them. However, the distance between people is usually determined by their relationship. The more intimate the relationship, the closer people will stand to each other. At times nurses may realise that either a colleague or patient is standing closer than they feel comfortable with. If the degree of proximity is not related to nursing care, the feeling of discomfort will be because the other person has broken the unspoken rule about distance and closeness. It is important that the nurse recognises and responds to this, as the closeness may indicate the potential for the perception of inappropriate behaviour or aggression. There will be situations where nurses providing physical care for someone will need to be physically close to them. This is part of care delivery and is considered acceptable. It is important to remember that this may feel uncomfortable for the patient who is less used to this level of proximity, though the way in which nurses orientate themselves to the patient can make the situation less intimate.

While the degree of distance is important, so is the way in which nurses orientate themselves to the other person. First, when speaking to patients and service users, the nurse needs to decide whether it is better to stand or sit. Standing over someone can have an impact on communication, as the person standing is normally perceived as being in a more powerful position. To ensure communication is balanced, it is better that where possible the nurse's eyes are level with those of the patient. This is essential when working with children. As adults, nurses may appear more intimidating to children if they stand over them. It is best practice to get down to the level of the child. If communicating with another adult, the nurse would need to be aware that standing directly opposite someone can be interpreted as a sign of aggression and so it is more usual to stand at an angle to the other person. The closer the angle, again, the more intimate the relationship. When working with patients or service users who are aggressive and agitated, nurses need to keep themselves safe, by constantly monitoring distance and orientation. Crossing one's arms when talking to others may convey disinterest and being defensive.

Don't forget!

- Be sensitive to how proximity may be felt by the patient
- Use the way you orientate yourself to enhance communication
- Adapt styles to suit the patient, child, young person or service user.

Touch

Touch is essential in nursing. It can comfort, reassure and calm patients who are anxious and distressed. However, as with all aspects of communication, there are many different social and cultural rules about what is considered appropriate or not. As an example, some parts of the body are considered more acceptable to touch than others, e.g., the hands and arms. It is less usual to touch someone's face or legs unless you know them intimately (Gallace and Spence, 2010). Before touching someone, a patient, service user or colleague, the nurse always needs to ask themselves, is it necessary? It is also important to be aware of how it will be interpreted by someone watching. While touch can be useful when working with children and young people, to gain attention or to comfort, it is important to maintain safety for the staff and for the child or young person. In child and adolescent mental health services (CAMHS), a non-touch policy is often advocated, as many of the children and young people may have been physically or sexually abused. When working with this group of patients, nurses will need to remember that, for them, touch may not be safe and that touch can be misinterpreted.

Always ensure that touch is used for a therapeutic reason. It is a natural reaction for many people to want to put their arm around someone when they see that they are upset, but nurses should not make that assumption. It may seem unnatural to ask someone if they want a hug but it is important to remember that the use of touch should be for the patient's comfort. They may come from a family that is not tactile or from a culture that does not allow touch between different genders and rather than bring comfort, the physical contact may cause them to feel more distress. It is important that nurses familiarise themselves with the cultural aspects involved in relation to touch. For example, Hasidic Jews do not touch people outside of their faith and while in Western cultures, one way of greeting someone may be with a handshake, it would be inappropriate to do so in this instance.

Don't forget!

- Use touch in relation to the patient's needs
- Always think how other people may interpret it
- Be sensitive to cultural differences
- Ensure all touch is safe.

Listening skills

All of the above non-verbal skills need to be used when listening to patients, service users and colleagues, so as to demonstrate that the nurse is actively listening. To really listen to someone is not easy or simple. It is easy to become distracted, lose focus or start to make judgements in response to what the other person is saying. In order to listen well, it is important that the focus is on the other person. Ideally the environment would be appropriate, i.e. quiet and private with no interruptions. However, in nursing that may not often happen, as patients and service users may need to talk and express their concerns at any time. In order to listen well, the nurse needs to use the skills described above. Leaning forward and tilting the head indicate that the nurse is concentrating on what is being said. Nodding and eye contact show understanding. Most importantly it is important for the nurse to remember the qualities described by Rogers (1980) and listen to the reality of the patient or service user, they may become distracted by trying to think of answers or the most appropriate response and these will have as much an impact on the ability to listen as being in a crowded noisy room. If unsure of what has been said or the meaning, the nurse can ask the patient or service user to clarify what they have said and check that their understanding of the meaning is correct. The nurse will also need to 'listen' to the non-verbal language that is being used to aid understanding.

Perceptions

The skills required in verbal and non-verbal communication have been explored and discussed above. However, there still remains an important aspect of communication for discussion. It is how patients and service users perceive the nurses who are caring for them and the perceptions of their colleagues. The perceptions and judgements of others are formed after observing nurses as they go about their work. They will also base this on verbal and non-verbal communication skills, as well as personal characteristics, such as age, gender, behaviour and appearance. Characteristics, such as age or gender, cannot be altered but the nurse's overall professional appearance, e.g., the way they wear their uniform can be changed. Nurses need to be aware of how aspects in relation to themselves, that they may take for granted, such as their appearance, may influence how others perceive them.

Professional communication

Nursing is a rewarding but demanding profession and it is important that nurses communicate respect for each other. One simple example of this is punctuality, not only for the beginning and ending of shifts but also when returning from breaks. It communicates a great deal about how professional the nurse is as a person. For example, it is important that staff arrive in plenty of time to be able to change into their uniform before the shift starts. The reason why this is necessary is so that the team will be ready to take part in the handover where important information about patient and service user care is communicated between shifts. Being late can lead to miscommunication between shifts and patient safety can be compromised, which is not acceptable. For patients, a lack of punctuality may communicate to them that the nurse concerned cannot be trusted and is unreliable. For someone dependent on nurses for all their basic needs, such as Mr Basset in Case study 2.1, to be told by the nurse caring for them that they will return in 5 minutes, but in reality it is 30 minutes, can be very distressing. For children, this is especially important as their perceptions of time depend very much on their age and level of development. In order for nurses to gain their trust, it is important that they are consistent and reliable, and are perceived as such.

Case study 2.3

Nurse Ramsay has asked Student Nurse Adelele to escort Mr Netter, 80 years old who is on bed rest, to the X-ray department. The X-ray department is very busy and they have been waiting for 40 minutes for the porters to help take Mr Netter, on his bed, back to the ward. Student Nurse Adelele is sitting on one of the chairs and has not spoken to Mr Netter during the time they have been waiting together. She yawns several times and looks bored, which is noticed by the other patients and their families who are waiting to be seen. Mr Netter is becoming restless, saying that he needs to go to the toilet and that he is thirsty. She says she will go and get him a glass of water and be 'back in a minute' but does not return for 20 minutes.

Look at the answers in Box 2.4.

The most concerning aspect in Case study 2.3 is the lack of consideration shown towards Mr Netter. Equally concerning, is the impression Student Nurse Adelele's behaviour has on those observing her. It does not inspire confidence in other patients or members of the public who witness it. It is important for nurses to remember that while on duty they are constantly being observed and will need to think about what impact their behaviour is having on the people around them. When escorting patients or service users, it is important to check with them at regular intervals to see if there is anything they need, before going on the escort and throughout the duration. There will always be eventualities that cannot be planned for and in these instances, be as clear as possible about waiting times and apologise for any situation that causes distress. A simple explanation will help patients and colleagues understand. It communicates honesty and concern. Patients and service users should be told who they can call on for assistance should they need anything when the nurse who is allocated to call for them is not available. The nurse also needs to communicate with colleagues so that they are aware of the patient's needs.

Self-awareness: the nurse's responsibility

Some of the situations that influence patients' perceptions of nurses, and the judgements these can lead to, have been explored. However, one of the issues not yet dealt with is the perceptions and judgements of nurses towards patients and colleagues. It is essential that all nurses develop their sense of self-awareness so as to be aware of their own preju- dices and beliefs. The reason is so that they can put them to one side, as it is important

Box 2.4 Answers using the PER tool

Prepare

- It is difficult to know how long escorting a patient to another department will take
- Student Nurse Adelele could have taken a text book with her to read, in case she was there for a long time and in case Mr Netter did not want to converse.

Engage/Communicate

- It can be difficult to for nurses and patients to maintain conversation for a prolonged period of time
- However, Student Nurse Adelele made no attempt to engage Mr Netter while they were in the X-ray department
- Instead she sat away from him and spent her time yawning.

Reflect

- Student Nurse Adelele could have prepared Mr Netter by telling him that having the X-ray might take some time and asking if there was anything he needed before leaving the ward, such as using a urine bottle
- She could also have thought to bring some water in case he needed a drink while they were waiting
- Student Nurse Adelele should also have appreciated that even though she was not on the ward, she was still at work, and as such should have been aware of the impression she was making on the people observing her
- She should have ensured that she checked with Mr Netter regularly to see if there was anything he needed and to let him know that she was there. When going to get the drink, she could have given a more realistic time scale than 'one minute'.

that personal beliefs do not have a negative impact on professional relationships with patients and colleagues. Beliefs can relate to different cultures, religions and lifestyles. If nurses do not develop awareness of their perceptions and judgements, they may lead to ineffective communication, either through verbal or non-verbal communication. The NMC (2015a) is clear that all people are to be treated equally when receiving health care. Nurses' judgements and perceptions do not have to be explicit. They can be as subtle as dismissing someone's religious beliefs because they are not religious themselves or are not the same as those of the nurse, or not respecting their customs. One example would be if nurses do not drink alcohol themselves; they may have difficulties accepting the reality of patients or service users who have problems with alcohol and blame them for their addiction. Another situation may include patients who have contracted HIV, they may be judged by nurses who consider it be their own fault for being promiscuous or deviant. Whatever the reason for the patient or service user needing health care, the nurse needs to be aware of their own beliefs so as to ensure they do not let them influence the way they communicate with patients.

It is also good practice for nurses to introduce themselves to other members of the team they are working with, especially the first time they meet each other.

Table 2.1 presents the key principles of communication for nurses.

Table 2.1 Key principles of communication

- All nurses, whether caring for adults, children, young people or service users with mental health problems will need to know how to communicate effectively with each of these groups, even if they are not the primary group of patients or service users being cared for in any setting
- Nurses need to think back to the basis of all nursing communication, the Rogerian or humanistic approach and to see each person and family as individuals with their own special needs and way of communicating
- The nurse will need to communicate with all the family of the person they are caring for, as they are part of the team as described by the NMC in the Code of Conduct (2015a)
- Nurses need to note things that may have an impact on communication such as the age, gender and culture of the individual
- Nurses ought to consider:
  - If the person has a physical problem that may have an impact on their ability to communicate; are they wearing a hearing aid?
  - If they have a physical or learning disability
  - If English is their first language or not. If not, they will need to assess how good their understanding is and ensure that verbal communication is adapted as required
  - Whether written information will be understood (language, reading, level).
- Each patient and service user will have their own unique way of communicating and it is necessary to be aware and sensitive to it. Some may talk quickly, others more hesitantly and it will be necessary for nurses to adapt their style to suit that of the patient
- The nurse must always introduce themselves, stating their name and their position when first meeting the patient and their family
- Always ask how the patient wants to be addressed.

Adult nursing

Adult or general nursing covers a wide age range, from 18 years of age through to someone who may be 90 years old or older. As with each field of nursing, each patient has to be seen as an individual and the style of communication adapted accordingly.

Ask the patient what they want to be called; do not assume that everyone wants to be called by their first name. How will the reason for admission or treatment impact on the patient's ability to communicate? At times nurses will be required to care for patients who are unconscious or have lost their ability to communicate verbally or non-verbally. In situations like these, the responsibility for effective communication is the nurse's. As patients who are non-verbal may not be able to communicate what their needs are, the nurses caring for them will need to plan care so that all basic needs are met. However, they must also make sure that they communicate what they are doing to the patient and not assume that they should carry out their care in silence or talk across them to other nurses.

Nurses and other professionals can at times forget that some discussions are not appropriate in front of patients or their families. As nurses work together in caring for a patient they may forget to put the patient at the centre of the communication and talk to each other over the patient. This is not acceptable practice, and again if they put themselves in the patient's position, the nurses would appreciate how uncomfortable this is. It is also important for nurses working with children and young people to recognise that they may be listening even though they look as they are distracted by play or television. Similar situations can occur in all fields of nursing, when nurses forget that other patents or clients may be listening. Even if nurses are talking in the office, if the door is open, their conversations can be overheard. This needs to be taken seriously as patient confidentiality can easily be compromised.

Mental health nursing

The NMC (2010a, p. 24) states that those nurses working in the mental health field need to develop communication through 'the therapeutic use of self'. This means that the nurse has to have excellent skills in how they use their communication skills but also how the interpret them: communication in all its forms is central to every aspect of care in mental health nursing. While this can be said about all fields of nursing, the service users who are being cared for by mental health professionals are particularly vulnerable. This vulnerability is related to their ability to communicate and understand communication, which may be affected by their mental state. Depending on their presenting problem, the client may often need help in clarifying their thoughts and communication. This skill carries a great deal of responsibility on the part of the nurse and this is one of the main differences in the level and complexity of communication in relation to the other fields. When working in mental health nursing or with any person with a mental illness, it is important to read the non-verbal communications carefully, not only in order to recognise that a service user may become violent but also to recognise service users who may be at risk of self-harm or become actively suicidal. For service users who are experiencing psychotic episodes, in which they may have delusions or hallucinations, the nurse has to be sure not to collude with them by agreeing and reinforcing them. They need to use their communication skills to reassure and comfort the service user through what can be a frightening and unpleasant experience. Service users who feel suicidal may have difficulty in expressing their distress and it may be the responsibility of the nurse to help them find the language to do so. The nurse would also need to be able through careful observation of verbal and non-verbal communication to recognise when a service user may be suicidal and so know when to intervene safely. There is no one set of behaviours that a service user may exhibit to aid the nurse, as each will have a different way of expressing their distress, and this is the particular skill in reading communications that mental health nurses need. Being able to read the signs expressed through verbal and non-verbal behaviour will enable them to take the appropriate actions to keep the service user and others safe.

Children and young people's nursing

Nursing children and young people requires an in-depth knowledge of child development, particularly in relation to children's language and understanding so that verbal communication can be adapted to their level of development. It is not only an understanding of verbal communication that is necessary but also how to use non-verbal communication skills appropriately. For infants and babies, touch and handling are very important as they communicate caring and comfort. Facial expressions are also important as babies respond positively to smiles and the nurse can use facial expressions to engage the infant or baby. However, from the age of about 6 months, babies become wary of strangers and so the nurses need to understand that the way they interacted with a younger baby may not be appropriate with an older one. The level and type of communication are very much set by the child and young person and the nurse needs to respond to their cues. However, it is the nurses' responsibility to set boundaries so that they do not come to harm. It is particularly important for nurses to be aware of the amount of physical contact they have with children and young people and ask themselves if it is necessary or appropriate. This is not only to protect the nurses from accusations of unprofessional behaviour but to protect the child, as they may not be able to recognise the difference between appropriate and inappropriate touch. However, touch can be a very powerful method of offering reassurance to a distressed child and it is the responsibility of the children and young people's nurse to know how to use it wisely. Working with young people can be difficult as they may appear to have a good understanding of their condition or what is required of them, but the nurse needs to check this rather than accept it. This is particularly important for young people who may physically look like an adult but have not yet developed the emotional and cognitive and communications skills of an adult. Young people may have difficulty in reading facial expressions the same way as an adult does and this will need to be taken into consideration (Blakemore and Choudhury, 2006). As children develop, the nurse will need at times to act as their advocate and communicate on their behalf in relation to other professionals in situations where their parents or carers are not present. As they grow older, the nurse will need to adapt their communication style to help the young person express their own needs and discuss their treatment with the team. This is especially important as they reach the age of consent and transition into adult services when it is expected that they will need to take a more active role in making decisions about their health (Kelsey and Abelson-Mitchell, 2007).

Don't forget!

- Whichever of the three fields of nursing one works in, there will be times when you will meet and care for people with learning disabilities
- Find out how to communicate best, i.e. by interpreting facial expressions and movements, by using the vocabulary the patient uses to describe their condition or through the use of technology where appropriate.

Communicating

Communicating with other professionals

Some of the most important professional relationships a nurse will have throughout their career are with their colleagues. For student nurses, one of the most important will be with their mentors, as it is expected by the NMC (2010a) that student nurses will work with their allocated mentor for at least 40 per cent of their time while in practice. The reason for this is so that the mentor will have the opportunity to communicate regularly and effectively. As with all relationships, students and mentors need to think about the first impression they want to make. It is important to remember that this is a two-way process, with both parties having equal responsibility in it. For students, it is important that their mentor perceives them as being interested, motivated and professional at all times. This means being prepared for the area by reading about what the service provides, asking relevant questions, being proactive at work, wearing the correct uniform/clothes, being punctual, communicating effectively and being safe. This relationship can begin with the first contact with the practice area and the initial meeting between the mentor and student. For the mentor, their responsibility is to see the student as an individual and to ensure they provide a supportive and rewarding learning environment. The first meeting between mentor and student is important as this is when they agree learning outcomes, it is the responsibility of the student to communicate the experiences they have had before arriving in that area so the mentor has realistic expectancies about what level of skills they can expect the student to have.

Other professional relationships that are equally important are with the wider members of the team, such as doctors, pharmacists, porters and any other person involved in the care of the patient or service user. Regardless of the perceived status of the other team member, communication must be professional and respectful. It is important to have a clear understanding of each of the team roles in the care of patients and service users, so as to be aware what needs to be communicated to them, as information needs to be communicated as appropriate. In situations where there are concerns about a patient's well-being, the nurse needs to be particularly clear so that other professionals know how to respond effectively. One tool to help focus communication between the nurse and the other members of the team is the SBAR technique (Thomas *et al.*, 2009). This was first developed in the armed forces but has been adapted for the nursing and medical profession. This technique can help nurses organise their thoughts and therefore be more effective when calling doctors or handing over care to another nurse:

- **S**ituation: what is the situation? Why are you calling the doctor or pharmacist?
- **B**ackground: what background information do you need to give?
- **A**ssessment: what is your assessment of the problem?
- **R**ecommendations: how should the problem be dealt with?

The reason for using this technique is that at times communication can be poor, especially when nurses are anxious or under pressure and in situations where patients' or service users' safety may be compromised, there is no room for error.

Telephone calls

Wherever a nurse works in the health service, throughout the day and night they will need to use the phone and answer the phone. While this seems a simple task, often it is not done well. When calling someone, the nurse should always state their name, position and area that they are in and be clear about what it is they want. When answering, they should again state their name, position and area they are in and then they should ask who is speaking and how they can help. Some calls may be simple enquiries and easily dealt with, others may be much more complex. What is important is not to give confidential information over the phone if unsure who it is being given to. Because there are no visual means of communication, there is more emphasis on the words used and paralanguage. Keep the message clear and repeat information if necessary, to be sure it has been understood correctly. If the call is in relation to a patient or service user, and help is required, the SBAR technique outlined above can be used to give the relevant facts. It is best practice that the nurse have these readily and at hand before starting the call.

Practice areas are busy environments and messages can be forgotten and misplaced if not written in the correct place. The most important fact is that messages are communicated so that patients' and service users' safety is not compromised.

Documentation

Communication skills involve more than verbal, non-verbal skills and perceptions. In the nursing profession there is a need to complete documentation on a daily basis. The NMC (2010b) have given guidelines on how nursing documentation should be completed. The reason that the guidelines are so prescriptive is because of the legal implications, the consequences of poor communication and the need to ensure safety. Errors in communication have led to patients' safety being compromised, for example, unclear prescriptions on drug charts have led to drug errors, poor notes in medical files have led to the wrong operation being carried out. While nurses may not be responsible for completing these documents, they do have a responsibility in following the instructions written in them. When written communication is unclear, it is important to approach the person who made the entry and ask them to re-write it. Should there be an investigation into poor care or in relation to child protection, the facts need to be clear and unambiguous. In nursing notes it is necessary to make sure entries are clearly written and remarks such as 'doing well' are avoided. Nurses writing the documentation need to be specific, to document things as they happened and be comprehensive. It is also important to record specific conversations where the content may impact on a patient's or service user's care (Dimond, 2005).

For student nurses, as well as contributing to the patient's nursing documentation (which should be agreed and counter-signed by a qualified nurse), there is also the need to complete practice learning documentation and course work, to record and demonstrate their development over the three years. This record of learning communicates to mentors which practice experiences the student has had. It is important when completing this documentation to maintain confidentiality at all times, and ensure that the information is correct and original. As a reflection of professional development, it is important that it is given as much attention as the record keeping on the ward.

Top tip

- Before completing documentation, ensure you know what you want to say
- Make sure the information is correct
- Record the facts
- Avoid general statements such as 'doing well'.

Social networking

There has been a rapid growth in the development of social media networks over the past few years. While they in themselves may be useful means of communicating with friends, they can be potentially problematic for nurses who post information that crosses professional boundaries. It is important that nurses remember that they are accountable for their behaviour to the NMC (2015b) in their personal and private lives. When using social media, it is important to think carefully before posting messages. The following top tips are taken from the NMC guidance on social networking (www.nmc-uk.org).

Top tip

- Do not share confidential information on social media
- Do not post inappropriate comments
- Do not bully or intimidate colleagues
- Do not use sites to develop personal relationships with patients or service users.

Summary

The ability to communicate effectively is the most basic skill that all nurses require. Without it, all other aspects of nursing, such as the development of therapeutic relationships, carrying out care and ensuring patient safety, will be compromised. For nurses, communication in all its forms has to be a conscious activity. The patient or service user has to be the focus of all aspects of communication: verbal and non-verbal must complement each other so that they and their colleagues understand what is being communicated without confusion. Communicating effectively is a skill that will need to be adapted and developed throughout the nurses' career in order that each patient and service user is treated in the way that suits their needs. It is also the means by which the nurse can display empathy, caring and compassion, which are the basic qualities required for all fields of nursing.

References

Blakemore, S. and Choudhury, S. (2006) Development of the adolescent brain: implications for function and social cognition. *Journal of Child Psychology and Psychiatry*, 47(3/4): 296–312.

Dimond, B. (2005) Exploring common deficiencies that occur in record keeping. *British Journal of Nursing*, 14(10): 568–570.

Ekman, P. (1999) Facial expressions. In T. Dalgleish and M.J. Power (eds) *Handbook of Cognition and Emotion*. Chichester: John Wiley & Sons Ltd.

Gallace, A. and Spence, C. (2010) The science of interpersonal touch: an overview. *Neuroscience and Biobehavioral Reviews*, 34: 246–259.

Kelsey, J. and Abelson-Mitchell, N. (2007) Adolescent communication: perceptions and beliefs. *Journal of Children's and Young People's Nursing*, 1(1): 42–49.

Knapp, M.L., Hall, A.J. and Morgan, T.G. (2014) *Nonverbal Communication in Human Interaction*, eighth edn. Boston: Wadsworth Cengage Learning.

McCarthy, A., Lee, K., Itakura, S. and Muir, D. (2006) Cultural display rules drive eye gazing during thinking. *Journal of Cross Cultural Psychology*, 37(6): 717–22.

NMC (Nursing and Midwifery Council) (2010a) *Standards for Pre-registration Nursing Education*. London: NMC.

NMC (Nursing and Midwifery Council) (2010b) *Record Keeping*. London: NMC.

NMC (Nursing and Midwifery Council) (2011) *Guidance for Students of Nursing and Midwifery*. London: NMC.

NMC (Nursing and Midwifery Council) (2015a) *The Code: Professional Standards of Practice and Behaviour for Nurses and Midwives*. London: NMC.

NMC (Nursing and Midwifery Council) (2015b) *Guidance on Using Social Media Responsibly*. London: NMC.

Rogers, C.R. (1980) *A Way of Being*. Boston: Houghton Mifflin Company.

Thomas, C.M., Bertram, E. and Johnson, D. (2009) The SBAR communication technique: the nursing students' professional communication skills. *Nurse Educator*, 34(4): 176–180.

Williams, S. and Stickley, T. (2010) Empathy and nurse education. *Nurse Education Today*, 30: 752–755.

Chapter 3

Personal care

Mariama Seray-Wurie

The amount of relief and comfort experienced by the sick after the skin has been carefully washed and dried is one of the commonest observations made at a sick bed. If a nurse declines to do this because it was not her business, I should say that nursing was not her calling.

(*Florence Nightingale, 1860*)

Key concepts

Integumentary system

Personal care: hair and skin care

Mouth and oral care

Eye and eye care

Learning outcomes

By the end of this chapter you will be able to:

- Discuss the main functions of the skin and its relevance to meeting personal care needs
- Conduct a comprehensive assessment of the patient to identify the care or advice needed to promote their individual personal care needs (including skin, mouth, hair and eyes)
- Identify factors that influence personal care practices for an individual
- Explain how nurses can provide specific personal care to a patient and specific client groups e.g. the elderly and child
- Demonstrate the correct procedures to perform personal care.

Introduction

Although in practice the task of meeting personal care needs is now being delegated to healthcare support workers, it remains an essential aspect of nursing care for registered nurses, as it is often during the procedure of meeting personal hygiene needs that the nurse/patient relationship can develop as it is highly personal and very intimate. Not only does this procedure aim to promote patient comfort, it also provides one of the best opportunities to observe the patient and perform a detailed assessment of their skin, hair, eyes, mouth, nose, feet and nails. There could be some challenges in addressing and meeting the personal care needs of some patients, e.g. those with mental disorders such as depression and low mood. This chapter will discuss the techniques required to address the patient's personal care needs.

The skin, hair, glands and nails

To appreciate the significance of this skill, it is essential that there is an understanding of the importance of the role of the integumentary system. The skin (see Figure 3.1) is one of the largest organs of the body and its derivatives, hair, glands and nails make up the integumentary system.

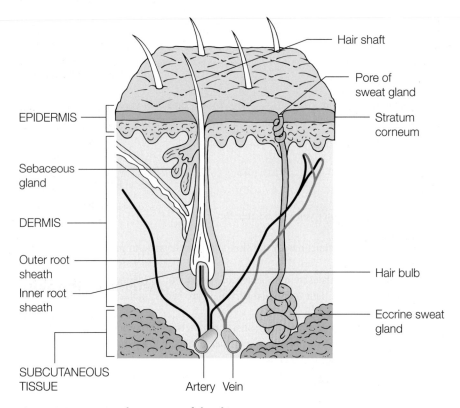

Figure 3.1 Layers and structures of the skin

In an attempt to prevent invasion from infection the skin has certain properties that help it in its protective role, e.g. keratin, which is a tough protein found in the epidermis, hair and nails. Keratin contributes to the protective functions as it waterproofs the skin, hair and nails, providing resistance to friction and thus bacterial invasion. Other properties include the intercellular junctions which hold the skin cells tightly together. It must be noted that that in healthy individuals the skin has transient and resident micro-organisms that cause no harm (known as normal flora).

Hair also provides protection, but this is minimal. It guards the scalp from injury and the sun's rays; eyebrows and eyelashes protect the eyes from foreign particles. Hair in the nostrils and ear canals also offers protection to these organs from dust and insects.

The glands associated with the skin are the sudoriferous (sweat glands), of which there are two types: eccrine glands and apocrine glands. These glands produce sweat or perspiration in an attempt to maintain body temperature and eliminate waste. However, sweat contains the enzyme lysozyme that is acidic, with chemicals making the skin hostile to pathogens (by digestion of the cell walls of certain bacteria), thus increasing its protective function. The sebaceous gland secretes sebum, which moisturises hair and forms a protective layer waterproofing the skin, keeping the skin soft and supple and preventing the growth of certain bacterial and fungal infections.

Rationale for meeting personal care needs

The apocrine glands develop during early to mid-puberty, producing sweat containing fatty materials. Found mainly in the armpits and around the genital area, they are the main cause of body odour (contact with the skin bacteria and chemical substances in the sweat giving off a distinct odour). This is one of the reasons why children in general tend not to have any body odour until they reach puberty.

As the skin ages, each layer is affected in terms of structure. The epidermis becomes thinner, making the skin more susceptible to tissue breakdown; the dermis atrophies and the skin loses its elasticity; the subcutaneous tissue diminishes, especially in areas like the face, shins, hands and feet. There is also a reduction and shrinkage in the eccrine and apocrine glands, therefore sweating is reduced, affecting the thermoregulation of the skin. The nail bed tends to become thinned and there is reduction in the density of the hair follicles. A study undertaken by Schofield *et al.* (2009) estimated that 28 per cent of the over-75s age group seek medical advice for a skin disease each year. Box 3.1 details the functions of the skin.

Box 3.1 Functions of the skin

- Protection, acting as a physical barrier to infection and injury, considered the body's first line of defence against infection
- Maintains body temperature
- Secretion of sebum
- Receiving stimuli
- Excretion of water, salts and several organic compounds
- Vitamin D synthesis.

Activity 3.1

There is an anecdote that somebody has said: 'The graduate nurse is too posh too wash.' Reflect on what this anecdote implies and think about why maintaining personal care should be a significant aspect of the nurse's role.

Personal hygiene care is:

> The physical act of cleansing the body to ensure that the hair, nails, ears, eyes, nose and skin are maintained in optimum condition. It also includes mouth hygiene which is the effective removal of plaque and debris to ensure the structures and tissues of the mouth are kept in a healthy condition. In addition, personal hygiene includes the appropriate length of nails and hair.
>
> (DoH, 2010)

This physical act of cleansing removes transient micro-organisms, dead skin as well as secretions, and excretions from the body which may be causing unpleasant odour. At the same time the skin will be stimulated, increasing circulation and, as stated by Florence Nightingale (1860), it provides comfort and a sense of well-being to the individual. The amount of assistance required to meet this function will vary, be it an adult (with physical and/or mental health needs) or child. Personal care needs and preferences should be met according to individual and clinical requirements; the individual is assessed to identify the advice or care required to maintain and promote their personal care (DoH, 2010). The assessment of personal care is usually included in most nursing care models, e.g. Roper *et al.* (2000), Orem (2001), and should include individual skin care practices, self-care abilities and skin conditions. It is also important to physically assess the condition of the skin, as healthy skin should be supple to touch with a good degree of elasticity, have an even colour that is unblemished and be clear of lesions.

Clinical significance

The skin also has resident micro-organisms that cause no harm, the normal skin flora. The physical act of washing removes the transient micro-organisms. Over-washing with harsh products or too hot water can cause the skin to become dry, changing the normal skin flora which can lead to the skin losing its antibacterial abilities.

Having completed an assessment of the skin (Box 3.2), in addition to a physical assessment, the nurse can identify how much assistance the patient will require, based on the condition of the skin, and other factors that influence individual hygiene practices.

Case study 3.1

Mrs Mildred Brown, aged 61, is a patient on the ward who is totally dependent on all aspects of nursing care, as she is unconscious, resulting from hypoxic brain injury following a cardiac arrest. She is breathing spontaneously (on her own), her heart rate and blood pressure are within normal limits. She has a urinary catheter in situ and is passing adequate amounts of urine. Her nutritional and hydration needs are being maintained via percutaneous endoscopic gastrostomy (PEG) feeding. She is being nursed in a profile bed with an alternating pressure relieving mattress, but still requires two-hourly changing of her position. She has two daughters who visit regularly and at times participate in her care. They state their mother had always paid attention to her hygiene and personal appearance when she was well.

- Why is assessment of the skin important for Mrs Brown?
- Identify factors that can affect the health of the skin and its appearance.

Think of a patient whose skin you have had to assess and with your mentor reflect on the following questions:

- Did the patient have healthy skin and were you able to identify any potential problems that might affect the condition of their skin?
- If the patient did not have healthy skin, what were the identified problems and how were these problems addressed?

Now compare your answers to the information in Box 3.2 and the relevant text in this chapter.

Clinical significance

Healthy skin is defined as: even skin colour, smooth texture, well hydrated (not dry) and with a normal sensation (no itching, burning or stinging).

Other factors that may affect the health of the skin include nutritional status, circulation, certain medications, the environment, smoking, exposure to sunlight and the ageing process.

Findings from the assessment should be documented in the patient's care plan. If from the assessment it is evident that meeting an individual's personal care needs has identified a nursing problem, then further information needs to be documented in the care plan and should include:

- Level of dependence/independence/physical ability of the patient/client
- What specific assistance the patient/client requires to meet hygiene needs, such as a full bed bath, help with showering or taking a bath, oral care or hair washing

Box 3.2 Assessment of the skin

The skin can provide a great deal of information about a person's general health, age, internal functioning of the body and emotional well-being.

- *The colour of the skin* can indicate an underlying disease – pallor, blanching or redness will depend largely on the person's blood flow and may indicate underlying circulatory problems; yellowish skin (jaundice) signifies liver disease; red skin (erythema) is linked to disorders that can cause inflammation/infection; violet skin (bruising) is also linked to circulatory/blood clotting problems or possible signs of physical abuse
- *Temperature of the skin* – can denote underlying disease. Heat could indicate local or systemic infection (fever), cold may imply circulatory problems
- *Skin type and texture* – the skin of an African/Afro-Caribbean person tends to have thicker cartilage with very little or fine wrinkling and signs of ageing appear very late; Anglo-Saxon or Northern European people tend to have fair, dry thin skin and signs of ageing appear earlier. Mediterranean skin types tend to be oily with a dark olive complexion, again ageing signs appear later
- *Scars* on skin should be noted. Anglo-Saxon, Northern European and Asian skin types tend to have scars that heal well and are thin; scarring in Mediterranean skin tends to be thicker and darker and in African/Afro-Caribbean skin, formation of keloids is possible
- *Abnormal skin conditions* such as rashes, lesions, pigmentation, crusting, bullae, pustules (to name a few) of the skin could be caused by underlying pathophysiological problems
- *Integrity* of the skin for any excoriations, abrasions or superficial breaks for risk of pressure ulcer formation.

- Skin care requirements, such as use of soap, emollients, moisturising lotions/creams
- Presence of areas that need to be kept dry, such as wounds, stoma sites, plaster cast
- Cultural and religious practices, e.g. washing before prayer (Islam, Hinduism).

Don't forget!

The level of dependence/independence required with personal care may change as dictated by the patient/client's condition (physical/psychological) and therefore the care plan will need to be reviewed daily as the assessment of the patient's/client's needs is an ongoing process.

Having completed this initial assessment, the activities of personal care will include:

- The physical act of washing or bathing, including skin care and shaving
- Oral hygiene
- Eye care.

Skin care

Procedure for assisting with bed bathing

Preparation is essential for you and the patient, therefore you must ensure that all the equipment required is available and within easy reach when performing this procedure. Maintaining privacy is essential, therefore, doors should be closed/curtains around the bed area closed and pinned if necessary; any blinds/curtains on windows must also be closed and in addition a privacy sign can be put up outside the door or on the curtains. Do ensure that the temperature in the room environment is comfortable for the patient as well (this will help prevent hypothermia). Nurses should wear a disposable apron and may wear non-sterile gloves to prevent cross-contamination if indicated in the local policy.

Don't forget!

Verbal consent needs to be gained before carrying out any aspect of care with a full explanation of what you will be doing at all times, no matter what the condition of the patient is and how responsive they are.

Equipment needed at the bedside

- Two towels
- Washbowl and hand-hot water
- Skin cleanser – soap or soap substitute/shower gel/foam wash
- Disposable wipes/wash cloth
- Non-sterile gloves and apron
- Clean linen
- Slide sheets
- Linen bag and rubbish bag
- Clean clothing for the patient
- Moisturiser, deodorant, make-up (if required)
- Shaving equipment (if required)
- Brush or comb.

If it has been identified that the patient requires assistance but they have some degree of mobility and are allowed to get out of bed, then if possible take the patient to the bathroom where there will be a wash basin with running water. Alternatively, the patient can sit out of the bed and be provided with a bowl of water that is at a comfortable temperature for the patient or hand-hot. If the patient is able to sit upright, they are more likely to participate. There will be some patients who are on bed rest but have some degree of mobility while in bed, such as the ability to sit up in bed and roll from side to side and therefore assistance by one person only will be required.

If the patient requires analgesia, ensure that this is administered before assisting them as this may help with mobility and involve a less painful experience overall.

For the patient confined to bed with limited or no mobility, then the assistance of two people will be required to reduce unnecessary over-exposure of the patient with one person on either side of the bed.

Watch out

For skin that is thin and fragile, extra care should be taken, as this can break down very easily with delayed healing.

Procedure for washing the patient

Stage 1 Preparation

1 Explain the procedure to the patient and gain consent.
2 Wash your hands and put on protective clothing as required in line with Standard Procedures (NICE, 2012).
3 Remove the top bedding covers, keeping the top sheet on the patient, assist with removal of the patient's clothing as necessary underneath the sheet. Patients who have weakness/paralysis of one limb should have the clothing removed from this limb last, i.e. for right arm weakness – remove the top from the left arm first and vice versa.
4 If the patient is wearing any items of jewellery, seek permission to remove if required and keep in safe place in line with local policy. This will ensure that access can be gained to skin surfaces.
5 Once undressed, keep the patient covered with the top sheet as this will ensure that the patient is kept warm and you continue to maintain privacy and dignity.

Stage 2 Washing the face and neck

1 Start from the face, working the way down to the lower parts of the body. Starting with the face first will minimise cross-infection from genitalia.
2 Wash the face and neck area, place a towel across the patient's chest and check what type of skin cleanser they use on their face.
3 Remove any glasses or hearing aids at this point. If the patient is able to, they can wash their own face using a disposable wipe to encourage patient participation.
4 If the patient is not able to wash their own face, using a disposable wipe and cleansing agent, if used, start with the eyelids first, then forehead, cheeks, nose, ears and jaw, ending at the neck.

5   Rinse off any cleansing agent and gently pat face dry using the second towel.
6   If the patient uses facial moisturiser, then this can be applied at this stage before replacing any glasses or hearing aids on the patient if required. Ensure that no soap/cleanser gets into the patient's eyes.

Stage 3 Washing the upper body

1   This includes washing the arms one at a time and the chest.
2   Placing the towel under the arm and using a new wipe with preferred cleansing agent, wash the whole of the arm from the shoulder down to the fingertips and armpit.
3   Wash the arm furthest away first.
4   Rinse off the cleansing agent and pat dry, using the second towel and repeat this for the next arm.
5   If the patient wishes the use of deodorant, this can be applied once skin is dry.
6   Remove towel to expose the chest area to wash and rinse. Particular attention needs to be paid to underneath the breasts in female patients checking this area for any redness and ensuring that the area is dried thoroughly and then cover the patient to protect their dignity.
7   If patient can sit forward, assistance can be given to wash and dry the back area and, once completed, the patient's top clothing can be replaced. This will ensure that the patient is not left exposed unnecessarily.
8   Use this opportunity to check skin on back for any redness especially the pressure point areas such as the shoulder blades.
9   For the patients with weakness/paralysis of one side, put the affected arm into the nightdress/pyjama first. Patients with intravenous lines – put the bag and tubing in first through the sleeve, followed by the patient's arm. Hang the bag on the drip stand, then put the unaffected arm in the other sleeve and pull garment down covering the patient's torso.

Stage 4 Washing the lower body

1   The lower part of the body includes washing both legs one at a time (furthest away from genitalia first), the genital area and back if the patient is not able to sit forward.
2   If the patient still has pyjama bottoms on, remove them. Anti-embolic stockings must also be removed.
3   Place the towel under the leg; and wash, rinse and dry the leg from the hip to the toes washing and drying between the toes and examining the condition of the skin, also checking the pressure points on heels.
4   Repeat the same again for the other leg.
5   Take extra care and vigilance with patients who have diabetes – as they may develop the complication of peripheral neuropathy – where foot injuries do not heal very well.
6   Having completed washing and drying the legs for the patient, change the water and disposable wipe and gain consent from the patient to wash the genital area.
7   Ask the patient if they are able to wash this area themselves, if they are not able to

do this, ensure that you are wearing disposable gloves and using a new disposable wipe, wash, rinse and dry the area carefully.

8   For female patients, irrelevant of age, start from the pubic area working downwards to the labia and perineum, also known as cleaning from front to back, to minimise infection risk from anus to urethra.

9   For male patients, if they are uncircumcised, it is important to clean the glans penis by washing underneath the foreskin, gently pulling the foreskin back to clean the glans penis area and ensuring that the foreskin is pulled forward.

10 Dispose of the wipes and water, once finished.

11 If the patient is not able to sit forward, you will now need to wash their back and bottom. The patient should be asked or assisted to roll onto one side (Figure 3.2).

12 If the patient is not able to roll independently, appropriate equipment for moving and handling such as a slide sheet should be used.

13 Once the patient has been rolled onto their side, place the towel along the length of the patient's back and using clean water and a new disposable wipe thoroughly wash, rinse and dry the back from the shoulders to the sacral area.

14 Check the skin for any red areas, assessing the main pressure points on the back, the shoulder blades.

15 Using gloves, wash, rinse and dry the bottom area and check the sacrum and surrounding skin.

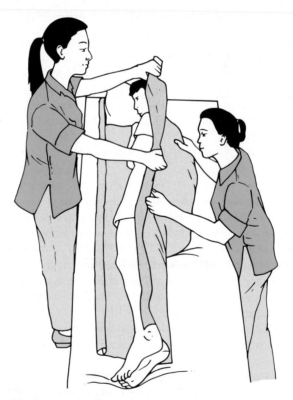

Figure 3.2 **Bed bathing and rolling a patient**

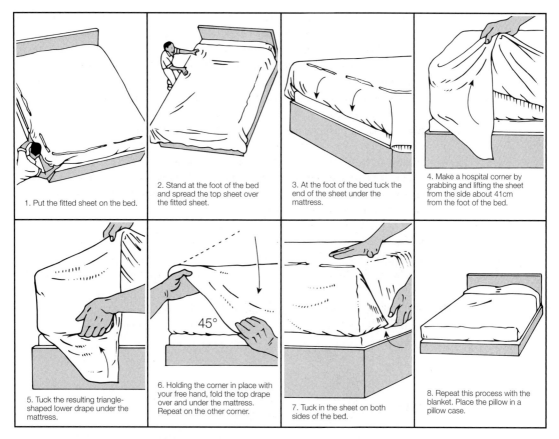

Figure 3.3 **How to make a bed**

16   For patients who are restricted to their bed, you will need to change the bottom bed sheet at this point (Figure 3.3).
17   Put on the patient's pyjama bottoms or appropriate clothing, comb/brush hair and shave the patient if required.
18   If appropriate, sit the patient out of bed (see Chapter 11).
19   Document any findings and care in the care plan as all aspects of care given to patients must be documented, as should any changes in line with hospital policies and the Nursing and Midwifery Council (NMC, 2015).

Procedure for shaving the patient

Shaving the male patient will need to be done if the individual is too ill to carry out the procedure.

1   Explain the procedure and where possible gain consent.
2   To prevent infection, if the patient's family can provide a razor, ask them to do so, if not, use a disposable razor.

3   Wash your hands.
4   Moisten the patient's face with a warm wet washcloth, then put soap or shaving lotion on the patient's face.
5   Shave gently, following the direction of the hair.
6   While shaving the patient, be careful of the skin creases near the mouth and nose. These areas are best shaved in short strokes while carefully stretching the skin flat with your free hand.
7   When finished, rinse the patient's face thoroughly with warm water and disposable wipe.
8   Dispose of razors in sharps bin and wash your hands.
9   Document any findings and care in the care plan, as all aspects of care given to patients must be documented, as should any changes in line with local policies and the NMC (NMC, 2015).

Top tip

Some patients like to moisturise their skin or need to have their skin kept moisturised if they have a skin condition. Remember to check for this and apply moisturising cream or ointments as required by the patient to their body once you have completed their wash.

Watch out

Be extra careful with patients who have blood clotting problems and those with very thin fragile skin as their skin will cut very easily and they will bleed profusely.

Hair care

This is an aspect of personal care that is sometimes overlooked. It is a basic aspect of personal care that should be performed when a patient is not able to do this independently or their condition does not permit. Keeping hair clean minimises odour, prevents infection and promotes patient comfort as it can impact on how the patient feels with regard to self-image and well-being, irrespective of age. It provides an opportunity to check the scalp for any dry skin conditions, infestations and hair loss.

For patients who will require some assistance, where possible, take them to the wash area. If there is a wet room with shower facilities, this procedure can be carried out there. Alternatively hair can be washed in the bath or in a wash basin. For patients who are restricted to the bed, then hair will need to be washed in bed and the procedure will be explained.

Washing the hair of a patient who is confined to bed involves time and preparation, but this should not be an excuse not to do it. Choose a time when it is convenient for the patient and staff for example in late afternoon when all activity is minimised and lunchtime is over. A hair washing tray is a convenient piece of equipment that can be used to facilitate this skill (see Figure 3.4).

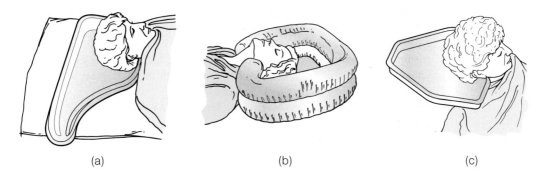

(a)   (b)   (c)

Figure 3.4 **Examples of hair washing trays**

Procedure for performing hair care at the bedside

Equipment needed at the bedside

- Two towels
- Jug
- Large wash bowl for water x 2 (second bowl only required depending on type of hair washing tray used. Figure 3.4 (a) will require two bowls, the second bowl is used as a receptacle.)
- Hair washing tray
- Bedside table
- Shampoo and conditioner as required by patient
- Comb, brush and hairdryer (optional)
- Incontinence pads
- Slide sheet
- Disposable plastic apron.

Stage 1 Preparation

Preparation is vital to prevent unnecessary movement away from the patient once you start and to avoid causing harm to the patient. Communication, an important part of the procedure that is often forgotten, and assisting the patient with their hygiene needs provide the opportunity to get to know the patient and for them to confide in you.

1 Have all the equipment prepared, within easy reach and explain procedure to the patient and where possible gain consent.
2 Wash hands and put on required protective clothing.
3 Check the temperature of the water (warm).

4   Pull the bed away from the wall and remove the back rest to facilitate access to wash the patient's hair with them being in the supine position.

5   Adjust height of the bed and position the bedside table behind the patient at the head end of the bed. Cover the table with the incontinence pads; put the hair washing tray on the table and position receiving wash bowl beneath the drip outlet if required on the side.

6   Assist the patient to move up the bed using the slide sheet, so that their head is resting in the hair washing tray. For a patient who has limited mobility or is unconscious, this will have to be done by two people with the slide sheet and correct moving and handling techniques (Chapter 11).

7   For the unconscious patient – MONITOR THE AIRWAY AT ALL TIMES for signs of obstruction.

8   Place one of the towels around the patient's chest and neck area. Before starting, check that the patient is comfortable and the head is resting in the head washing tray to collect the water.

Stage 2 Washing the hair

1   Assess the condition of the hair and scalp for any abnormalities.

2   Wet hair using the jug with water poured over the patient's hair.

3   Apply shampoo and wash the hair and rinse thoroughly.

4   If required, apply conditioner and gently rinse.

5   Wrap the other towel around the patient's hair to dry and move the patient back down the bed to make them comfortable to avoid having the patient positioned in the hair washing tray longer than necessary.

6   To reduce clutter around the bed area, move the table with the hair washing tray to one side.

7   If a second person is helping, they can start disposing of this equipment.

8   Now that the patient has been positioned back in bed, continue with ensuring that the hair is dried thoroughly, using the comb/brush and hair dryer if available. To promote patient comfort, hair must be dried thoroughly.

9   Once hair is thoroughly dry, clean and tidy around the bed area; dispose of all equipment; remove apron and wash hands to minimise cross-infection.

10 After washing the patient or performing hair care, wash bowls must be decontaminated with antibacterial solution and dried thoroughly before storage to minimise infection risk.

11 Ensure that the patient is comfortable.

12 Document any findings and care in the care plan as all aspects of care given to patients must be documented as should any changes in line with local policies and the NMC Code.

Oral care

Oral (mouth) care is another basic requirement that should be carried out as part of meeting the personal care needs of the patient. It involves care of the lips, the mucosal lining of the mouth, the tongue, the teeth and the gums, which are the parts of the oral cavity. The aim is to promote patient comfort and maintain a clean and healthy mouth. Carrying out this skill involves assessment of the mouth and the physical act of cleaning the mouth. In order to do this, you have to have some understanding of the structure and function of the mouth (Figure 3.5) and salivary glands as they have several functions that can affect health.

Mouth (oral cavity)

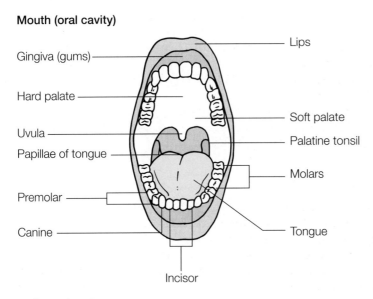

Figure 3.5 The oral cavity

The main functions of the mouth are ingestion, mastication and swallowing of food, speech, and breathing when the nasal passage is blocked. The salivary glands are part of the oral cavity and there are three major salivary glands around the mouth (Figure 3.6). The salivary glands produce saliva which is important for the health of the mouth as: (1) it provides lubrication, preventing the mouth from drying out and therefore preventing infection by controlling bacteria; (2) it protects the teeth from decay; and (3) it contributes to the digestion of food as saliva helps the food that has been chewed stick together to form a bolus to ease swallowing and it also contains enzymes which help break down the starch in food. The salivary glands produce 1–2 litres of saliva a day. When there is a reduction in the flow of saliva, the oral cavity becomes dry, the tongue will become coated with dried mucous saliva and dead cells, making the mouth susceptible to infection.

Assessment of the mouth

A healthy mouth will be moist and the gums, oral mucosa and tongue should be clean, have a reddish pink appearance and the tongue should be covered in papillae which contain the taste buds (Figures 3.7 (a) and (b)). The teeth should also be clean, and if the individual has dentures, these should fit properly in the mouth. Assessment of the mouth

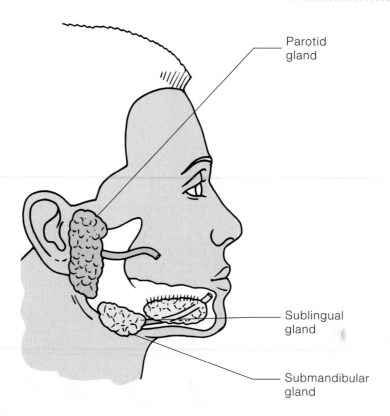

Parotid
gland

Sublingual
gland

Submandibular
gland

Figure 3.6 The salivary glands

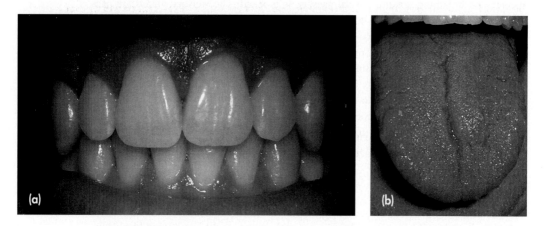

Figure 3.7 (a) Healthy gums and teeth; (b) a healthy tongue (see Plate section at end of chapter for colour photos)

Activity 3.2

What is the impact of an unhealthy mouth on a patient (adult, baby, child or young person)?

Read Case study 3.1 again; which factors may impact on Mrs Brown's oral hygiene?

is an essential part of personal care assessment in order to identify any actual or potential problems and the frequency of mouth care that will be required. Box 3.3 outlines the procedure for oral assessment.

A mouth that is unhealthy and dry can impact on the main functions of the mouth. Certain groups of patients are more prone to mouth problems; these groups will be patients who are immunosuppressed, diabetic, who are dehydrated, are receiving oxygen therapy, are unconscious and having treatments such as chemotherapy or radiotherapy. Box 3.4 outlines the main problems that you can identify when you carry out an oral assessment. Figures 3.8 (a)–(c) present problems with the mouth.

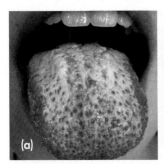 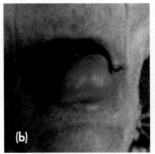 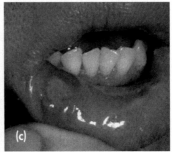

Figure 3.8 (a) Oral thrush; (b) a dry mouth; (c) mouth ulcer (see Plate section at end of chapter for colour photos)

Box 3.3 Oral assessment

■ Is the patient (adult, child or young person) complaining of pain in their mouth?

■ Does the mouth and throat have a sticky dry feeling?

■ Has the patient complained of problems with taste?

■ Does their breath smell?

■ Are the lips red, peeling, dry in appearance or cracked?

■ Is the tongue dry, inflamed, furry in appearance, cracked or ulcerated?

■ Do the teeth look decayed or have debris, and if wearing dentures, do they fit well?

■ In the case of children, are there any loose teeth?

■ Are the mucous membranes and gums inflamed, bleeding or blistered?

■ Are there any thick white patches on the mucous membranes and tongue?

Box 3.4 Problems linked to an unhealthy mouth

- Fungal infection and a common example is oral candidiasis (thrush)
- Bacterial infection
- Xerostomia (very dry mouth)
- Mouth ulcers.

See Figures 3.8 (a), (b) and (c).

Children and young people need to understand the importance of good oral hygiene as they can be affected in the same way as adults when ill and can develop similar problems with poor oral health. As with meeting the personal hygiene needs of babies, children and young people, oral hygiene can often be overlooked, as it may be assumed that the parent/carer will do this.

From a total of 133,516 clinical examinations it was found that overall, 27.9 per cent of 5-year-old children in England had experienced dental decay. On average, these children had 3.38 teeth (out of an average of 20 primary teeth) that were decayed, missing or filled (Davies *et al.*, 2013). Therefore, it is important that nurses encourage good oral care within the hospital setting and check that it has been carried out as not all parents/carers will carry out this basic care.

Procedure for performing oral care

Having completed the assessment of the mouth, it is important to document your findings and submit a written care plan of how the oral hygiene needs of the patient will be met and the frequency for providing this care. In general, to maintain good oral health, teeth should be cleaned twice a day.

The main aim in performing oral care is to ensure that the mouth is clean and moist, free of debris, to prevent or limit infection and to promote patient comfort, irrespective of age. Where possible, this is an activity that the patient should be encouraged to do independently, and if possible, take the patient to the wash area where they will have access to a sink and running water. If the patient cannot be taken to the wash area

Watch out

Check if the patient has a latex allergy, and if they do, use latex-free gloves. An allergic reaction may cause the patient to develop an itchy, red, mildly swollen skin rash at the site of contact. In some cases if the reaction is severe, the rash will be widespread, the patient will complain of tightness of the throat, wheezing or difficulty breathing, and these are all symptoms of anaphylaxis which can lead to death if not recognised and treated.

and have some degree of independence, then provide the patient with the necessary equipment to perform this activity by the bed area. If the patient is totally dependent on nursing care, then you will have to carry out this activity.

Privacy and dignity of the patient must be maintained at all times. For those patients who are totally dependent, gain consent and explain the procedure.

Equipment needed at the bedside

- A soft toothbrush
- Toothpaste (fluoride) (DoH, 2014). For adults, a large amount; children under 3 years, a smear; children aged 3–6, a pea-sized amount of toothpaste.
- Water
- Disposable cup
- Receiver such as a disposable kidney bowl (Figure 3.9 (a))
- Foam sticks (Figure 3.9 (b))
- Towel
- Tissues
- Lip balm if needed
- Non-sterile gloves and disposable apron
- Suction machine (for patients who are unconscious).

Procedure for mouth care

1   Explain the procedure to the patient, to allow the patient to feel at ease with you carrying out the procedure. Where possible, gain consent.
2   Wash hands and put on protective clothing.
3   Where possible, sit the patient in an upright position in bed or a chair and stand by the side of the patient. If the patient is in bed and cannot be sat upright or if they

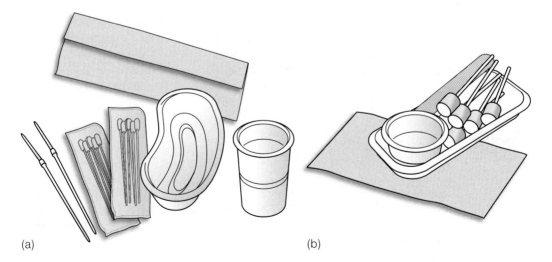

(a)   (b)

Figure 3.9 (a) and (b) Mouth care equipment

are unconscious, then roll them to their side and position yourself directly in front of them. This is to avoid the risk of the patient choking.

4   Position the towel around the patient's neck and chest area to protect the patient from getting wet.

5   Squeeze the recommended amount of toothpaste onto the brush (DoH, 2014) and wet the brush with some water poured into the disposable cup. Depending on the situation with the patient, less than the recommended amount may be used, as applying too much toothpaste on the brush can make spitting out difficult.

6   To ensure all surfaces of the teeth are cleaned and any plaque or debris is removed, first hold the brush at an angle of 45 degrees to the teeth and brush using a circular motion, cleaning the gums and outer surfaces of the teeth and then the inner surfaces of the teeth (Figures 3.10 (a)–(c)). Holding the brush at 90 degrees, clean the biting surfaces using the same circular movement of the brush and then the tongue.

7   Assist the patient to spit out toothpaste. Sips of water can be given after 30 minutes or so as it is recommended traces of toothpaste remain for a short time (ibid). Wipe

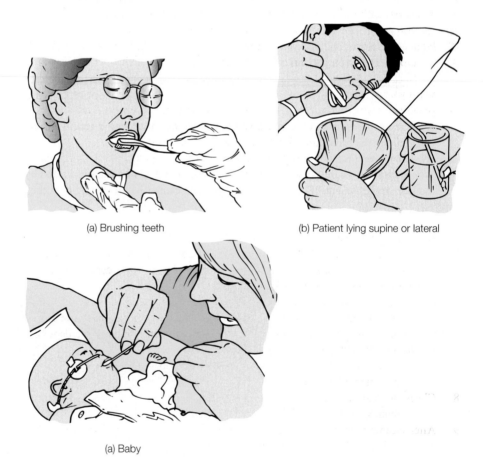

(a) Brushing teeth   (b) Patient lying supine or lateral

(a) Baby

Figure 3.10 (a)–(c) **Examples of how to give mouth care**

the patient's lips and chin area with tissue. It is important that all the toothpaste and debris is removed from the mouth.

■ For a baby or for the patient who is lying flat, or is unconscious and is unable to rinse out their mouth, then you can use the sponge foam sticks to do this. Wet a stick in some water (not too much) and apply a twisting movement in the mouth to absorb the toothpaste and any debris in the mouth, remove and dispose. This action must be repeated until all the toothpaste and debris is removed from the entire mouth using a clean foam stick with each repetition. If required, suction out excessive water using a yanker sucker. Care needs to be taken when giving mouth care to the unconscious patient or a patient with swallowing problems because of the risk of choking. ASSESS THE AIRWAY AT ALL TIMES DURING THE PROCEDURE.

8   Apply some lip balm or yellow soft paraffin to the lips sparingly as this will help soften and moisturise the lips and prevent them from cracking. Make sure that the patient is comfortable.

9   Rinse out the toothbrush under running water and store it in a clean disposable cup on the patient's locker to dry. Rinsing out toothbrush thoroughly and leaving it to dry will prevent the growth of bacteria and prevent cross-infection.

10 Equipment used has been contaminated with the body fluid, i.e. saliva, and will need to be disposed of as clinical waste, therefore dispose of all other equipment in the clinical waste bin, including your apron and gloves.

11 Wash your hands.

12 Document care in the patient's records and any changes observed in the condition of the mouth as all aspects of care given to patient must be documented, as should any changes in line with local policies and the NMC (NMC, 2015).

13 For patients with a dry mouth or underlying health problems, mouth care may need to be a carried out as often as one or two hourly.

Dentures

1   Explain the procedure and gain consent where possible.

2   Wash hands thoroughly before and after the procedure. Put on disposable gloves.

3   If the patient wears dentures, check what their practice is with regards to cleaning their dentures. The dentures will need cleaning, as will their mouth.

4   Remove the dentures, if the patient is able to do so, they can do this themselves.

5   If you need to remove the dentures, ensure that you are wearing non-sterile gloves and, using a piece of gauze, start with the top set to gently remove the dentures, followed by the bottom set (Figure 3.11 (a)).

6   Place dentures in the designated denture pot for the patient (Figure 3.11 (b)).

7   Clean the mouth of the patient.

8   Clean the dentures thoroughly using toothpaste and a brush to clean all surfaces under running water.

9   After cleaning, dentures should be left in water or soaking in a denture cleaning agent until ready for re-insertion into the mouth.

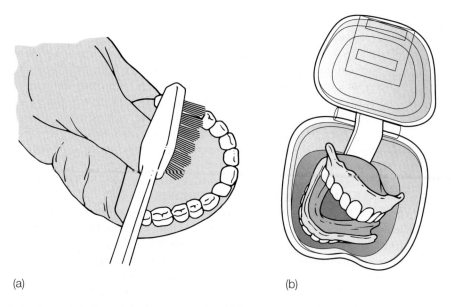

(a)   (b)

Figure 3.11 (a) Cleaning; (b) storage of dentures

Eye care

As part of maintaining hygiene needs, good eye care is important to prevent infection and promote comfort, as the eye is a very sensitive part of the body that can be damaged easily if not cared for adequately during illness. Eye care involves cleaning of the eyes for those patients who are unable to do this independently. An understanding of the basic structure of the eye is essential before undertaking this, as it is an organ that can be damaged very easily if care is not taken.

For protection purposes, the eye is located in a cone-shaped socket in the skull. Figure 3.12 shows the main structures of the eye. The eye is protected by the eyelid, the thin fold of skin and the conjunctiva, a thin lubricating mucus membrane that lines the eyelid. The action of blinking, the lubricating mucus and also tears, both produced by the lacrimal gland (see Figure 3.13), clean and lubricate the eye. This action prevents infection and drying out of the cornea as tears contain proteins and antibacterial properties beta-lysin and lysozyme. Blinking also protects the eyes from damage by irritants, with the eyelashes providing the first line of defence against irritants. If the reflex of blinking is absent or protection to the cornea is reduced, the patient will be prone to bacterial or viral infection of the cornea and the cornea can also become ulcerated if the eye is not cared for adequately.

During the ageing process, patients may develop problems affecting their sight, for e.g., cataracts, presbyopia (reading print at a distance further away), diminished central vision caused by retinal cells dying, or reduction in night vision.

Patients may require eye care for a range of reasons. The eye is a sensitive organ that can be damaged very easily, therefore, any abnormalities found with the appearance of the eyes must be reported. It is important to establish the condition of the eyes through assessment in the first instance to establish if there is a problem with the eyes and the

Activity 3.3

Reflect on the clinical scenario about Mrs Brown and her condition. What impact does her clinical condition have on her eyes?

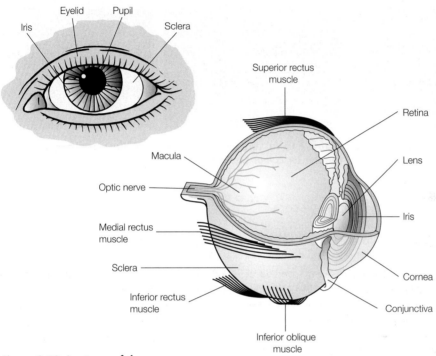

Figure 3.12 **Anatomy of the eye**

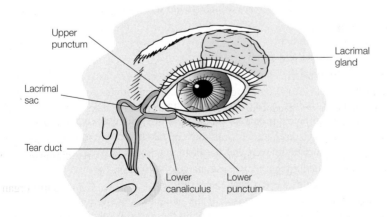

Figure 3.13 **Glands of the eye**

type of care that will be required. In normal eyes (Figure 3.14), the eyelid sits securely over the eyeball, lashes turned outwards. The conjunctiva should have a clear appearance and the sclera (white of the eye) must be visible. The eyes should be free from signs of infection such as inflammation, or yellow/green sticky discharge (Figures 3.15 (a) and (b)). Eye care should be seen as an essential part of nursing care when meeting patients' hygiene needs to promote comfort and prevent complications.

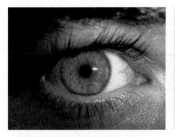 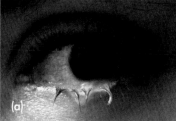 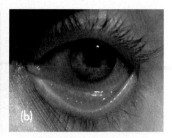

Figure 3.14 A healthy eye (see Plate section at end of chapter for colour photo)

Figure 3.15 (a) and (b) Infected eyes (see Plate section at end of chapter for colour photos)

Procedure for performing eye care

If there are any abnormalities identified from the assessment of the condition of the eyes, they must be reported and documented first, and a plan of care written on how to care for the problem with the eyes. Cleaning of the eyes at least twice a day is sufficient, however, if there is evidence of sticky discharge, then eye care may be required more often to promote patient comfort. Each eye must be cleaned separately to prevent cross-infection from one eye to the other.

Equipment needed at the bedside

- Clean trolley
- Eye care pack or dressing pack which should have two gallipots (one for each eye) and lint-free gauze
- Normal saline solution
- Non-sterile gloves and apron
- Hand-cleaning gel

1   Explain the procedure to the patient, even if they have a reduced conscious level, and have all the equipment prepared. Where possible, gain consent. Maintain privacy.
2   If there is any eye discharge, a swab must be taken and sent to the laboratory.
3   The patient must be relaxed and the head supported to avoid sudden movements during the procedure that may cause damage to the eye. Position the patient sitting upright (if possible, support head using pillows).
4   Remove glasses or contact lenses. If the patient is unconscious, position lying on back, but ONLY if the patient can maintain their airway, otherwise patient will have to be placed on their side.

5   Wash hands and have all the equipment opened and prepared on the trolley to prevent cross-infection and unnecessary movement away from the patient once started.

6   Moisten the lint-free gauze in the normal saline and gently cleanse the upper eyelid of the first eye from the inner part of the closed eye (closest to the nose) to the outer aspect in one movement and discard the gauze.

7   Repeat cleansing action until the eye is clean. Cleaning the upper eyelid first with eye closed from the inner aspect of the eye to the outer aspect prevents any discharge being forced back into the eye, and a thorough cleansing of the eye minimises complications, e.g. spread of infection.

8   Clean the lower eyelid, ask the patient to open eye and look up and clean the lower eyelid from the inner aspect outwards with one gentle movement and then discard the gauze.

9   Repeat cleansing action until eye is clean. If the patient is unconscious, you will need to gently open the eyelid to do this.

10 Dry the eye with a swabbing action from the inner to outer eye in one movement using dry lint-free gauze as drying the eyes promotes patient comfort.

11 Repeat the procedure for the second eye. *Before* cleaning the second eye, decontaminate hands and change gloves. Cleaning each eye separately and decontaminating hands between eyes minimises cross-infection from one eye to the other.

12 Once procedure has been completed, make sure that the patient is comfortable.

13 If the patient is unconscious, then eye drops or artificial tears may be prescribed to keep the eyes moist. This is also to promote patient comfort and protect the eye from becoming dry or damaged.

14 Clear the trolley and dispose of all equipment, wash your hands to minimise cross-infection.

15 Document care and any findings/changes in the care plan, as all aspects of care given to patient must be documented as should any changes in line with local policies and the NMC (NMC, 2015).

Children in hospital: hygiene needs

Children in hospital will also need to have their hygiene needs met as they would at home. It is important to work in partnership with the parent/carer or young person as they need to be involved in their care and the child will feel more secure in the presence of their carer. The parent/carer and young person may not always be in a position to meet the basic need of personal hygiene and therefore this will have to be met for them. There are some specific needs that must be applied when caring for children, such as the use of play which is therapeutic and emotionally enhancing, more so when performing personal care in a strange environment, especially when this is being carried out by the nurse who may be unfamiliar to the child. For the adolescent there is increased need for privacy and the need to be sensitive to ensure that they do not feel embarrassed. Table 3.1 outlines some of the specific needs for babies (age 0–1), toddlers (age 1–3) and children (age 4–11).

Table 3.1 Personal care needs for babies and children

Baby	Toddler/child
▪ Daily top and tail wash or bath	▪ Daily washing or bath
▪ Eyes to be kept clean with sterile water	▪ Hair care including brushing
▪ External ear care	▪ Washing of ears
▪ Hair/scalp care	▪ Twice daily brushing of teeth
▪ Face (including neck) cleansing	▪ Regular hand washing, e.g., after
▪ Nappy area care	using the toilet and before meals
▪ Umbilical care	▪ Nappy area care if applicable.
▪ Nails kept trimmed.	

Source: Roberts (2008).

Summary

A principal feature in caring for patients is assessing and meeting their personal care needs. Not only is this beneficial for nurses – enabling them to build a therapeutic relationship for the patient but it is a useful way of assessing the patient for problems/signs of underlying disorders. Throughout all procedures, privacy and dignity of the patient must be maintained. Where possible, patients must be involved in the procedures in an attempt to promote independence.

References

Davies, G., Neville, J. and Rooney, E. (2013) *National Dental Epidemiology Programme for England: Oral Health Survey of Five-Year-Old Children 2012. A Report on the Prevalence and Severity of Dental Decay*. London: Public Health England.

DoH (Department of Health) (2010) *Essence of Care 2010: Benchmarks for Personal Hygiene*. London: The Stationery Office.

DoH (Department of Health) (2014) *Delivering Better Oral Health: An Evidence-Based Toolkit for Prevention*, third edn. London: The Stationery Office.

NICE (National Institute for Clinical Excellence) (2012) *Health Care Associated Infections: Prevention and Control in Primary and Community Care*. CG139. London: NICE.

Nightingale, F. (1860) *Notes on Nursing: What It Is, and What It Is Not*. New York: Dover Publications.

NMC (Nursing and Midwifery Council) (2010) *Record Keeping Guidance for Nurses and Midwives*. London: NMC.

NMC (Nursing and Midwifery Council) (2015) *The Code: Professional Standards of Practice and Behaviour for Nurses and Midwives*. London: NMC.

Orem, D. (2001) *Nursing: Concepts of Practice*, sixth edn. New York: McGraw-Hill.

Roberts, S. (2008) Meeting the personal hygiene needs of a hospitalized child. *British Journal of Healthcare Assistants*, 2(5): 214–216.

Roper, N., Logan, W. and Tierney, A. (2000) *The Roper-Logan and Tierney Model of Nursing: Based on Activities of Living*. London: Churchill Livingstone.

Schofield, J.K., Grindlay, D. and Williams. H.C. (2009) *Skin Conditions in the UK: A Healthcare Needs Assessment*. Centre for Evidence-Based Dermatology. Available at: www.nottingham.ac.uk/scs/documents/documentsdivisions/documentsdermatology/hcnaskinconditionsuk2009.pdf (accessed 4 February 2016).

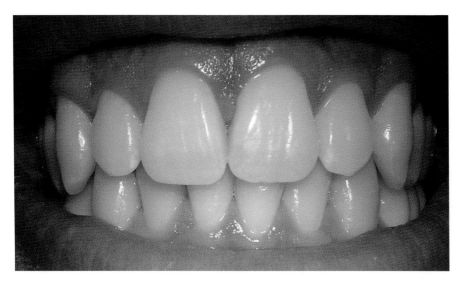

(a)

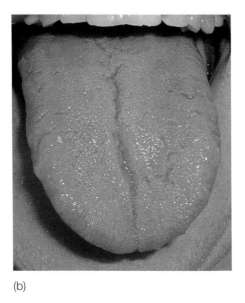

(b)

Figure 3.7 (a) Healthy gums and teeth; (b) a healthy tongue

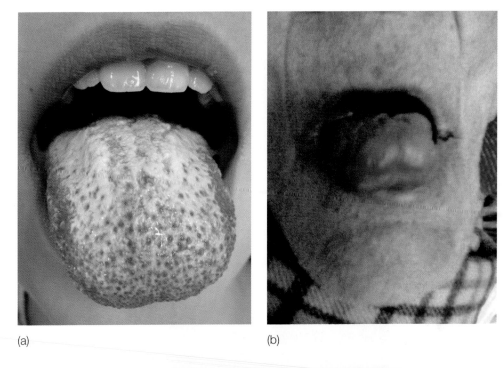

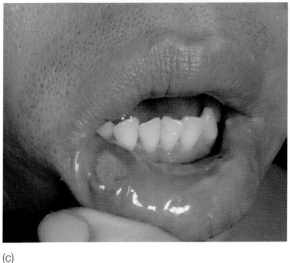

(a)

(b)

(c)

Figure 3.8 (a) Oral thrush; (b) a dry mouth; (c) mouth ulcer

Source: (a) Photo credit: James Heilman. Reproduced under the Creative Commons Attribution- Share Alike 3.0 Unported License; (b) Photo credit: Frivadossi. Reproduced under the Creative Commons Attribution- Share Alike 3.0 Unported License; (c) Photo credit: Project Manhattan. Reproduced under the Creative Commons Attribution- Share Alike 3.0 Unported License.

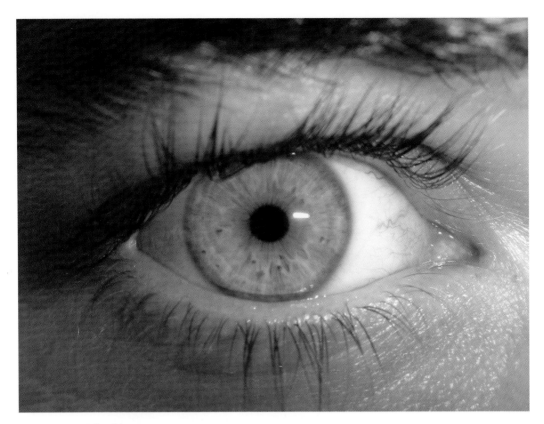

Figure 3.14 A healthy eye

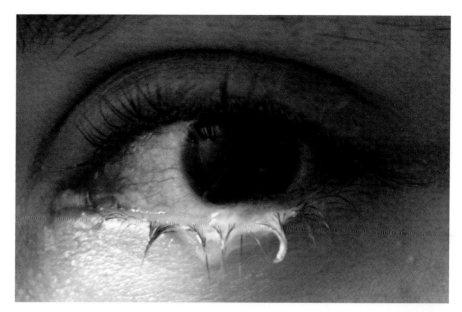

(a)

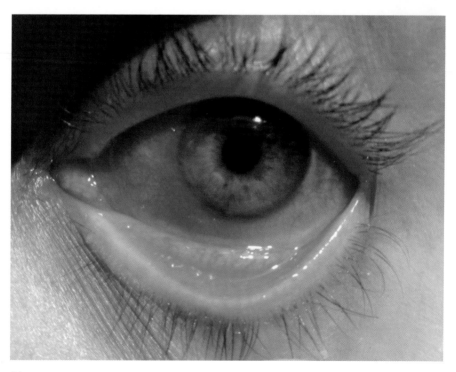

(b)

Figure 3.15 (a) and (b) Infected eyes

Chapter 4

Elimination

Marion Hinds and Sheila Cunningham

Elimination of urine and faeces is an essential bodily function. Nursing assistance with elimination is basic care, however, and as an activity of daily living, a very important one. The amount and type of nursing support required with elimination needs vary and depend upon a thorough assessment and should be undertaken with sensitivity and compassion to ensure patient privacy and dignity.

Key concepts

Continence
Incontinence

Catheterisation
Retention

Learning outcomes

By the end of this chapter you will be able to:

- Define elimination and continence
- Identify the different modes of elimination
- Explain and describe nursing assistance with urine elimination, specifically on:
    - bladder training
    - infant nappy changing
    - offering bedpans
    - catheterisation.
- Demonstrate knowledge and understanding of the assessment of urine and obtaining a specimen
- Explain and describe the role of the nurse in assisting with faeces elimination.

Introduction

Elimination can be described as the removal of the waste products of digestion from the body, a human function. These products will be in the form of urine or faeces (stool); the volume, amount, colour, frequency and consistency of these will depend upon a variety of factors such as age, patient condition, lifestyle factors, pain and any prescribed medications. Sweating and vomiting are also considered forms of elimination; however, this section will consider only the urine and faeces elimination process.

The purpose of assisting a patient with their elimination needs is to ensure that the patient is given prompt support in an ideal and appropriate setting. There are many reasons why a patient will need help with their elimination, such as frailty, cognitive impairment, poor mobility, injury, and incontinence. The Essence of Care benchmark for Bladder, Bowel and Continence Care specifies that an individual's bladder and bowel care needs are met, including providing a suitable environment that is compatible with the patient's needs and preferences (Essence of Care, 2010, p. 3). A safety risk assessment may also need to be undertaken on each patient to make sure that any issues can be identified and any necessary actions. For many patients, assistance with elimination can cause feelings of embarrassment or even distress, which in turn may lead to a delay in a patient reporting any abnormalities to nursing staff.

Clinical significance

A detailed set of standards for toilet provision were identified by the British Geriatric Society in 2007, which include the areas of accessibility, equipment, safety, timeliness, privacy, choice, cleanliness and hygiene. These still apply today.

Assessment of bladder and bowel activity

The process of elimination from the bladder is termed 'micturition' or 'voiding' and is both a voluntary and involuntary action. It is voluntary in the sense that control of where and when to empty the bladder occurs at around the age of 2 years old. The bladder fills with urine for excretion and a trigger or signal to empty it goes to the brain where it is then acted upon by relaxation of a muscle sphincter to release urine at a place and time which are convenient. This is termed 'continence'. Furthermore, there are conditions and factors which alter the process of urinary elimination and lead to a situation of lack of control or incontinence. The types of incontinence can be seen in Box 4.1. It is estimated that between 3 and 6 million people in the UK may have some degree of urinary incontinence (NHS Choices, 2014). You may wish to review the physiology of micturition and the organs involved in a good quality anatomy and physiology book.

Bowel elimination is termed defecation. The product is termed 'faeces'. This is a waste from digestion mainly. This process has an involuntary and voluntary phase aided by the movement of the faecal material along the bowel in waves of movement which occur periodically during the day and often culminating in one mass elimination daily. This can be controlled to ensure a suitable time and place but, unlike urine, there is a danger that avoiding defecation can lead to a build-up of faeces and retention which can cause a blockage called 'impaction'. This is uncomfortable and can be painful and

Box 4.1 Common types of urinary incontinence

- *Stress incontinence* – urine leakage when sneezing, coughing, laughing or exertion (SIGN, 2004). Can be experienced by people with a weak pelvic floor such as women following multiple births
- *Urge incontinence* – urgent need to urinate, may also be due to infection
- *Overactive bladder* – urgent need to urinate, usually with frequency and often occurring at night
- *Overflow incontinence* – leakage when the bladder is full and over-extended. A feature which may be seen in men with enlarged prostate
- *Reflex incontinence* – incontinence without warning
- *Functional/immobility incontinence* – leakage of urine when unable to access suitable facilities or location due, e.g., from mobility problems or dementia and forgetting.

dangerous. Individuals' elimination patterns vary and are 'normal' to them. However, assessment may indicate irregular elimination (constipation) or frequent elimination (diarrhoea) and the cause may need to be explored if recently occurring. This is not straightforward, as for some people faecal elimination may be daily and for others every third day. Assessment of the faeces may be more useful and reference to a picture chart such as the Bristol Stool chart may be useful and aid description and documentation. A person's pattern of defecation may be unique to them which is where skilled assessment and determination of patterns are necessary.

Box 4.2 presents a range of treatments for stress or urge incontinence.

Box 4.2 Range of treatment approaches for stress or urge incontinence

- Pelvic floor training (Kegel exercises)
- Bladder training – timed toileting, the relearning of the body to respond to cues
- Being near a toilet when away from home
- Lifestyle amendments – reduce weight, reduce caffeine intake and alcohol, use of absorbent pads
- Catheters – periodic self-catheterisation, indwelling urinary catheters or supra-pubic catheters
- Drug therapy – if necessary, e.g. Duloxetine to reduce spasmodic contractions of the bladder.

Source: Adapted from SIGN (2004); NHS Choices (2014)

Enuresis and encopresis

Enuresis is the term used when a child is unable to control their bladder during the day or night. Children become engrossed in play and may not respond to the urge to pass urine and thus leakage will occur and can be upsetting for them. Most children remain dry at night by the age of 5. If wetting continues, this is termed nocturnal enuresis, though the occurrences decrease with increasing age.

Faecal incontinence or faecal soiling in children is termed encopresis. This could be very embarrassing and may be due to constipation or faeces impacted in the bowel, psychological distress or emotional problems. It may also be induced by the child refusing to go to the toilet at school or nursery and eliminate faeces but that does not lessen the distress and potential physical pain it can cause.

Assessment

The key to assessment is to determine the patient's normal patterns and any recent changes. The nurse also needs to consider the current problem and medications or mobility issues and whether this will affect elimination. Since this is an activity of daily living (ADL), it is addressed in many nursing assessment documents and the key aspects to also consider are:

1   Ask about the patient's usual level of activity, mobility and lifestyle, medications or concerns over using public facilities.
2   Does the patient have any history of problems with elimination (urinary or bowel)?
3   Ask the patient about their usual nutrition and fluid intake (e.g. diet, hydration).
4   Ask the patient if they experience any of the following problems:
    dysphagia, nausea or vomiting, heartburn, flatulence, pain, jaundice, mass, distention, ascites, haemorrhoids, rectal bleeding, recent weight loss/gain, bowel sounds, change in character of stool (faeces), any change in bowel patterns or frequency, changes in urine appearance or volume (polyuria, oliguria, nocturia, dysuria, dribbling, pyuria, retention), infections, perineal rash, change in urgency, and character of urine.
5   Visually inspecting the faeces and urine as well as 'dipstick' testing will also aid in the assessment. When was their last stool? Check consistency of stool, e.g. hard or soft?
6   Ask whether the patient uses any devices or aids to urine elimination, e.g. bedpans, sheaths.

Environment suitable for elimination

Many patients experience bowel and urinary problems and this can be made worse by having to use bedside toilet methods. It may also be a cause of anxiety to many patients for a number of reasons such as personal embarrassment.

The toilet facility needs to be fit for purpose. That is they need to be accessible, fitted with any assistive equipment (wall bars for frail people, steps for children, correct height) or adjustments for disability. It also needs to be private with an adequate supply of toilet tissue and hand-washing facilities. Culturally sensitive care, dignity and anticipation of patient needs are necessary and determining cultural needs and preferences is important. For example, some faiths require the use of running water to wash hands or facilities to wash their genitalia following elimination (Essence of Care, 2010; RCN, 2012).

Odour elimination may be a concern for patients especially if they have diarrhoea and this also is an aspect to pre-empt and address discreetly. The ideal place for a patient to carry out their elimination needs is behind a closed toilet door. However, for certain patients, it may not be possible and therefore, the bedside area may be the most appropriate and safest place with in as near optimum conditions as possible and with due regard for dignity and privacy (Essence of Care, 2010).

Activity 4.1

Reflect on a time when you had to assist a patient with their elimination needs:

- How was this recorded at assessment and care planning?
- What aspects did you need to consider (e.g. environment, preference, noise, odour)?
- How did you demonstrate privacy and dignity for this patient when helping them with their elimination needs?
- What evidence do you have for this answer?

Assisting a patient with elimination

When patients call for assistance with elimination, it is imperative to respond to their request or call immediately and the rationale is dignity, comfort and the most appropriate support. However, it would be better to ask frequently before the urgency becomes extreme.

Providing a commode

Equipment needed at the bedside

- Clean commode with bedpan insert and cover
- Non-sterile gloves and apron
- Manual handling equipment if needed or additional nurse
- Toilet paper
- Wash bowl, water, soap and towel.

1 Ensure appropriate manual handling assessment has been completed prior to doing this procedure and if using, ensure the hoist is used in accordance with local procedures or manufacturer's instructions (see Chapter 11).
2 Wash hands and put on non-sterile gloves and apron.

3   Close curtains or screens around the patient – the commode ought not to be used by the bedside unless total privacy can be assured.

4   Explain the equipment and procedure to the patient and obtain consent.

5   Remove the commode cover and assist the patient out of bed or chair and onto the commode.

6   Ensure the patient is sitting securely on the commode with their feet touching the floor.

7   Ensure patient is comfortable, warm and draped with a towel to retain dignity.

8   Check there is sufficient toilet paper or wipes within reach.

9   Step away from the area ensuring patient has a call bell and privacy.

10   Once finished, check if the patient needs assistance with final genital cleansing or wiping. If assisting females, ensure the genital area is wiped front to back only. Offer the patient. water/wipes if the patient wishes to wash their genital area.

11   Assist patient to redress in underwear or pyjamas.

12   Offer patient water/soap to wash hands.

13   Help patient to walk to bed or chair and ensure they are sitting safely and comfortably, ensuring call bell is within reach.

14   Apply any odour-eliminating measures to the area if desired by the patient.

15   Replace the cover on the commode.

16   Take commode to dirty utility room or toilet and remove pan from the commode.

17   Examine contents if possible (urine volume or stool appearance).

18   Dispose of contents safely and place pan in cleansing/disposal unit unless abnormalities are detected and further examination is necessary.

19   Clean commode in accordance with the local policy.

20   Remove non-sterile gloves and apron and dispose.

21   Wash hands using bactericidal soap and document details of urine or faeces. observed/tested. Report any abnormalities immediately.

Clinical significance

The advantage of using a commode rather than a bedpan is that it allows a patient to assume a position with hips and knees flexed – the Valsalva manoeuvre – which aids elimination.

Don't forget!

Local infection control policy and procedures must be adhered to in order to prevent any possibility of cross-infection or contamination.

If patient is restricted to bed, they will then need to eliminate while in the bed. Bedpans are devices used for patients who are unable to get out of bed to use toilet facilities (Pellatt, 2007). A standard bedpan is metal or plastic and usually large in size, with a deep bowl and curved sides. It is ideal to use when a patient has some mobility and can balance themselves with no assistance. Bedpans should always be handled on the outside with the use of gloves.

A 'slipper' pan is notably flatter and is of benefit when the patient is unable to sit upright, it is usually made of plastic and has a handle for ease of use (Figures 4.1 (a)–(d)).

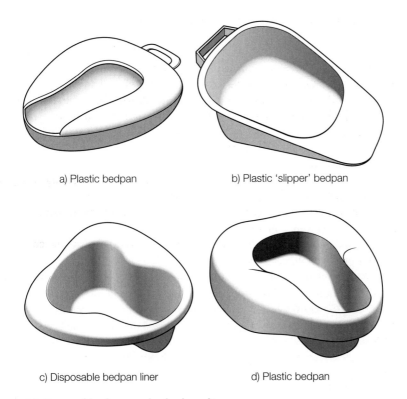

a) Plastic bedpan

b) Plastic 'slipper' bedpan

c) Disposable bedpan liner

d) Plastic bedpan

Figure 4.1 **Types of bedpan and a bedpan liner**

Don't forget!

A patient risk assessment is required before any attempt is made to assist a patient with their toileting needs and any manual handling equipment or extra staff should be made available.

Providing a bedpan

Equipment needed at the bedside

- Non-sterile gloves and apron
- Appropriate bedpan and holder, dependent on patient needs

- Bedpan cover
- Toilet paper
- Wipes
- Bowl
- Towel
- Air freshener
- Protective pad to place under the bedpan to protect the bed linen and if the patient prefers.

Follow steps 1–4 in Providing a commode (see above). Select the most appropriate bedpan.

1   Close the door/curtains around the patient bed space to provide privacy.
2   Remove the bedclothes and assist the patient to sit upright, unless this is contraindicated.
3   If the patient has some mobility, have him/her lift their bottom independently by flexing the knees and placing pressure on the heels to lift themselves and slide the bedpan under the pelvic area, with the widest part of the bedpan under the buttocks. With male patients, make sure that the penis and scrotum are free from the sides of the bedpan to prevent damage to the genital area.
4   Ensure patient comfort by using pillows to support the upper body and maintain a safe upright position.
5   Alternatively, if the patient is unable to mobilise or move independently into a sitting upright position; roll the patient onto one side and insert a slipper bedpan, ensure that the narrow flat end is correctly positioned underneath the buttock area and roll the patient back so that they are positioned directly on the bedpan.
6   Once the patient is safely on the bedpan, assist them to move their legs so they are slightly parted and the patient is in a squatting position, check that the bedpan is correctly situated to prevent any content spillages.
7   Ensure that the patient's lower body is covered to maintain privacy and dignity and that toilet paper and call bell are within the patient's reach; the nurse must remain nearby in case the patient needs help.
8   Follow Steps 8–10 of Providing a commode.
9   Assess the skin for any abnormalities such as skin breakdown or rashes.
10 Discreetly use the air freshener to reduce any strong odours and prevent patient embarrassment, unless this is contraindicated, e.g., if a patient has respiratory problems.
11 The patient should be offered hand washing facilities following elimination to maintain cleanliness.

For disposal of the contents, follow steps 15–21 of Providing a commode.

Don't forget!

The patient must be advised NOT to remove the bedpan themselves, but to wait for assistance, the nurse must wait nearby.

Activity 4.2

Gus is 15 years old. He was injured during a game of football and his femur is in a cast. He is strong and can use the monkey pole to lift himself onto a bedpan. In the next few days he can get out of bed to be wheeled to the toilet. In the meantime:

■ How do you think he will feel about using a bedpan?
■ How might you help to reduce the risk of constipation during his period of bedrest?

Sample collection: mid-stream specimen of urine (MSU)

There are times when a patient has a urinary problem which needs investigation and laboratory analysis, specifically if an infection is suspected. A urine sample which is relatively uncontaminated (from outside the urine tract) is requested, called a 'mid-stream' specimen. This is as it sounds. The urine 'stream' is split into three stages: beginning, middle and end. The urine is caught from the middle point or 'mid' point. The patient can do this themselves if able to do so. Alternatively the nurse can aid the patient with this. The skill is as follows:

Obtaining an MSU

Equipment needed at the bedside

If patient is collecting MSU:

■ Gauze cloth moistened with normal saline 0.9%
■ Sterile specimen jar
■ Pathology request form
■ Biohazard specimen bag
■ Plastic bag for disposal of waste.

If nurse is collecting MSU:

■ Personal protective equipment: plastic apron, gloves, eye protection
■ Pathology request form
■ Cotton balls/gauze squares
■ Sachet 0.9% sodium chloride
■ Sterile receiving bowl
■ Sterile specimen container
■ Biohazard specimen bag
■ Bedpan or urinal
■ Disposable plastic gloves
■ Plastic bag for disposal of wastes.

Procedure for collecting an MSU

1 Explain procedure to patient and obtain consent.
2 Ensure patient privacy.
3 Ensure patient washes hands. If the nurse is taking the specimen – wash hands and put on apron and gloves.
4 Advise patient how to undertake meatal cleansing (downwards motion FRONT TO BACK) with gauze. If nurse is assisting, then the nurse undertakes this aspect.
5 Ask patient to pass first part of urine stream into the toilet/bedpan/bottle
6 Catch mid-stream specimen in sterile specimen container or sterile receiving bowl.
7 Take care not to contaminate the specimen.
8 Allow patient to void remainder of urine.
9 Ensure lid is tightened on the container.
10 Label specimen correctly with patient's name, medical record number and time and date of collection. Do note on the request form if the patient is a female who is menstruating.
11 Place specimen container and request form in a biohazard specimen bag for transportation to the laboratory or store refrigerated for collection.
12 Remove gloves and apron and discard.
13 Wash hands.

Assisting young children

The changing of a nappy on the infant or young child is a skill that can take some practice to master, largely due to the fact that children will not necessarily respond as you would wish or can be resistant to being in a position to have their nappy changed. The rationale for this skills is that nappies can be worn by children up to the age of 5 years old though from 2 years it is more likely to be only at night until full bowel control is achieved. In some patients or young people with disability or impaired physical ability, it may mean they wear nappies either temporarily or longer term and this must be addressed sympathetically if embarrassment occurs.

Nappies in common use are either disposable or re-usable and made of material such as cloth or terry towelling (Johnson and Taylor, 2010). A wet or soiled nappy can cause misery in some children and should be changed every three to four hours. Prompt nappy changing should occur to prevent discomfort and the development of any skin irritation such as nappy rash (CKS, 2013). Skin irritation can be caused by a number of factors such as sensitivity to soap or baby wipes, prolonged contact with urine, stool or diarrhoea, rubbing and chafing. If skin irritation has occurred, the frequency of nappy changing should be increased. If circumstances allow, exposure of the genital/nappy area to the air during the day may be helpful though in a busy nursery or ward, this may not be possible.

Safe practice and standard infection control procedures must be followed in accordance with local policy to prevent undue harm to the infant and young child (NMC, 2010).

Activity 4.3

What aspects would you need to consider before starting the nappy changing procedure? Hint: consider:

- Safety
- Preparation
- Consent
- Comfort.

Changing a nappy

It is important that an appropriate firm, but comfortable surface or baby changing mat is used; if the baby is relaxed, then they are less likely to move about, making the changing process easier. The surface should be cleaned between each use in accordance with infection control procedures.

Watch out

Never leave a child unattended on a changing mat, if you must leave the changing area, then take the child with you, or ask someone else to continue the task.

Equipment needed at the child's changing area

- Bowl
- Warm water
- Non-sterile gloves and apron
- Changing mat
- Cleansing cloths/wipes
- Clean nappies
- Disposal bag/bin
- Change of clothing may be required
- Ointment/cream, if required. Where cream is used, the child should have their own named cream, and written permission must be obtained from the parent.
- Mobile/toy to distract the baby/infant during the nappy change.

Top tip

It is a good idea to have a named box or bag for each child containing these items and spare clothes in case of accidents.

Procedure for changing a nappy

Ideally the key worker or named nurse will do the procedure as they will have established a rapport with the child. Otherwise it should be a person the child knows associated with the key worker.

1   Wash and dry hands.
2   Put on gloves and apron. The nurse or carer should use a new set of gloves and apron for each nappy change.
3   Approach the child and say or sign that it is time for a nappy change. You may need to negotiate (e.g. say 'I see you enjoying this game but I need to change your nappy. Play for two more minutes, then we will change it'). Do not tell the child you will just start the procedure as you risk a resistant/uncooperative behaviour or frightening the child.
4   Place the child on a nappy changing mat or, if using steps, support the child if necessary to climb up the steps.
5   Remove the child's clothing to access the nappy. Remove the nappy and place it inside the nappy sack.

If the child's clothes are soiled, they should be bagged separately – check with the local policy what happens to these (i.e. sent home), they ought not be rinsed by hand. If there is excessive faeces, the child may be experiencing diarrhoea and this should be documented and reported.

6   Clean the child (girls wipe from front to back) and place the used wipes or cotton in the nappy sack. Tie the nappy sack and put it in a pedal-operated bin.
7   Ensure that the skin is clean and dry, particularly the skin folds of the groin and scrotal area as these are the areas where nappy rash may occur (Hale, 2007). Assess the genital area and skin condition for any abnormalities and document if present.
8   Put on a clean nappy and apply cream if necessary.
9   Take off the gloves and apron.
10   Dress the child.
11   Help the child to wash their hands using liquid soap, warm water and paper towels.
12   Wash your own hands.
13   Take the child back to the supervised room/area of play.
14   Return to the nappy changing area, clean the changing mat, surrounding area and underneath the mat before leaving to dry.
15   Then wash and dry your hands again.

Don't forget!

Where cream is used, the child should have their own named cream and written permission obtained from the parent if in a nursery/care environment.

Activity 4.4

You are preparing to change the nappy of 11-month-old Jas. You remember to engage and prepare Jas for this but she has recently become resistant and tries to crawl away. You think she might be bored – a few minutes might seem like an eternity to Jas. What can you do to make this less of an ordeal for Jas? List a few ideas:

Hint: You might consider songs or counting – what else?

Watch out

In small children, exposing nappy areas may stimulate urine, especially little boys! Do try to cover their genital area with a cloth or wipe during the procedure if possible to 'catch' any sprays.

Developing continence

The RCN (2013) paediatric continence guidance document identifies that normal urinary and faeces elimination in children alters with increasing maturity, ability to 'hold on' and response to triggers to 'void'. It is also linked to diet and hydration. Most babies stop opening their bowels at night before they become 1 year old and in fact soiling at night may not be diarrhoea but a sign of constipation (overflow). They provide an assessment tool for determining a child's readiness for toilet training which is especially useful for children with disability (physical or learning) when the usual development times maybe delayed. The One Step at a Time approach (CFA, 2010) was developed and is used successfully with families of children with a whole range of learning difficulties to help them become toilet trained. The steps are outlined in Box 4.3.

Box 4.3 One Step at a Time toilet training programme

Step 1: Setting the scene: location, time of day, sensation of wet/dry.

Step 2: Developing physical skills: sitting on the toilet, pulling pants up and down, washing and drying hands. Use of equipment or interventions to aid this.

Step 3: Raising awareness: how long the child is able to stay dry, moving the child out of disposable nappies into washable underwear or trainer pants.

Step 4: Using the toilet and wiping own bottom.

Step 5: Night-time control: if problematic, this may need referral to a continence service for further advice and support.

Adapted from CFA (2010).

Bladder training in adults

Nursing students may come across adults undergoing various forms of bladder retraining. These might be an approach for patients who have had a stroke, for example. It follows similar principles to that mentioned in the 'One Step at a Time' approach in Box 4.3 and will generally involve:

1   Regular visiting of the toilet with assistance if mobility is challenged.
2   Attending to timing and cues of bladder filling – increasing urine storage and timed voiding to promote bladder emptying. May need prompted voiding until habits develop.
3   Pelvic floor exercises to promote bladder and elimination control.
4   Manipulation of clothing.
5   Personal hygiene and self-cleaning.

Applying a penile sheath

A urinary sheath system is another method to manage urinary incontinence in men. This resembles a condom with an exit point which connects to a tubing system and the rationale for this skill is that it is non-invasive. There are many brands available made from different materials and in a wide range of sizes. The correct size is important. This should be done using a specially designed measuring guide to ensure that the sheath is neither too tight, (which could result in discomfort or even sore skin) nor too loose in which case the sheath is more likely to fall off.

Equipment needed at the bedside

- Bowl of warm water and soap
- Non-sterile gloves
- Selection of appropriate penile sheaths
- Anti-bactericidal alcohol hand rub
- Disposable plastic apron
- Drainage bag and stand or holder
- Hypo-allergenic tape for securing tubing or leg strap
- Catheter leg bag.

Procedure for applying a penile sheath

1   Explain and discuss the procedure with the patient and gain consent.
2   Screen the bed if in shared area or ensure do not disturb notice on bedroom door.
3   Assist the patient to get into the supine position with the legs extended – do not expose their genital area until ready to apply sheath.
4   Wash hands and put on apron.
5   Prepare equipment and have it all readily accessible.
6   Remove cover that is maintaining the patient's privacy and position a disposable pad under the patient's buttocks and thighs.

7   Using the measuring guide supplied, correctly measure the penis around the glans (head of the penis).

8   Wash the area with soap and water, ensuring that the area is dried thoroughly.

9   Do not use talcum powder or creams as this will prevent the sheath from sticking to the penis. It may be necessary to trim the pubic hair to ensure an adequate seal and to prevent the discomfort that this otherwise may cause.

10 Place the rolled end of the sheath over the glans, leaving a small gap between the end of the penis and the cup of the sheath. (If the patient is not circumcised leave the foreskin forward, do not retract it.)

11 Slowly unroll the sheath down the shaft of the penis ensuring that there are no creases and the sheath has stuck evenly to the area. Try not to leave any unrolled sheath at the base of the shaft of the penis.

12 Extra security can be given if needed with the use of Urifix tape or sheath liners.

13 Connect to leg/night bags to ensure there are no kinks in the tubing and the bag is positioned correctly on the leg or on a stand at the bedside to ensure good drainage.

14 Discard equipment.

15 Remove apron and wash hands.

16 Document the procedure including: the reason for applying penile sheath, date and time of application, sheath type, length and size, manufacturer, any problems negotiated during the procedure, a review date to assess the need for reapplication.

Procedure for removing the sheath

1   This should be done carefully, either in the bath or shower or wrap a warm flannel around the sheath to help loosen the adhesive.

2   Roll the sheath gently down the penis, easing the skin away from the sheath Adhesive remover wipes or sprays are also available to help with removal. The sheath should be changed every 24 hours.

3   Do note a sheath can be worn for up to three days provided that the sheath is intact and the skin appears to be in good condition.

4   Leg bags should be used for five to seven days. Disposable night bags should be used for one night only and then discarded.

Urinary catheters

Urinary catheterisation refers to the aseptic insertion of an artificial hollow tube into the bladder usually for elimination or instilling of fluids. It may also be used for blockages, post-surgery or situations when the accurate monitoring of urine is needed. Urinary catheterisation is not without risks and can makes patients vulnerable to hospital associated infection (HAI) as it is invasive, with the risk increasing the longer the patient remains catheterised. The procedure can only be performed under strict aseptic conditions by those with additional training and competency. Catheters can be left in place (or 'in-situ'), intermittent or long term. They can be inserted by nurses and doctors or the patient themselves. Generally catheters are passed into the bladder via the urethra but occasionally they are inserted directly through the mid-suprapubic region in the abdominal wall. This is a surgical procedure and one reserved for patients with either long-term requirements or those following pelvic injury or disease. The principles of care for catheters whatever route is used are similar and are outlined in the following section.

Activity 4.5

Revisit your preferred anatomy and physiology book. List the key structures involved with urine production – perhaps draw a diagram and label it – do look for the terms:

- Kidney
- Ureter
- Urethra
- External sphincter
- Prostate gland (in males)
- Bladder
- Pelvic floor muscles (looks like a 'hammock').

Clinical significance

Catheterisation should only be used as a last resort as a method of bladder emptying, as it is an invasive procedure and is associated with an increased incidence of urinary tract infection (UTI); if inserted, the catheter should be removed at the earliest opportunity.

A catheter can be inserted short term (up to seven days) and long term (six weeks–three months) and will be dependent upon the individual case (Hart, 2008). Intermittent catheterisation (IC) may be considered as an option, particularly in women who experience bladder dysfunction (NICE, 2013). The process allows the individual to insert and remove the catheter at regular intervals. Box 4.4 lists the types of catheter and Figures 4.2 (a) and (b) show the female and male insertion and a normal catheter.

Risks associated with female catheterisation

- *Bacteriuria and urinary tract infection* – using an aseptic technique will minimise the risk
- *Haematuria (bleeding)* – patients taking medication such as aspirin or warfarin will increase the risk of haematuria; recent catheter-related trauma, recent urinary tract surgery, and known bladder cancer will also increase this risk
- *Urethral stricture* – occurs when a part of the urethra becomes narrowed and scarred. The length of the female urethra is 3–4 cm. Any section of the urethra may be affected
- *Loss of bladder tone*
- *Altered body image* due to urethral catheterisation may impede sexual intercourse.

Box 4.4 Types of catheter

Intermittent

- *Polyvinyl chloride (PVC) non-coated*: are quite rigid and require lubrication prior to insertion
- *Hydrophilic-coated catheters*: impregnated with a coating, which lubricates the catheter throughout the entire catheterisation process.

Short to mid term (up to 28 days)

- *Latex*: latex is a purified form of rubber and is the softest of the catheter materials. Its surface is smooth and has a tendency to form a crust. NOTE: Some patients have allergies to latex
- *Polytetrafluoroethylene (PTFE)*: the coating is applied to a latex catheter to render the latex inert and reduce irritation.

Long term (up to 12 weeks)

- *Silicone elastomer-coated latex*: resistant to crusting on the surface
- *Hydrogel-coated latex*: a latex core catheter, coated with a hydrophilic polymer coating
- *All-silicone*: a thin-walled catheter, which has a large D-shaped lumen. Suitable for those with a latex allergy. However, they are relatively stiff and some patients find them uncomfortable. Because silicone permits gas diffusion, balloons may deflate and allow the catheter to fall out prematurely.

Look these up on the internet to see the difference. Ask about the choice of catheter when you are on placement.

Catheterisation is not a comfortable procedure. Ensure that privacy and dignity are maintained throughout. Cover all parts of the body not requiring exposure, and keep checking for any signs of distress throughout the procedure. Stop immediately if any extreme discomfort is expressed and seek advice from a senior nurse or doctor.

Inserting a female catheter

Equipment needed at the bedside

A catheter pack contains:

- Sterile drape (fenestrated, disposable)
- Cotton gauze balls
- Gallipot (for cleansing solution)

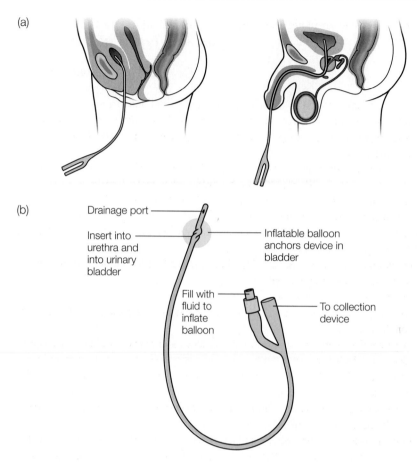

(a)

(b)

Drainage port

Insert into urethra and into urinary bladder

Inflatable balloon anchors device in bladder

Fill with fluid to inflate balloon

To collection device

Figure 4.2 (a) Insertion of female and male catheter; (b) the workings of a catheter

- Gauze surgical swabs
- Collecting receiver or kidney bowl.

In addition:

- Two 10 ml sachets of 0.9% saline (for cleansing)
- Urine collection bag, or urometer for more frequent measuring
- Catheter (start with 12cH, or may require larger, e.g. 14cH if post surgical in some circumstances). For short-term use (under 28 days), use an uncoated latex, PVC, polytetrafluoroethylene (PTFE) or silver alloy catheter. For longer-term state, use an all-silicone, silicone elastomer or hydrogel-coated catheter. Check the patient has no latex allergies. Check for length too (male versus female lengths).
- Sterile lidocaine (6 ml, 2%) gel (for lubrication, dilatation and analgesia) if needed
- 10 ml sachet of sterile water for injections to inflate balloon (10 ml used for standard catheters, check catheter label for correct volume)

- 10 ml syringe and green needle (to aspirate water for balloon inflation)
- Two pairs of sterile gloves.

Procedure for inserting a female catheter

1 Ensure environment is well lit, warm and private.
2 Explain procedure to patient, including risks and benefits, and gain informed consent. If patient unable to give consent, act in patient's best interests by following local Consent Policy.
3 Offer patient a chaperone and document the decision in health records.
4 Wash and dry your hands, and put on an apron.
5 Check for any allergies, e.g. latex or anaesthetic gels. If patient is allergic to latex, then a silicone catheter should be used.
6 Open the catheter pack carefully, exposing the sterile field onto the top shelf of the trolley using an aseptic technique.
7 Open all other packs onto the sterile field now stretched out on the trolley, pouring the 0.9% saline into the gallipot.
8 Ensure the patient has privacy.
9 Assist the patient in the supine position with the knees flexed and separated and feet flat on the bed, about 60 cm apart (Figure 4.3 (a)).
10 Place protective sheet under the patient's buttocks and adjust lighting as necessary
11 Re-wash and dry your hands.
12 Put on a pair of sterile gloves from the trolley, taking care not to contaminate the sterile field.
13 Hold the labia open exposing the urethral meatus with your dominant hand for the remainder of the procedure.
14 With your other hand, cleanse the urethral meatus, using saline-soaked gauze balls. Use each gauze for a single downward movement (i.e. towards the anus) only (Figure 4.3 (b)).
15 If using anaesthetic or lubricating gel, place a small amount onto a sterile gauze which you then dip with the tip of the urinary catheter. Place the fenestrated sterile drape appropriately.
16 Place the collecting bowl for urine between the patient's legs.

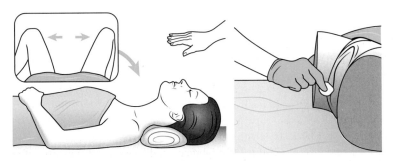

Figure 4.3 (a) Position of patient for catheterisation; (b) position for cleaning the urethral meatus

17 Using the blue sterile sheath to hold the catheter, tear a small hole in the perforations near the tip and gently pass it into the urinary meatus.

18 Introduce the catheter into the urethral opening in an upward and backward direction. Advance the catheter until 5 or 6 cm have been inserted and urine begins to flow, then advance the catheter a further 1–2 cm, thus 6–8 cm in total). Never force the catheter if resistance is felt.

19 If there is no urine present, remove the catheter gently and start the procedure again with a new catheter.

20 Attach appropriate urine-collecting product.

21 When the catheter is successfully placed and urine is flowing, inflate the catheter balloon with 10 ml of sterile water (NICE, 2012) according to the manufacturer's instructions (or as printed on the catheter). Withdraw the catheter slightly to ensure the balloon is inflated and secure.

22 Ensure the patient is dry and made comfortable by assisting with clothing or nightwear

23 Secure a support for the catheter, either a leg strap support or a urine-collecting bag stand. Ensure the catheter does not become taut or occluded.

24 Dispose of gloves and materials in appropriate clinical waste bag, and wash hands.

25 Document the procedure (NMC, 2015) including:
   a   date and time;
   b   catheter type and batch number – catheter may have an adhesive label to stick in the notes;
   c   amount of water used to inflate balloon;
   d   any problems during the procedure;
   e   urine volumes observed.

26 Send a urine sample, if requested – this is called a 'catheter specimen of urine' (CSU).

Watch out

Rapid drainage of large volumes of urine may cause hypotension so do observe the patient throughout this procedure for signs of this.

Top tip

Catheters come in different lengths – the female ones are shorter (26 cm) than male ones (43 cm) – do not mix them up as short ones can cause damage to males!

Catheter care

Over time if not kept clean, encrustation can occur, especially if patients have long-term catheters. The need for catheter care is important because, as micro-organisms colonise a catheter surface they multiply rapidly, forming a living layer, known as a biofilm, which becomes increasingly thicker as multiplication continues. Patients especially in the community are encouraged to do the following to reduce the risk of encrustation and infections occurring from a catheter:

1   Wash hands before touching their catheter and after emptying or changing the drainage bags and after every bowel motion. Explain procedure to the patient and obtain consent.
2   Personal hygiene: it is advisable for the patient to have a bath or shower daily, always emptying the drainage bag beforehand. If baths/showers are not possible, then men should wash under their foreskin, then wash the area around the indwelling urethral catheter using a clean cloth and some mild soap and water and dry thoroughly. Women should ensure they wash from front to the back passage to keep bacteria away from the catheter. If supra-pubic – the abdominal entry point – wash with cooled boiled water or in a shower.
3   If this is a supra-pubic catheter, the care outlined earlier is also required to avoid pulling at the catheter with clothing.
4   Fluid intake is encouraged, e.g. up to 1.5 to 2 litres of fluids daily and observe urine to ensure it is clear and straw-coloured.
5   Educate the patient in relation to avoiding becoming constipated, e.g. diet to contain vegetables and fibre. Constipation can block catheters which dangerously impeded urine flow.
6   Changing drainage bags: only disconnect from the indwelling urethral catheter when absolutely necessary to reduce the risk of introducing infection. Maintain hand hygiene and use gloves
7   Patients should observe all the advice above and be aware that activities such as exercise, swimming, holidays and sexual activity are still possible with some adjustments to position of the catheter, drainage bags, and perhaps with lubrication.

Don't forget!

Observe the catheter for signs of blockage or poor draining – this can be dangerous for the patient.

Care of the supra-pubic catheter

A supra-pubic catheter is an alternative way for urine to be continuously drained from the bladder cavity. It is indicated in situations such as trauma to the urinary tract (Kumar and Pati, 2005), neurological conditions, acute or chronic retention, palliative care, urological investigations, urinary incontinence, post-operative care or patient choice (NHS Quality Improvement Scotland, 2004). Due to the invasive nature of this type of catheterisation, the procedure, known as a supra-pubic cystostomy is usually performed under general or local anaesthesia (Robinson, 2004) by a qualified professional. The patient should be fully informed of the procedure and appropriate pain relief administered prior to and following the insertion.

Watch out

Should the catheter become expelled from the bladder, there is only a short time frame of approximately 30–45 minutes in which it needs to be replaced before the tract will begin to granulate and re-insertion may prove difficult.

Following the initial insertion, the cystostomy wound should be cleaned using the aseptic technique and a dry dressing applied. The entry site will heal in seven to ten days and then may be cleaned with cooled boiled water in a direction away from the insertion site. The nursing care of a patient with a supra-pubic catheter will include daily visual assessment of the urine as well as monitoring the amount of urine drained. Ensure that the patient washes their hands thoroughly before and after coming into contact with the catheter drainage system. The patient should be encouraged to drink plenty of fluids, usually 1.5–2 litres daily to encourage an adequate urine flow and output and to maintain hydration, as long as there are no contraindications of the patient condition. It is the nurse's responsibility to ensure that documentation is completed (NMC, 2015).

Emptying a catheter bag

Equipment needed at the bedside.

- Non sterile gloves
- Apron
- Appropriate container for urine (disposable or heat-resistant)
- Paper towel to cover
- Alcohol swabs.

Procedure for emptying a catheter bag

1   Explain procedure to the patient and obtain consent.
2   Ensure privacy.
3   Wash hands and put on gloves and apron.
4   Ensure the drainage pot of the catheter bag is visible and accessible (may need to be removed from the leg strap); if on a stand, this does need altering, just place over collecting container or toilet if at home.
5   Clean the outlet port with the alcohol swab and allow it to dry.
6   Open the drainage port and allow the urine to drain into the collecting container during which do not let the port touch the inside of the container.
7   Close the port and clean with an alcohol swab.
8   Reposition the catheter bag as before or for the comfort of the patient – ensure the catheter is not occluded or taut.
9   Cover the container and take to the clinical room for measuring and then document this.
10 The container then should be disinfected or disposed of according to the local policy.
11 Remove gloves and apron and wash hands.

Removal of an indwelling catheter

Catheters are removed as soon as they are not needed. The rationale is so bladders can resume their role and to minimise bladder weakness.

Equipment needed at the bedside

- Non sterile gloves and apron
- Syringe – minimum 10 ml to remove water from balloon
- Appropriate container for urine (disposable or heat-resistant)
- Disposable absorbent pad
- Waste bag.

If catheter specimen of urine (CSU) is required, also:

- Specimen pot
- 20 ml syringe
- Needle
- Alcohol swabs.

Procedure for removing an indwelling catheter

Follow steps 1–4 in the procedure for female catheterisation:

1. If requested by the doctor or senior nurse, obtain a specimen of urine from the catheter sampling port.
2. Ensure privacy and dignity.
3. Assist the patient in the supine position with the knees flexed and separated and feet flat on the bed, about 60 cm apart (see Figure 4.3 (a)).
4. Place a collecting bowl between the patient's legs and place an absorbent pad underneath the patient's buttocks.
5. Examine the balloon label for volume and select the appropriate size syringe. Then connect and withdraw the correct volume of water from the balloon. If the volume is different, i.e. less, then seek advice.
6. Ask the patient to relax and focus on breathing – in and out. On expiration gently pull the catheter out. This should have no resistance. If there is, then stop and make the patient comfortable and seek advice for the nurse or doctor in charge.
7. If the catheter comes out smoothly, place it in the receiving bowl. Ensure patient is covered and comfortable.
8. Remove gloves and wash hands.
9. The patient may feel the need to urinate – ensure a toilet or commode is near at hand and the patient is supported to the toilet safely according to their mobility assessment.
10. Document the date and time of removal of the catheter and any urine volumes.
11. Advise the patient to drink fluids to enable urination to proceed as normal.
12. Do monitor the patient's pattern of urination afterwards: frequency, amount, any pain or discomfort and report.

Obtaining a catheter specimen of urine (CSU)

This is a common nursing procedure in which a specimen of urine is obtained from a urinary catheter for reasons such as diagnostic purposes in the case of a suspected urinary tract infection (UTI) or sepsis/pyrexia of unknown origin. Taking a CSU must be a non-touch, aseptic technique and must be taken from the sampling port on the drainage bag.

Clinical significance

Do not obtain a CSU from a drainage bag/when changing a drainage bag (such as, straight out of catheter and into a specimen bottle) or by running the urine straight through a new drainage bag and into a specimen bottle. This potentially aids the spread of microbes and risk of infection.

Equipment needed at the bedside

- Non-sterile gloves and apron
- Sterile 10 ml syringe
- 70% alcohol swabs suitable for equipment use
- Single-patient use disposable clamp
- Specimen containers
- Laboratory request form
- Detergent wipe for equipment.

Procedure for obtaining a CSU

1   Explain to the patient what you are doing and obtain their consent.
2   Wash hands and put on gloves and apron
3   If there is no urine in the catheter bag tubing, clamp tubing 5–10 cm below the sampling port using a single-patient use, scissor-style clamp. Decontaminate hands.
4   Clean sampling port prior to attaching the syringe with a 70% alcohol wipe suitable for equipment use for 30 seconds contact time.
5   Attach a sterile 10 ml syringe to the needleless sampling port to aspirate urine:
    - If a needleless port is not used, add a 23 gauge needle to the syringe and insert into the specified port at a 45 degree angle to prevent going through the tubing. Withdraw the required amount of urine. Dispose of needle and syringe in a sharps box immediately, following the local policy.
6   Clean the sampling port with 70% alcohol wipe after removal of the syringe.
7   Place some urine in appropriate specimen container for urinalysis.
8   Place remaining urine in appropriate specimen container to send to laboratory.
9   Remove clamp from catheter bag tubing and decontaminate with an alcohol.
10 Remove gloves and apron.
11 Wash hands with soap and water.
12 Label specimen.

13 Complete laboratory request.

14 Promptly transport to laboratory or if out of hours, hold safely in a designated specimen refrigerator for up to 24 hours only.

Bladder lavage/irrigation/washout

Bladder washouts should never be routinely administered to catheterised patients without a therapeutic intervention and should not be used as a substitute for re-catheterisation. Catheter maintenance solutions are prescription only medication (POM) and should be treated in the same way as any POM medication. Nurses should undergo further training to do this. A bladder lavage can be described as the use of a sterile fluid to manually wash out the bladder, whereas bladder irrigation is a continuous washout with sterile fluid, usually 0.9% sodium chloride. The rationale for either procedure can be for the removal of blockages, the breakdown of blood clots and debris or, for medicinal reasons.

Constipation

Constipation refers to a symptom whereby bowel movements are infrequent or hard to pass. The severity of constipation varies from person to person. Many people only experience constipation for a short time, but for others, constipation can be a long-term (chronic) condition that causes significant pain and discomfort and affects their quality of life. It can be severe and cause bowel obstruction and become life-threatening and, if it persists, it should be investigated further. As a symptom, it has many causes but two main ones: obstruction and slow colon mobility (or movement). Constipation in childhood is common.

In adult patients, the Norgine Risk Assessment Tool for constipation is a useful tool which asks questions on medication, condition, diet, mobility, toileting facilities and fluid intake and calculates the risk of constipation and suggests appropriate action. It can be found at: www.movicol.com.au/file/Constipation%20Risk%20Assessment%20Tool.pdf.

For children, NICE guidelines indicate a rating tool offering 'red flags' for certain changes in bowel habits and associated investigations and treatments. This can be serious for very young children and may indicate an underlying condition. See: www.nice.org.uk/guidance/cg99/chapter/guidance.

If patients are constipated, then they may be prescribed a laxative given orally or for more immediate effect medication given rectally, i.e. solid gel-like (suppositories) or fluid-based (enemas). The rationale for this skills is that nurses need to know this process to either manage constipation or administer these medications which can be given via this route. The procedure for suppositories is outlined in Chapter 16. In children, the NICE CG99 (2010) guidelines warn professionals not to use rectal medications for disimpaction of faeces unless all oral medications have failed and only if the child or young person and their family consent.

Clinical significance

Manual evacuation or removal of faeces is an invasive procedure and should only be performed when necessary after an individual assessment such as impacted faeces in a patient with spinal cord lesion. Manual evacuation should be avoided if at all possible since it is a distressing, often painful and a potentially dangerous procedure for the patient. Cultural and religious beliefs as well as age and reason should be considered prior to performing this procedure.

Stomas

The word stoma originates from the Greek and means 'mouth' or 'opening' and it is the part of the ostomy (the surgical opening of an organ to the outside of the abdominal wall to allow for the removal of waste products) that is attached to the skin The name will identify which part of the bowel has been used. A colostomy is the most common stoma.

Generally, stomas can be divided into three groups:

Colostomy: opening from the colon (large intestine)
            formed stool requiring closed pouch unless diarrhoea
Ileostomy: opening from the ileum (small intestine)
            liquid stool requiring drainable pouch
Urostomy: a stoma formed to divert urine
            urine requiring pouch with tap.

A temporary stoma may also be formed to promote healing, in the case of bowel disease. At a later date (minimum of 6 weeks), following healing, the temporary stoma will be closed by an anastomosis (joining) and the intestine can return to normal functioning.

Stoma care

Stoma care is provided to maintain a healthy stoma and its surrounding skin, to monitor for any signs of complications, such as stoma retraction, sore skin or parastomal hernia and to provide patient comfort and security. In many clinical areas a stoma care nurse specialist (SCNS) provides support and is a good resource for students.

Don't forget!

Caring for a patient with stoma requires great sensitivity as the patient may not yet have come to terms with the change in their body image.

To observe the stoma appliance and function you should check that:

- A clear pouch is in place
- The appliance is intact
- The closure is correctly applied/fastened
- The pouch is positioned vertically
- The clear drainable pouch remains in place for 24 hours post-surgery (if new), then change and assess stoma and peristomal skin (around stoma).

Note the following:

- The colour should be pink and the stoma should visibly appear moist due to the mucous coating. A newly formed stoma is usually oedematous due to bowel handling during surgery and this should minimise over time.
- Faecal consistency and volume will vary dependent upon the type of ostomy and all output should be clearly documented. Any abnormality such as discoloration or skin excoriation must be reported, as this may indicate complications which may require further intervention.

The stoma and surrounding skin should preferably be gently cleaned with dry wipes and plain warm water and rinsed. Ensure after cleaning that the surrounding skin is intact, clean and dry. If preferred, specific skin cleansers may be used in accordance with the manufacturer's guidance. The use of non-specific cleaning agents, disinfectants or wipes should be discouraged as this may cause skin soreness and can leave a film on the stoma, which may hinder the application of stoma appliances to the skin.

Changing a stoma appliance

Ensure that you are able to carry out this procedure in a suitable environment, free from distractions. Inform the patient to gain consent and their cooperation. Promote patient privacy and dignity.

Equipment needed at the bedside

- Pouches (clear, drainable pouches for first few days after surgery; then the type may change according to individual needs) (Figure 4.4)
- Pouch clips (if required)
- Small bowl for water
- Disposal bags
- Wipes/swabs (non sterile) – to clean and dry skin
- Adhesive remover
- Ostomy deodorant spray
- Barrier wipes – to protect skin
- Additional accessories as specified in care plan
- Template/measuring guide see Figure 4.5
- Paper towel/pad to protect clothing.

Procedure for changing a stoma bag

1   Wash and dry hands thoroughly and put on apron and gloves.
2   If the stoma has a drainable bag, empty the contents into the toilet or a jug.
3   Reassure patient throughout.
4   If drainable pouch is being used and faecal fluid or urine is evident, empty and dispose of prior to removal of pouch.
5   Use a wipe/tissue to protect waistband/underwear.

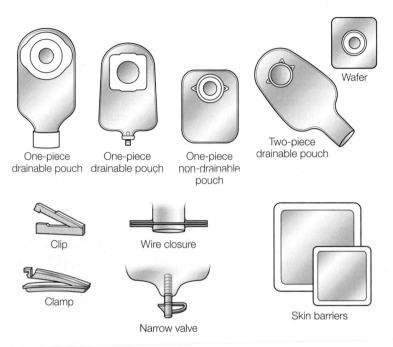

One-piece drainable pouch   One-piece drainable pouch   One-piece non-drainable pouch   Two-piece drainable pouch   Wafer

Clip   Wire closure   Clamp   Narrow valve   Skin barriers

Figure 4.4 **Types of ostomy appliances**

6   Using adhesive remover, gently peel appliance from skin and discard in disposable bag.
7   Wash stoma and peristomal skin using disposable soft wipes and tepid water.
8   Mild soap/non-perfumed soap can be used if patient wishes.
9   Dry skin with a soft disposable wipes.
10   Observe/assess the peristomal skin and document observations.
11   If there are problems or concerns – this should be reported to the nurse in charge and SCNS.
12   Use a clean gallipot/disposable medicine pot to protect the stoma.
13   Cut a hole in the flange of a stoma bag (using a previously created template).
14   Remove the backing paper and apply to gently stretched skin.
15   Gently press into place. Press close to stoma and also the outer edges of the flange.
16   If appropriate, ask the patient to press the palm of his/her hand over the appliance for a few minutes.
17   Remove gloves before leaving patient's area or bathroom.
18   Wear new gloves to dispose of soiled items in sluice area or disposal system if in the community.

Patients can do this for themselves and have their own routine so do be aware of their preferences and support if needed.

Equipment to create a stoma template

- Piece of paper or card
- Measuring guide (optional)
- Scissors.

Procedure to create a stoma template

1   Take a piece of card or paper and cut out the stoma template (Figure 4.5). Or use the disposable measuring guide found in most boxes of appliances.
2   Place the template over the stoma and check that there is a small allowance of approximately 1–2 mm around the stoma for a 'snug fit'.

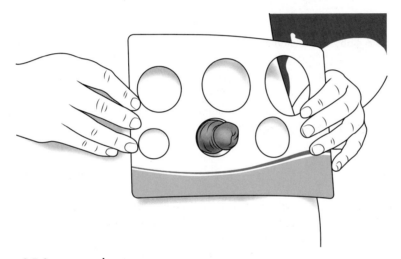

Figure 4.5 Stoma template

Smaller templates are available for babies, see Figure 4.6.

Clinical significance

There can be wide variety of different beliefs and practices even within the same religious group and this will affect attitudes to and care of stomas. How strictly practices are observed can also vary, so it is important not to make assumptions but to make sure you understand the needs of each patient as a unique individual.

Summary

Elimination is a sensitive issue and providing effective care can be challenging. There is the potential for a person's dignity to be compromised and it is essential that this is foremost in nurses' minds when discussing, assessing or assisting with elimination

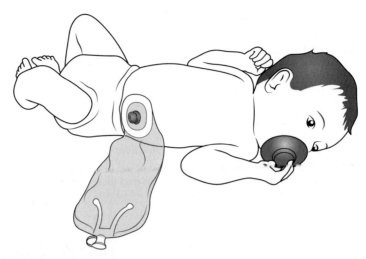

Figure 4.6 Baby with a stoma

processes. This is a key skill which needs to be accompanied by a skilled assessment of the patient as soon as possible after admission to a care facility or into a community setting. This will form a baseline of elimination function and identify any underlying issues, as well as address any patient concerns and preferences.

References

British Geriatric Society (2007) *Behind Closed Doors: Delivering Dignity in Toilet Access and Use*. Available at: www.bgs.org.uk/campaigns/dignitypress.htm (accessed 12 February 2016).

CKS (Clinical Knowledge Summaries) (2013) Nappy rash. Available at: http://cks.nice.org. uk/nappy-rash#!scenario (accessed 10 February 2016).

Continence Foundation of Australia (2010) *One Step at a Time: A Parent's Guide to Toilet Skills for Children with Special Needs*. Victoria, Australia: Continence Foundation of Australia.

Essence of Care (2010) *Essence of Care: Benchmarks for Bladder, Bowel and Continence Care*. London, HMSO. Available at: www.gov.uk/government/uploads/system/uploads/ attachment_data/file/216693/dh_119971.pdf (accessed 10 February 2016).

Hale, R. (2007) Newborn skincare and the modern nappy. *British Journal of Midwifery*, 15(12): 785–787.

Hart, S. (2008) Urinary catheterisation. *Nursing Standard*, 22(27): 44–48.

Johnson, R. and Taylor, W. (2010) *Skills for Midwifery Practice*. London: Elsevier.

Kumar, P. and Pati, J. (2005) Suprapubic catheters: indications and complications. *British Journal of Hospital Medicine*, 66(8): 466–468.

NHS Choices. (2014) Urinary incontinence. Available at: www.nhs.uk/Conditions/ Incontinence-urinary/Pages/Introduction.aspx (accessed 20 February 2016).

NHS Quality Improvement Scotland (2004) *Urinary Catheterisation and Catheter Care: Best Practice Statement*. Edinburgh: NHS Quality Improvement Scotland.

NICE (National Institute for Clinical Excellence) (2010) *Constipation in Children and Young*

People: Diagnosis and Management of Idiopathic Childhood Constipation in Primary and Secondary Care. NICE Guidelines, no. CG99. London: NICE.

NICE (National Institute for Health and Care Excellence) (2012) *Urinary Incontinence in Neurological Disease: Management of Lower Urinary Tract Dysfunction in Neurological Disease.* London: NICE.

NICE (National Institute for Health and Clinical Excellence) (2013) *Urinary Incontinence: The Management of Urinary Incontinence in Women.* London: National Collaborating Centre for Women's and Children's Health.

NMC (Nursing and Midwifery Council) (2010) *Essential Skills Clusters: Standards for Pre-registration Nursing Education.* Oxford: Wiley-Blackwell.

NMC (Nursing and Midwifery Council) (2015) *The Code: Professional standards of practice and behaviour for nurses and midwives.* London: NMC.

Pellatt, G.C. (2007) Anatomy and physiology of urinary elimination, Part 1. *British Journal of Nursing,* 16(7): 406–410.

Robinson, J. (2004) A practical approach to catheter-associated problems. *Nursing Standard.* 18(31): 38–42.

RCN (Royal College of Nursing) (2012) *Catheter Care: RCN Guide for Nurses.* London: RCN.

RCN (Royal College of Nursing) (2013) *Assessment of Toilet Training Readiness and the Issuing of Products: An RCN Care Pathway.* London: RCN.

SIGN (Scottish Intercollegiate Guidelines Network) (2004) *Management of Urinary Incontinence in Primary Care.* Edinburgh: SIGN.

Chapter 5

Pain assessment and management

Sheila Cunningham

Pain is a multidimensional and complex phenomenon that requires comprehensive and ongoing assessment and effective management (IASP, 2012). Nurses play a key role in assessing but also successfully managing pain, after all, no-one should be left to suffer in pain.

Key concepts

Pain classification

Pain pharmacology

Pain assessment

Pain management

Non-pharmacological approaches

Barriers to effective pain management

Learning outcomes

By the end of this chapter you will be able to:

- Outline the classification of pain and pain types
- Identify methods to assess pain and determine the effect of interventions
- Describe pharmacological approaches to pain relief
- Demonstrate knowledge and practice of non-pharmacological approaches to pain relief
- Identify the skills needed to manage pain in vulnerable patients and patients with challenging pain
- Self-evaluate your own practice in knowledge of pain physiology, assessment and management skills and develop an appropriate self-development plan.

Introduction

Pain is a common experience throughout life yet one that few people experience in the same way. It can be seen as a burden which must be endured and in some cases accepted as a consequence of the ageing process or 'wear and tear' associated with general degeneration. However, this can severely limit the quality of life and is not necessarily helpful, given the advances in knowledge and understanding of the multidimensional nature of pain and advances in treatment approaches available. Pain is recognised as a useful indicator of tissue damage or injury but it is not always useful, e.g. cancer pain may be feared and associated with advanced disease and poor or no resolution. Pain is multidimensional, it is complex and requires complete and ongoing assessment and effective management (IASP, 2012). It is also a subjective personal experience. It is variously described as an unpleasant sensory and emotional experience associated with actual or potential tissue damage, or described in terms of such damage or, more simply, pain is what the patient says hurts. It is a sensation termed 'nociception', referring to the noxious or unpleasant nature of it. These definitions make it clear that tissue damage is not necessarily required to experience pain and also that it can lead to physical or even psychological and emotional consequences.

A relatively recent pain audit in the UK reported that each year over five million people in the United Kingdom develop pain, specifically chronic pain, but only two-thirds will recover (Price *et al.*, 2012). An estimated 11 per cent of adults and 8 per cent of children suffer severe pain, representing 7.8 million people in the UK. It was also identified that there were some significant predictors of chronic pain in the community, i.e. older age, female, poor housing and type of employment. Such information as this helps assessment and management.

Nurses play a critical role in effective pain assessment and management because they are in close contact with patients in a variety of settings, such as hospital wards or clinics, homecare settings, residential settings or the community. This places the nurse in a unique position to do the following:

- Identify patients who may be experiencing pain
- Assess patients in pain for cause, duration, location and effect. This may include the patient's family and significant others
- Plan and initiate interventions to manage the pain
- Evaluate the effectiveness of those interventions.

As nurses are so central in the assessment and management of pain, they need to be knowledgeable about pain mechanisms, the epidemiology of pain and barriers to effective pain control. They should be aware of frequently encountered pain conditions, variables which influence the patient's perception of and response to pain, valid and reliable methods of clinical pain assessment, and the available methods for relieving pain. The goals of pain management are to a large extent determined by those experiencing pain themselves.

Box 5.1 Planning pain management

The following aspects could be considered in planning pain management (e.g. Turk *et al.*, 2008):

- Emotional well-being
- Range and level of reported and directly assessed activity, including physical performance
- Social activities and social role
- Pain experience
- Changes in healthcare use (e.g. medication, consultations and treatment visits) where possible
- Changes in work status, where relevant
- Quality of life.

What is pain sensation?

The experience of pain results from interrelated process involving the nervous system (nerve fibres, receptors, spinal cord and brain), neurotransmitters (nerve chemicals). Knowledge of pain transmission can enable the nurse to understand how pain travels to the brain, how it is understood and, importantly, how it can be modified and relieved. There are four main processes:

- Transduction
- Transmission
- Modulation
- Perception.

Transduction literally means the translation of a stimulus into a pain message to be taken along nerve fibres. Pain initiation can be by any number of triggers, e.g. tissue damage which releases inflammatory chemicals, severe pressure or temperature, visceral change and release of tissue enzymes. This then triggers the nerve fibres which transmit the message along toward the spinal cord and brain. The key fibres which do this are A delta fibres (myelinated, fast conducting) and C fibres (slightly slower and unmyelinated). Modulation then refers to the inhibition of pain transmission by descending influences from the brain on the spinal cord 'gate'.

The transmission process involves ascending routes via the spinal cord (tracts) alongside all other sensory fibres such as those carrying touch or pressure sensations. Thus, the 'traffic' can be competitive and some fast fibres influence the transmission of the 'pain' fibres, at times blocking the slow fibres or sometimes the faster ones, thereby only letting dominant sensory messages through. This 'traffic' then is alluded to as going through a 'gate' with the dominant ones taking priority. This can help explain how rubbing an affected area or massage stimulates dominant touch fibres and thus impedes the transmission of pain fibres. This theory proposed by Melzack and Wall in 1965 helps to explain several of the traditional approaches to pain management and is a useful model on which to pin drug and non-drug approaches. There is no scope to explain further here and readers are referred to the references at the end of the chapter. Many of the pharmacological treatments act by interfering with the transmission or perception of pain sensations from the site of initiation to the brain, e.g. local anaesthetics temporarily 'block' transmission.

Understanding types of pain

Understanding pain types can aid in assessment and management approaches. In short, there are many ways to classify pain and classifications may overlap (Figure 5.1). It can be understood in a number of ways including:

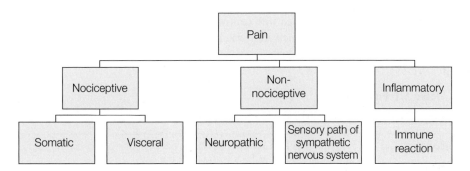

Figure 5.1 Pain classification

- *Nociceptive pain:* represents the normal response to noxious insult or injury of tissues such as skin, muscles, visceral organs, joints, tendons, or bones. It arises from the stimulation of specific pain receptors. These receptors can respond to heat, cold, vibration, stretch and chemical stimuli released from damaged cells. Examples include:
  - *Somatic*: tissues such as skin, muscle, joints, bones, and ligaments – often known as musculo-skeletal pain;
  - *Visceral*: internal organs of the main body cavities and smooth muscle; it is often poorly localised, and may feel like a vague deep ache, sometimes being cramping or colicky in nature. Often described by patients as 'referred' meaning the pain sensation produces referred pain distant to the site; pelvic pain refers pain to the lower back.
- *Non-nociceptive or neuropathic pain*: caused by a primary lesion or disease in the somatosensory nervous system;
- *Sensory abnormalities*: these sensations are interpreted by the brain as pain, and can be associated with signs of nerve malfunction, such as hypersensitivity (touch, vibration, hot and cold, also termed *hyperalgesia* or *allodynia*) to paraesthesia such as tingling, numbness, and weakness. Causes include:

- Nerve degeneration: multiple sclerosis, stroke, brain haemorrhage, oxygen starvation
- Nerve pressure: trapped nerve
- Nerve inflammation: torn or slipped vertebral disc
- Nerve infection: shingles and other viral infections. Examples include, but are not limited to, diabetic neuropathy, postherpetic neuralgia, spinal cord injury pain, phantom limb (post-amputation) pain, and post-stroke central pain.
- *Inflammatory pain*: a result of activation and sensitisation of the nociceptive pain pathway by a variety of chemicals released at a site of tissue inflammation:
  - The immune system chemicals (mediators) that have been implicated as key to this inflammation include interleukins, vasoactive amines and other factors released by infiltrating leukocytes or tissue mast cells. Examples include appendicitis, rheumatoid arthritis, inflammatory bowel disease, and herpes zoster (shingles).

There are several terms associated with pain which may be used in the communication between health professionals which are worth knowing. A few are given in Table 5.1.

Table 5.1 Pain terms

Term	Explanation
Allodynia	Pain due to a stimulus that does not normally provoke pain, e.g., heightened sensitivity following burn
Hyperalgesia	Increased pain from a stimulus that normally provokes pain
Neuralgia	Pain in the distribution of a nerve or nerves
Neuritis	Inflammation of a nerve or nerves
Nociception	The neural process of receiving and interpreting a sensation as a noxious stimuli
Pain threshold	The minimum intensity of a stimulus that is perceived as painful
Pain tolerance level	The maximum intensity of a pain-producing stimulus that a person is willing to accept in a given situation
Time course of pain:	I. Acute pain: pain of less than 3–6 months duration II. Chronic pain: pain lasting for more than 3–6 months, or persisting beyond the course of an acute disease, or after tissue healing is complete III. Acute-on-chronic pain: acute pain episode on top of underlying chronic pain.

Source: IASP (2012).

There are clinical implications of pain classification but nurses ought be aware that pathological processes do not generally occur in isolation and, as such, more than one pathology process may be present and more than one type of pain may be detected by a single patient; e.g., the inflammation processes and neuropathic pain which can be sudden and acute or slowly evolving.

There are well-recognised pain disorders that are not easily classifiable. While an understanding of their mechanisms might be unclear, there might be specific therapies established for those disorders. They include cancer pain, migraine and other primary headaches and widespread pain of the fibromyalgia type.

Top tip

The language of pain description enables communication of assessment and interventions to colleagues and aids multi-disciplinary care.

Box 5.2 Clinical example of pain: neuropathic pain after herpes zoster infection (shingles)

This is also termed post-herpetic neuralgia (PHN), which is chronic in nature, often causing some distortion of sensation and can impair the quality of life if not well managed. It does not occur in all people post-shingles but it is estimated that approximately 20 per cent of people will experience PHN after the initial shingles rash has cleared.

- Locations affected include: the trigeminal area, especially the ophthalmic division, and also the brachial plexus
- Hyperalgesia may be present, that is, increased sensitivity to painful stimuli
- Pain can be debilitating. It can interfere with sleep, the activities of daily living, and can also be so severe that it leads to depression and social isolation
- Symptoms may be present for a few months or even years.

Assessment of pain

Accurate assessment is a key rationale in the process of pain management. The aim is to identify factors (physical and non-physical) which affect the patient's perception of pain, in order then to select the most appropriate management approach. Nurses play a pivotal role in the assessment of pain, owing to the nature of their relationship with patients. Pain has been previously identified as the fifth vital sign in an attempt to enable accountability for pain assessment and management (Chronic Pain Policy Coalition, 2007) with a call for scores to be incorporated into patient assessment.

Pain assessment can be challenging because of the subjectivity and multi-dimensionality of the pain experience. There are several key principles to pain assessment for nurses to consider and they are included in the following skill:

Who should assess and what is assessed? Using pain scales

Self-reporting is the most appropriate. The patient knows what their pain feels like to them. In the first instance you should choose the most appropriate pain scale for your patient. Pain measurement tools can be unidimensional (measuring the quantity of one dimension of the pain experience, for example, intensity) or multidimensional (measuring a combination of dimensions) (Box 5.2). Examples include:

- *Visual Analogue Scale (VAS):* this is a 10 cm line with 'no pain' at one end and 'worst pain imaginable' at the other. The patient indicates on the line where they believe best fits their experience of pain. Some scales include words at set interval to help such as 'slight', 'moderate' or 'severe'
- *Verbal Numerical Rating Scale (VNRS):* this is similar to the VAS, however, on this scale, 0 represents 'no pain' and 10 'worst pain imaginable'. The patient selects the number which best represents their pain
- *McGill Pain Questionnaire:* consists of groupings of words that describe and locate pain. Some examples of the words used are tugging, sharp and nagging. Once the patient has selected their pain words, the nurse assigns a numerical score, called the Pain Rating Index
- *Abbey Pain Scale:* this is an observational pain tool for people with dementia who cannot verbalise and is completed by the nurse or observer.

Decide when pain should be assessed

This depends on the individual's circumstances, e.g., post-operatively or on movement. This will guide when to assess but in the main consider the following:

- Ask at every encounter if the patient has pain – even before surgery or procedures for surgical patients. Beliefs or negative previous experiences or worry about surgery or test results may affect how patients experience pain. It is advisable not to ask only during medicine rounds or when you think the patient looks like they are in pain. This discourages patients from reporting pain or discussing it. It is recommended that this question is asked more regularly
- Ask about the severity of pain with level of activity or movement. Assessing during rest may not provide a clear picture but enquiring about movement, position, coughing, etc. and activities which aggravate or alleviate pain would
- Ask about the type of pain management – assessment frequency will aid in determining how effective any interventions are, e.g. before or after administering analgesia
- Ask if any procedures occurred which may initiate pain. This may necessitate more frequent assessment of pain experience, e.g. surgery or invasive procedures
- Ask about the effect of any pain relief measures to determine if they are working or not for example heat or massage
- Ask if patients with pre-existing pain use any measures which relieve or exacerbate pain. Put assessment into the context of a 'pain history', so appropriate measures to manage the pain are chosen and evaluated.

What is assessed?

- *Location, duration, intensity and characteristics of pain.* This is important to determine as different pains may have differing treatment approaches. The location would enable identification of the spread or the worsening of pain, similarly, terms which define the quality of pain may indicate what improves or aggravates or what course it is taking. Terms to describe pain may include sharp, stabbing, continuous, gnawing, etc. They may also indicate whether the pain is acute or longer-term (chronic) or changing in its characteristics
- *The underlying condition.* For example, an acute injury may cause acute pain for some time, then as this reduces, it will indicate an improvement in the injury. Or worsening pain in a joint may indicate a flare-up of inflammation at a joint. For some patients, the goal is palliation (to improve symptoms) and assessment monitors this
- *Precipitating or aggravating factors.* This includes activities such as movement, eating and drinking or time of day. This provides information on approaches to care and treatment. However, if, for example, coughing aggravates pain, the post-operative patient may still need to cough and practise breathing techniques, and the goal therefore is for them to be pain-free when they do this
- *Related symptoms.* This may include nausea, vomiting, breathlessness, etc. These are important not only in aiding diagnosis of any underlying condition but also point to factors which may cause the patient distress and their ability or manage their pain
- *Coping strategies.* Alongside pharmacological approaches there are numerous non-pharmacological approaches which patients may adopt to aid relief of pain and its stress. Simple measures can be effective such as positioning of limbs or support when seated or even ice packs on inflamed joints and assessment should include this
- *Meaning and significance of pain for the patient.* The experience of pain can be distressing but patients may assign meanings such as death, helplessness, punishment, etc. to the experience. This creates anxiety and fear which impact on their self-control and experience of pain
- *A complete picture cannot be derived solely from a pain scale.* Ongoing communication with the patient is needed to reveal and manage any psychosocial factors affecting the pain experience.

Assessment for those who have difficulty communicating

Some groups of patients may have difficulties expressing pain, for example, because of language barriers, or because they are children, the older person, those with cognitive impairment, learning disabilities or mental health problems. This requires skilled nursing communication and observation which may involve family and carers of patients remembering the total pain experience and effects on all aspects of patient functioning (emotions, behaviours and daily activities).

Procedure for assessing pain

1   Provide privacy for the patient.
2   Assess patient for the ability to communicate.
3   For patients who can communicate clearly, explain the procedure and gain consent. Ask the patient the following:
   a   If they are in pain using words like 'pain', 'hurt', and 'discomfort'
   b   About the patient's ability to sleep and perform ADLs, and how the pain is affecting work, relationships, and enjoyment of life (see mnemonic OPQRST below)
   c   About previously used interventions and whether they relieved pain
   d   What triggers pain
   e   What the pain feels like
   f   To show you where the pain is located
   g   If the pain increases or decreases at different times of day
   h   If they experience moaning, crying, reduced activity, grimacing, change in usual behaviour or in movement
   i   If they experience guarding, sweating, nausea, vomiting, constipation, muscle tension, sleep disturbances, headache, and increased blood glucose level.
4   Inspect site of pain for discoloration, swelling, drainage.
5   Select the most appropriate pain assessment tool to determine the patient's pain intensity.

Activity 5.1

Think of the many ways that patients describe a pain.

▪   What type of language do they use, e.g. part of the body, sensation, duration?
▪   Do they use metaphors?
▪   What measures or features do YOU consider when assessing whether patients are in pain or not?

How to approach assessing pain: assess, record, treat (continuous cycle)

The mnemonic OPQRST is useful. Observe and ask the patient about the following:

Onset of the pain and what they were doing when it started (active, inactive, stressed), and whether the onset was sudden, gradual or part of an ongoing chronic problem.
Provocation or palliation: whether any movement, pressure (such as rubbing) or other external factor makes the problem better or worse.
Quality of the pain: ask the patient to describe it using their own words. They may use various words such as sharp, dull, crushing, burning, or some other feeling, along with the pattern, such as intermittent, constant, or throbbing.

Region and radiation refers to where the pain is on the body and whether it radiates (extends) or moves to any other area. This can provide clues to underlying medical causes.

Severity: ask the patient to assign a pain score (usually on a scale of 0–10) to each pain site. See the scales mentioned above (e.g. the Visual Analogue Scale, VAS). This may also be assessed for pain then, compared to pain at time of onset, or pain on movement. There are alternative assessment methods for pain, which can be used where a patient is unable to vocalise a score. One such method is the Wong-Baker faces pain scale.

Time (history): ask the patient how long the condition has been going on and how it has changed since onset (better, worse, different symptoms), whether it has ever happened before, whether and how it may have changed since onset, and when the pain stopped if it is no longer currently being felt.

Do not forget to document: complete the records or patient notes with the assessment. Communicate the assessment to the nurse in charge or the medical staff.

Administer any treatments or analgesia and re-assess. Note any analgesia given (route, dose and response). Ask the patient what their pain level was prior to taking pain medication and after taking pain medication. If the patient's pain level is not acceptable, what interventions were taken?

In summary, there are three main aims when assessing pain:

1   To determine the patient's experience of pain and aid in either diagnosis, extent of disease process or treatment options.
2   To aid in decision-making of intervention and outcomes.
3   To evaluate any intervention or treatment or change in symptoms or features of the associated disease or injury.

Assessing pain for those unable to self-report

There are several groups of patients who potentially will be unable to self-report but will experience pain. These groups include infants and pre-verbal children, critically ill and unconscious patients, people with dementia or cognitive impairment, people with intellectual disability and those in end-of-life stages. In patients who are unable to self-report pain, other strategies must be used to determine pain and evaluate interventions. However, it must be noted that no single objective assessment strategy, such as interpretation of behaviours, pathology or estimates of pain by others, is sufficient by itself. It is recommended you try the following:

■   Assess for potential causes of discomfort (e.g., infection, constipation, or emotional distress)
■   Attempt to use a clinically-validated pain assessment tool that is easy to use with nonverbal, alert and oriented patients, such as the Visual Analogue Scale (VAS) or the Faces Pain Scale (Box 5.4)
■   If self-report is not possible, document in the patient's record why this is so.

Box 5.3 A clinical example

Eric is 40 years old and this is his second day following abdominal surgery. Your assessment reveals the following information:

BP = 140/86 mmHg; HR = 90 bpm; R = 22/min; Pain score on a scale of 0–5 (where 0 = no pain/discomfort, 5 = worst pain/discomfort)

Eric rates his pain at the surgical site as 4. Your assessment then proceeds as:

O – onset has been continual since surgery but is increasing in intensity
P – provocation of the pain occurs on movement and coughing, so he is then reluctant to do either of these
Q – quality of the pain is described as sharp and penetrating or stabbing and building up in intensity
R – region is around the surgical site below the umbilicus which does look red but not inflamed
S – severity is scored at 4
T – the pain builds up after some time after medication has been given. It appears to worsen on movement and coughing or sitting on the toilet.

Your assessment, above, is made four hours after Eric received morphine 10 mg Intramuscular (IM). You look at his prescription and see he is due for regular administration of a pain reliever which is prescribed to be given four hourly. Twenty minutes following administration you reassess Eric's pain ratings which are now ranged from 2 to 3 and he appears more relaxed and can manage to do his deep breathing exercises and cough.

Pasero and McCaffery (2011) propose a hierarchy of pain assessment techniques to guide assessment techniques. It outlines five principles:

1   Obtain self-report if possible, even if a simple yes/no.
2   Search for potential causes of pain (pathology, e.g. arthritis or procedures, recent surgery, physiotherapy or other rehabilitation treatment, pressure sores or other skin injuries).
3   Observe patient behaviour (restlessness, grimacing, moaning, crying, or rubbing a body part) though this may not indicate intensity or pain.
4   Consider a 'proxy report' from those relatives/carers who know the patient well indicating change in behaviour/habits. Ask family members or carers whether the patient seems to be in pain. They may identify subtle changes in behaviour that typically indicate pain for this patient.
5   Attempt an analgesic trial. If the patient's behaviour improves, assume pain was the cause.

Box 5.4 Children: pain assessment tools

Neonates

- All are observer-rated
- All require familiarisation and training
- Most include a measure of facial response to painful stimuli
- Most require a measure of physiological response.

Preverbal children

- Observer-rated tools have been validated.

Verbal children

- Several valid self-report tools are available for use, including the Faces Pain Scale, OUCHER (photographic or numeric), visual analogue scales and Wong-Baker FACES.

Non-verbal children or those with cognitive impairment

- Face, Legs, Activity, Cry, Consolability (FLACC) tool (including a revised version of the FLACC tool)
- Paediatric Pain Profile (PPP)
- Non-communicating Children's Pain Checklist (NCCPC).

Source: Modified from RCN (2009).

Following the assessment, document the procedure and the documents/contributors to the assessment process for ongoing assessment:

- Date and time of pain assessment
- Pain assessment scale used
- Any observable indications or patient self-report of pain
- Pain score obtained
- All patients/family involved and any advice or interventions suggested or given.

Children vary greatly in their cognitive and emotional development, medical condition, response to painful interventions and to the experience of pain, as well as in their personal preferences for care (RCN, 2009). Health professionals and parents have a responsibility to learn the language of children's pain expression, to listen carefully to children's self-reports of pain and to be aware of behavioural cues. Children's pain assessment can be improved by approaches and tools appropriate to their cognitive development, some of which are outlined in the RCN guidance (RCN, 2009).

It is important that children are listened to and believed in their self-reports. Parents or guardians also need to be listened to and their views respected and supported, especially if their child has difficulty expressing their emotions or they lack the language skills. It is useful to bear in mind culture and language too in assessing pain. Examples of signs that may indicate pain include changes in children's behaviour, appearance, activity level and vital signs. No individual assessment tool is recommended for pain assessment in all children and across all contexts as some may be more appropriate in post-operative situations in hospital or in residential situations. Pain assessment is not a one-off event but an ongoing and integral part of pain management.

The British Pain Society (www.britishpainsociety.org) publishes pain scales in a variety of languages (free of charge) to assist and encourage improved assessment both by the healthcare professional and the patient, for whom English is not their first language (Table 5.2). Difficulty in assessing pain is one common barrier that can inhibit effective treatment.

Table 5.2 Pain assessment tools

Unidimensional measurement tools (selection)

Visual analogue scales	Verbal descriptor scales
Verbal rating scales	Body diagrams
Graphic rating scales	Computer graphic scales
Numerical rating scales	Picture scales
	Coin scales.

Multidimensional pain measurement tools (selection)

McGill pain questionnaire (short and long)
Brief pain inventory (short and long)
Behavioural pain scales
Pain/comfort journal
Multidimensional pain inventory
Pain information and beliefs questionnaire
Pain and impairment relationship scale
Pain cognition questionnaire
Pain beliefs and perceptions inventory
Coping strategies questionnaire
Pain disability index
Hospital anxiety and depression questionnaire (HAD scale)
Neuropathic signs and symptoms (Leeds assessment of neuropathic symptoms and signs (LANSS)) (Bennett, 2001) now the self-report Leeds assessment S-LANSS (Bennett *et al.*, 2005)
Cognitively impaired/dementia pain scales (Abbey pain assessment check list for seniors with severe dementia (PACSLAC)) (Royal College of Physicians *et al.*, 2007).

Pain ought not be dismissed as a consequence of ageing. Incidences of surgery, injury and painful degeneration increase with advancing age, however, it appears that reporting of pain decreases with advanced ageing, indicating that experience of pain, and psychosocial responses towards pain are not altered. The key points in assessing pain are

Case study 5.1

Norma is a 66-year-old lady who presents with thoracic pain. While on holiday in Spain two months ago, she developed a painful vesicular rash. She visited a local doctor who diagnosed shingles and prescribed anti-viral medication and analgesics.

Although this doctor told her that her pain should subside over time, it has not resolved and is impacting her greatly. She is visiting her GP to find out why her pain is continuing and if there is anything that can be done to alleviate it. You are on placement with a practice nurse.

Assessment

- Pain intensity is reported as 7/10 to 8/10
- Severe allodynia
- Hyperalgesia
- Loss of self-worth and depressed as not able to wash and dress to her usual standard.

The patient is especially concerned with the difficulties she is having with washing and dressing herself, as this is something she was previously very meticulous about. She wants to get back to being able to go out and meet friends without having to worry that she will be in pain and not enjoy herself. She has complained about feeling 'down' and cannot be bothered to eat or go out since all her clothes hurt her skin. Her GP said something about antidepressants but you are not sure what this would do for pain.

Answer the following:

- How would you assess her pain?
- What at her key priorities and long-term needs?
- What advice would you give about pain relief?
- What is the purpose of antidepressants here?

outlined above (OPQRST). Chronic pain does require a comprehensive assessment of all the factors mentioned but also of the degree of functional impairment in activities of daily living and the social impacts of pain. Useful tools for this are available including the Pain Disability Index, and the Multidimensional Pain Inventory. Figure 5.2 shows the Brief Pain Inventory. The basic principles still apply, though in some older adults, pain self-report due to cognitive impairment (e.g. dementia) can interfere with self-report and there are other observer-rated scales in existence.

Case study 5.2 Procedural pain

Alice is a 9-year-old child admitted to the surgical ward for a procedure to insert grommets into her ears. She is does not want any 'needles' because they hurt.
    What might you do? Consider:

- Allaying anxiety – be truthful – establish trust
- Information – discussing what will happen and how long any 'hurt' might last
- Distraction   show her what equipment might be used or diagrams/cartoons, some form of distraction.

Don't forget!

Pain assessment is not a one-off event but an ongoing and integral part of pain management.

Pain management

The rationale of pain management is to relieve and if possible prevent pain. This can be achieved by drawing on skilled nursing practice, effective assessment and use of pharmacological (medication) or non-pharmacological means. The World Health Organisation's pain ladder is the most widely known model for pain management and provides a stepwise approach to treat mild, moderate and severe pain (WHO, 2015). The ladder recommends a hierarchy of medicines (analgesics) to be used. The ladder, while originally intended for treatment of cancer pain, can be applied to all pain including chronic pain, providing practitioners with guidelines rather than a rigid set of rules.

Acute pain (sudden onset)

1   Assess pain using the skill outlined above. This determines the level to measure any relief.
2   Check the patient's prescription sheet for prescribed medication. Using the five fundamental 'R's administer the analgesia (see Chapter 16). Ideally this will follow the World Health Organisation's stepwise or ladder approach.
3   Monitor the effect of the prescribed analgesia and report the effect.
4   Offer non-pharmacological interventions: distraction, massage, depending upon patient preference and condition.
5   If analgesia is ineffective, consider alternatives with the patient and healthcare team: other analgesia including patient controlled analgesia (PCA) or trans-cutaneous electrical nerve stimulation (TENS) or local anaesthetic.

STUDY ID #:_____ DO NOT WRITE ABOVE THIS LINE HOSPITAL #: _____

Brief Pain Inventory (Short Form)

Date:____/____/____   Time:_____

Name:_____ _____ _____
              Last   First   Middle Initial

1. Throughout our lives, most of us have had pain from time to time (such as minor headaches, sprains, and toothaches). Have you had pain other than these every-day kinds of pain today?

         1.   Yes   2.   No

2. On the diagram, shade in the areas where you feel pain. Put an X on the area that hurts the most.

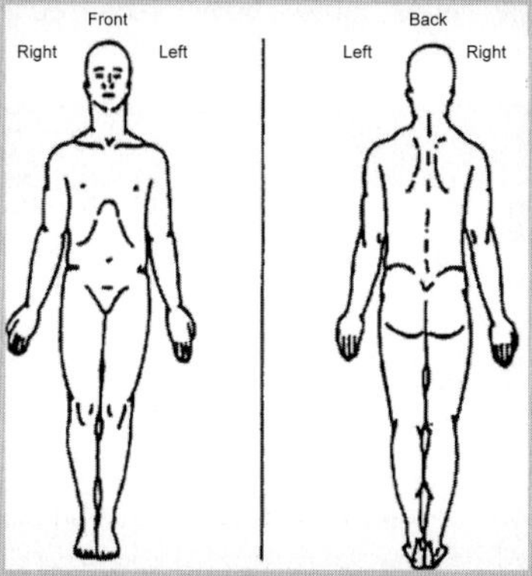

3. Please rate your pain by circling the one number that best describes your pain at its worst in the last 24 hours.

    0   1   2   3   4   5   6   7   8   9   10
    No   Pain as bad as
    Pain   you can imagine

4. Please rate your pain by circling the one number that best describes your pain at its least in the last 24 hours.

    0   1   2   3   4   5   6   7   8   9   10
    No   Pain as bad as
    Pain   you can imagine

5. Please rate your pain by circling the one number that best describes your pain on the average.

    0   1   2   3   4   5   6   7   8   9   10
    No   Pain as bad as
    Pain   you can imagine

6. Please rate your pain by circling the one number that tells how much pain you have right now.

    0   1   2   3   4   5   6   7   8   9   10
    No   Pain as bad as
    Pain   you can imagine

Page 1 of 2

Figure 5.2 Brief Pain Inventory

STUDY ID #:_ _ _ _ _ _ _ _ _ _   DO NOT WRITE ABOVE THIS LINE   HOSPITAL #:_ _ _ _ _ _ _ _ _

Date:_ _ _ /_ _ _ _ /_ _ _ _   Time:_ _ _ _ _ _ _
Name:_ _ _ _ _ _ _ _ _ _ _ _ _ _ _ _   _ _ _ _ _ _ _ _ _ _ _ _ _ _ _   _ _ _ _ _ _ _ _ _ _ _ _ _
                     Last   First   Middle Initial

7.   What treatments or medications are you receiving for your pain?

8.   In the last 24 hours, how much relief have pain treatments or medications
     provided? Please circle the one percentage that most shows how much relief
     you have received.

     0%   10%   20%   30%   40%   50%   60%   70%   80%   90%   100%
     No   Complete
     Relief   Relief

9.   Circle the one number that describes how, during the past 24 hours, pain has
     interfered with your:

     A.   General Activity
     0   1   2   3   4   5   6   7   8   9   10
     Does not   Completely
     Interfere   Interferes

     B.   Mood
     0   1   2   3   4   5   6   7   8   9   10
     Does not   Completely
     Interfere   Interferes

     C.   Walking Ability
     0   1   2   3   4   5   6   7   8   9   10
     Does not   Completely
     Interfere   Interferes

     D.   Normal Work (includes both work outside the home and housework)
     0   1   2   3   4   5   6   7   8   9   10
     Does not   Completely
     Interfere   Interferes

     E.   Relations with other people
     0   1   2   3   4   5   6   7   8   9   10
     Does not   Completely
     Interfere   Interferes

     F.   Sleep
     0   1   2   3   4   5   6   7   8   9   10
     Does not   Completely
     Interfere   Interferes

     G.   Enjoyment of life
     0   1   2   3   4   5   6   7   8   9   10
     Does not   Completely
     Interfere   Interferes

Page 2 of 2

Figure 5.2 **Brief Pain Inventory (continued)**

Source: used with permission from Pain Research Group

Chronic pain (lasting a long period of time)

1 Ensure pain is assessed as earlier.
2 Ensure analgesia is provided using the same stepwise approach mentioned above. If necessary, give written guides on analgesia to aid regular administration and pain control.
3 Explore lifestyle, behaviours and aspects which cause stress and anxiety, suggesting means to relieve these.
4 If analgesia is ineffective, consider alternatives with the patient and healthcare team: PCA, TENS or local anaesthetic (useful if reduced movement or inflamed joints).
5 Multi-disciplinary team interventions to treat underlying pathologies or accompanying depression or anxiety.
6 Suggest to the patient some non-pharmacological interventions, such as massage, relaxation techniques, aromatherapy or acupuncture, giving them choice and power over their pain relief. Ensure an open communication and a supportive environment to create trust and reduce stress.
7 Reassess pain after any intervention or therapy and adjust if appropriate. Observe for reluctance to take analgesia and explore any reasons for this (fear of addiction, etc.).

Clinical significance

Be aware of the side effects of analgesics. They should be prescribed and administered with care, e.g., NSAIDs may cause gastric problems or opioids may cause sedation, particularly in the elderly or young.

Pharmacological treatments

Medications can be prescribed or on a regular basis or on an as-needed basis. Research (Cregg et al., 2013) does show that response to analgesia may vary due to genetic differences. A patient may experience better relief or more adverse effects with one certain opioid or NSAID versus another. Thus if one product does not appear to have the desired effect for a patient, a different product should be prescribed.

The first step for patients with mild pain is the use of non-opioid medication such as paracetamol or non-steroidal anti-inflammatory medications (ibuprofen). The second step for patients with moderate pain might require the use of a weak opioid medication alone or in combination with a non-opioid or an adjuvant. Adjuvants are medications which enhance the action of other medications sometimes called 'co-analgesics', and will be addressed later. For patients with severe pain, this may require the use of a strong opioid with or without an adjuvant. For acute pain management, the WHO guidelines can be used in reverse, starting with step 3 for immediate post-operative pain and moving to step 2 and then step 1 as the pain improves (Figure 5.3). Although non-pharmacological strategies are often omitted in an acute setting because of time constraints, they do have a value. Complementary strategies (non-invasive ones) for pain relief provide an opportunity for the patient to play an active role in achieving a higher level of comfort and in some instances a reduction or relief from pain.

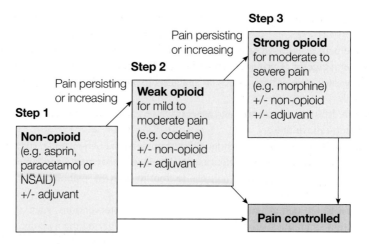

Figure 5.3 Pain management

Regular persistent chronic pain should be treated with regular medication (to maintain adequate blood levels of analgesia) remembering that pain is easier to prevent than to treat. Consideration of extra back-up analgesia in the event of pain 'breaking through' ought also be considered. Episodic pain can be treated with analgesia on an 'as-needed' basis. Too often pain is underrated due to inappropriate use of type and regularity of analgesia. At times healthcare workers or patients fear tolerance or addiction to the medication used. Patients using analgesics to manage chronic pain should be reviewed frequently if pain is poorly controlled (SIGN, 2013, p. 136).

Non-opioid medications

These include groups of medications termed non-steroidal anti-inflammatories and paracetamol. These have analgesic, anti-inflammatory and anti-pyretic properties and are commonly used as an effective analgesia, especially for musculoskeletal and visceral pain.

Opioids

Opioid analgesics interact with receptors called opioid receptors which occur naturally in the body to produce pain relief at the spinal and central (brain) level. These substances mimic the action of naturally occurring peptides, collectively termed endogenous opioids. Their pharmacological actions on cells account for some of the other (side) effects too – the reader is recommended to review this in a good pharmacological textbook. Suffice it to say an *agonist* such as morphine blocks the pain transmission and other transmissions, resulting in several side effects including respiratory depression and reduced gastrointestinal motility (constipation).

Examples of opioids for moderate pain include codeine, dihydrocodeine, tramadol and low-dose oxycodone (Table 5.3). These are used when pain is not relieved by non-opioid products and can often be found in combination with other formulations, e.g. cocodamol (= paracetamol and codeine). If these medications are ineffective, the next type of opioids would be those recommended for moderate to severe pain including: morphine, oxycodone, fentanyl, diamorphine, hydromorphine and alfentanil. Opioids are available in a variety of formulations and can be administered through a variety of routes, the most common being oral (PO), subcutaneous (SC) and intravenous (IV). Oral opioids are available in both short-acting and long-acting (modified, controlled or extended release). Intravenous patient-controlled analgesia allows patients to manage their own pain by self-administering opioid doses and is one of the most commonly used methods to treat acute pain post-operatively. Other routes for opioid use are epidural or intrathecal.

Don't forget!

When reading prescription charts, be attentive to whether the patient is taking short or extended release medication as the pain relief may not be immediate with the latter.

Watch out

In March 2015 a new 'drug driving' law came into force, which makes it an offence to drive with certain drugs or prescription medicines above specified limits in the body. The medicines covered by the law include morphine. Codeine is converted into morphine by the liver, which means it may be an offence to drive while taking this medicine.

Adjuvant drugs (co-analgesics)

These are a wide range of drugs whose primary action is for conditions other than pain but may be useful in aiding pain relief. Examples in this category include steroids, antibiotics, antidepressants, antispasmodics or muscle relaxants. The WHO analgesic ladder recommends the use of adjuvant medications with opioids or non-opioids to aid pain relief.

Local anaesthetics

These are locally (at the site) acting drugs. They may be used to block the impulses of individual or a group of peripheral nerves, e.g. during surgical procedures. They may also be useful when used topically to 'numb' a site for a procedure such as inserting an IV line in a child or local pain or hypersensitivity (chronic neuropathic pain).

Table 5.3 Actions and side effects of analgesia

Drug	Action	Side effect
Non-Opioids		
Paracetamol	Unclear but reputedly inhibits COX-1 and COX-2 and eventually prostaglandin (peripherally and centrally). Does not damage gastric mucosa like other NSAIDs. Most effective for reducing pain and fever (pyrexia) but not as effective for inflammation. Can be found used in combination with other products (caffeine or aspirin or codeine)	Liver toxicity (due to excessive doses)
Aspirin	COX enzyme inhibitor and blocks prostaglandin production. This blocks inflammation, swelling, pain and fever more effectively than paracetamol. Also irreversibly inhibits platelet aggregation (reduced clotting). Useful for mild to moderate pain. Can be found used in combination with other products (caffeine or aspirin or codeine)	Reduced clotting (platelet inhibitor) Gastric irritation Hypersensitivity (bronchospasm and anaphylaxis) Exceeding daily the dose can result in toxicity of liver, kidneys and central nervous system. Not to be used in children under 16 (due to adverse effects and link to Reyes syndrome causing liver and brain damage)
Non-steroidal anti-inflammatory drugs (NSAIDs)	Inhibit COX enzymes and prostaglandins, and effective for inflammation and useful in post-operative, infection or trauma pain. Various types may differ in their action and side effects, e.g. ibuprofen inhibits both COX-1 and COX-2 (non-selective) and has severe effects on gastric mucosa. Diclofenac is more selective to COX-2	Gastric irritation and ulceration Some hypersensitivity (e.g. Diclofenac) or liver toxicity
Opioids		
Codeine	Short-term relief of mild to moderate pain in adults over 18 years of age, in adolescents aged 12–18 years, when other painkillers such as paracetamol and ibuprofen have not been effective. Mimics the action of natural endorphins (painkillers) by combining with the opioid receptors in the brain and spinal cord. This blocks the transmission of pain signals	Several – people vary in response and reactions: ■ Sleepiness or dizziness ■ Slow, shallow breathing ■ 'Pinpoint' pupils ■ Lack of appetite ■ Constipation ■ Nausea and vomiting ■ Maybe reduced levels of consciousness ■ To avoid alcohol at the same time ■ Not for use in pregnancy.
Tramadol	An opioid for moderate to severe pain. Extremely strong and available in short-acting and extended release. Works on opioid receptors as above.	Similar to the above
Morphine	Agonist 'gold standard' Severe nociceptive pain combining with the opioid receptors in the brain and spinal cord. Given orally, intramuscular injection or subcutaneous may be intravenous Short duration of action (3–4 hours)	Several including: ■ Sedation ■ Nausea and vomiting ■ Respiratory depression ■ Bradycardia ■ Postural hypotension ■ Euphoria ■ Constipation ■ Rash/itchiness.
Diamorphine	Synthetic morphine-like derivative Same as morphine with wider range of receptors in the brain and spinal cord	Similar to above but more euphoria and nausea

Breakthrough pain

This refers to the emergence of pain in a patient who usually has been adequately controlled with analgesia before, often with the use of slow or extended release drug formulations. This has been known as an on-demand prescription to 'rescue' or manage this surge of pain. This should be assessed as to the cause and frequency and may need a review of the analgesia dosing regime. It may be that the breakthrough pain only occurs at specific events, e.g. procedure or wound dressing, and thus a short-acting analgesia with minimal side effects and short duration of action would be appropriate. This may require different routes of administration to address this short-term need, e.g., buccal.

Medication routes

These are varied and will depend upon the medication, any other physical abilities of the patient, preference and speed of action:

Oral analgesia

This is the main route used for non-opioid and at times opioid analgesia. This may also be the route used subsequent to another, such as post-surgery, the patient may need intramuscular analgesia which would be replaced with oral analgesia when they are able to swallow or tolerate oral products.

Intravenous analgesia

This route is used if patients require infusions or continuous administration of analgesia. This route is restricted to areas where patients are closely monitored (high dependency units) due to the potential risk of respiratory depression. An alternative to this in general wards is patient-controlled analgesia (PCA). This method is where analgesia (often morphine or diamorphine or fentanyl) is infused using an infusion pump and timing device and is self-controlled by the patient so adequate amounts of analgesia can be self-administered 'on demand'. When in pain the patient presses a button and a set dose of analgesia is administered. There is a 'lock-out' so patients cannot overdose by accident. Available routes for PCA administration include subcutaneous, intravenous (IV – the most common) and epidural. Monitoring for levels of sedation are needed with this form of analgesia administration.

This has the advantage of giving the patient control over their pain relief, however, it is still important that patients understand how, why and when to administer their medication. There are several advantages to PCA: constant blood levels of analgesia and pain control; patients receive better pain relief and fewer side effects. Failure to achieve pain relief may be due to misunderstanding by the patient of how this system works, pump failure or giving control of the drug administration over to a family member. There are of course potential issues with nursing staff not understanding how to set up PCA correctly or incorrectly calculating the dose concentration. This is the domain of the qualified nurse practitioner but students need to be aware of these issues and, if they see them, to report them immediately.

Procedure for care of a patient with patient-controlled analgesia

1   Explain what you will do and where possible gain patient consent.
2   Maintain hand hygiene.
3   Check the prescription of the PCA and the equipment: the patient label on the syringe, the drug dose, the concentration, the date and time. Note how much is left in the syringe.
4   Check the PCA programme (loading dose, lock-out duration, basal rate of infusion, and bolus dose (patient demand dose)).
5   Record the history from the PCA device (requests for doses and how much given). This indicates pain level and efficacy of pain relief.
6   Check the IV site for signs of redness, swelling or discomfort.
7   Check the IV line is functioning and correctly labelled for date/time of line change.
8   Assess the patient for pain and determine the level of pain relief. Ask the patient if they are confident in using the PCA and, if not, consider what advice you might give (i.e. timing of doses such as before procedures or moving).
9   Observe for alterations in pulse or blood pressure or respiration rate and any altered consciousness. If any observed, report immediately.
10 Document the findings reporting any concerns (NMC, 2015).

Watch out

Some patients do not use PCA to its maximum effect and experience pain – they may fear overdosing, or becoming addicted. This needs to be discussed and clarified with them sensitively.

Clinical significance

If opioids are used in PCA, this can cause sedation or respiratory depression. Nurses must watch out for altered breathing or levels of consciousness.

Subcutaneous analgesia

This route is often used to manage cancer pain. As seen above, it can be a route for PCA also. The advantage of giving analgesia subcutaneously is that it avoids the problems associated with maintaining intravenous access.

Intramuscular analgesia

Since other forms of analgesia are available, intramuscular analgesia is used less often today. Since this involves an invasive technique inserting a needle into a muscle, it relies on an adequate blood supply for drug absorption and distribution. In patients where there is poor muscle mass, poor mobility or poor perfusion, this is not an ideal route since the drug may not reach the systemic circulation. For the technique, see Chapter 16.

Nasal analgesia

There is some evidence that nasal administration of opioids is effective and particularly useful for some patients, e.g., children (Bendall *et al.*, 2011). It may also be useful in specific departments to achieve rapid pain relief, such as in emergency departments or managing traumatic incidents when no cannula is in-situ, or when other methods of pain relief are not suitable or adequate, e.g. rectal medications in the older child.

Epidural analgesia

This is a route whereby analgesia is administered into the epidural space via a small indwelling catheter. In babies under six months or weighing less than 5 kg the epidural catheter is sometimes inserted via the sacral hiatus (caudal) and performed in theatre. Only appropriately trained staff may care for epidural infusions.

This route is valuable for the control of pain following certain surgical procedures (thoracic, abdominal, lower limb or trauma) since it blocks pain transmission via the spinal cord. It has been associated with pain relief in childbirth or surgical procedures where a general anaesthetic is not appropriate. The most common opioids used for epidural administration are fentanyl or diamorphine which may be used alongside anaesthetics epidurally for optimum pain relief. There are advantages to epidural analgesia: improved pain relief; fewer side effects, e.g. sedation, post-operative nausea and vomiting; allowing the patient more involvement in their recovery; reduced complications following major surgery, e.g., deep vein thrombosis, pulmonary embolism, chest infection, nausea and vomiting and delayed bowel function. Disadvantages of epidural analgesia include: it requires a competent practitioner for insertion and management (anaesthetist) and its effectiveness is sometimes variable as well as having side effects.

Procedure for care of a patient with an epidural

1   Explain what you will do and where possible gain the patient's consent
2   Wash and dry hands.
3   The epidural infusion is prescribed, with full instructions. Check all the connections are intact, if not, report immediately. Ensure the equipment is on and working. Do not move or alter them.
4   Observe the patient: monitor respiratory rate, depth and pattern. Note any signs of respiratory alterations such as depression.
5   Monitor the blood pressure as frequently as indicated by the type of epidural and prescriber.
6   Observe the pulse rate and rhythm, as a high rate of epidural block can cause alterations.
7   Monitor and record the patient's temperature, reporting any signs of alteration.
8   Assess the patient's sedation score (use the tool or document indicated by the local policy).

9   Assess the patient for pain and determine the level of pain relief. Ask the patient if they are confident in using the PCA and, if not, consider what advice you might give (i.e. timing of doses such as before procedures or moving)

10 Assess the patient's level of lower limb strength and sensation (motor ability) before getting out of bed if permitted

11 Observe and record urine output

12 Observe and record any nauseas or vomiting or skin rash or itchiness

13 Document the findings, reporting any concerns (NMC, 2015).

Watch out

Epidural bags and infusion rates must be changed by a registered nurse, who is competent in the administration of IV drugs and the management of epidural infusions. This is potentially a dangerous route and one which needs further training.

Non-pharmacological methods of managing pain

A variety of non-pharmacological pain relief methods are available to lessen a patient's pain in a healthcare setting. These are used alongside pharmacological approaches and not as an alternative. Many non-pharmacological approaches trigger a relaxation response (stimulating the parasympathetic nervous system), but not all. In the main, the action of some of these approaches is unknown. However, some patients find these appealing and useful as it enables them to take control of their pain relief and can reduce other feelings such as anxiety or worry which can exacerbate pain. This is an excellent opportunity to add to the pain relief measures and the benefits should not be underestimated. The Pain Management Team in clinical areas will have more details and expertise in the range of interventions. The ranges of methods include emotional, psychological, physical and complementary/alternative approaches.

Emotional and psychological interventions

- Information/education – building trust
- Breathing exercises
- Visual imagery
- Cognitive behavioural therapy (CBT)
- Yoga
- Tai chi
- Music relaxation
- Distraction (guided imagery)
- Relaxation
- Spiritual or reflective activities related to the patient's belief system.

These cognitive strategies do require the patient's full participation. Progressive breathing or imagery is useful for chronic pain and provides a sense of well-being, reduces muscle tension and changes the awareness of pain. The use of gentle humour is also a possibility to aid coping or aid in withstanding a painful procedure.

Physical interventions

- Heat or cold therapy
- Exercise
- Rest
- Body position/movements
- Art therapy
- Massage.

These approaches work in a variety of ways such as providing comfort to a body part (heat), reducing spasms or localised joint pain. They could also provide basic comfort or body support or, in the case of exercise, loosen stiffened joints/limbs and strengthen muscles and provide a sense of well-being. Massage should be provided by someone with knowledge of the skill to avoid damage to skin or muscles. It can block pain impulses and improve circulation and the elimination of wastes stored in muscles. This ought not to be performed on bruised, swollen or inflamed areas. Of course, a gentle hand massage and physical contact can have benefits for relaxing a patient of any age, especially if very tense and frightened.

Complementary/alternative interventions

- Acupuncture
- Acupressure
- Biofield therapies, which include Reiki, therapeutic touch, and healing touch
- Reflexology
- Electrostimulation (TENS)
- Herbs (topical capsaicin).

Watch out

Advise using herbs with caution, some have unknown effects.

These interventions owe much to a holistic view of the patient. Some are reputed to stimulate the body's own opioid system (acupuncture). These are popular and do have a role to play in pain relief. Table 5.4 details some common myths about analgesia.

Table 5.4 Common myths about pain

Common myths	Explanation
Pain is a natural side effect of ageing.	Sometimes it can be. As we age, some 'nuisance pain' from physical wear and tear is normal. That differs from chronic pain.
It's better to tough it out and just live with pain.	Ignoring pain can have serious consequences, especially if you choose to self-medicate in unhealthy ways rather than see a healthcare professional.
You can injure yourself further if you exercise when in pain.	Exercise can cause further injury – it depends on the cause of the pain. If it is not traumatic, then exercises such as walking can be key to successful rehabilitation.
You can become addicted to painkillers if you take them too long.	The risk of addiction is exaggerated. The incidence of opioid addiction among chronic pain patients is about the same as in the general population. A pain management specialist will ensure that patients receive the right dose for the right amount of time.
You can get a heart attack from taking COX-2 inhibitors for pain.	Heart attacks and other vascular problems occur in only a fraction of patients using these anti-inflammatory medications. The benefits may outweigh the risks for chronic pain patients.
Chronic pain can kill you.	It can have a profound effect on quality of life. Certain severe situations may prompt suicidal feelings if pain seems unbearable. It is critical patients seek help from a pain management professional early.
Dwelling on pain won't make it worse than it already is.	The psychological suffering that comes with physical pain can certainly make patients more miserable. Dwelling on the pain can serve to emphasise it and distraction or other approaches can make it feel less intrusive.

Summary

Pain is a complex phenomenon. The key is early and frequent skilled assessment and sensitive patient-centred management. The patient is key to determining what will aid or aggravate pain as they are the ones experiencing it. Nurses do need a broad understanding of causes and types of pain but more importantly how to approach each individual patient to understand their pain and their specific needs they need to know to effectively manage their pain.

References

Bendall, J.C., Simpson, P.M. and Middleton, P.M. (2011) Effectiveness of prehospital morphine, fentanyl, and methoxyflurane in paediatric patients. *Prehospital Emergency Care*, 15(2): 158–165.

Bennett, M. (2001) The LANSS pain scale: the Leeds assessment of neuropathic symptoms and signs. *Pain*; 92(1–2): 147–157.

Bennett, M.I., Smith, B.H., Torrance, N. and Potter, J. (2005) The S-LANSS score for identifying pain of predominantly neuropathic origin: validation for use in clinical and postal research, *Pain*, 6(3): 149–158.

British Pain Society and British Geriatric Society (2007) The Assessment of Pain in Older People: National Guidelines. Available at:_www.gloucestershire.gov.uk/extra/CHttpHandler.ashx?id=45208&p=0 (accessed 10 February 2016).

Chronic Pain Policy Coalition (2007) *A New Pain Manifesto*. Available at; www.paincoalition.org.uk/ (accessed 10 February 2016).

Cregg, R., Russo, G., Gubbay, A., Branford, R. and Sato, H. (2013) Pharmacogenetics of analgesic drugs. *British Journal of Pain* 7(4): 189–208.

IASP (International Association for the Study of Pain) (2012) IASP taxonomy: pain terms. Available at: www.iasp-pain.org/Education/Content.aspx?ItemNumber=1698 (accessed 10 February 2016).

Melzack, R. and Wall. P.D. (1965) Pain mechanisms: a new theory. *Science*, 150(3699): 971–979.

NMC (Nursing and Midwifery Council) (2015) *The Code: Professional Standards of Practice and Behaviour for Nurses and Midwives*. London: NMC.

Pasero, C. and McCaffery, M. (2011) *Pain Assessment and Pharmacologic Management*. St. Louis, MO: Mosby.

Price, C., Hoggart, B., Olukoga, O., de Williams, A. and Bottle. A. (2012) *National Pain Audit 2010–2012*. London: The British Pain Society.

RCN (Royal College of Nursing) (2009) *Recognition and Assessment of Acute Pain in Children*. London: RCN.

Royal College of Physicians, British Geriatrics Society, British Pain Society (2007) *The Assessment of Pain in Older People: National Guidelines*. Concise Guidance on Good Practice Series, No. 8. London: RCP.

SIGN (Scottish Intercollegiate Guidelines Network) (2013) *Management of Chronic Pain*. Edinburgh: SIGN. Available at: http://sign.ac.uk/guidelines/fulltext/136/index.html (accessed 10 January 2016).

Turk, D.C., Swanson, K.S. and Gatchel, R.J. (2008) Predicting opioid misuse by chronic pain patients: a systematic review and literature synthesis. *Clinical Journal of Pain*, 24(6): 497–508.

WHO (World Health Organisation) (2015) WHO's cancer pain ladder for adults. Available at: www.who.int/cancer/palliative/painladder/en/ (accessed 10 January 2016).

Chapter 6

End of life care

Kirstie Dye

End of life care (EoLC) is support for people who are in the last months or years of their life. People who are approaching the end of their life are entitled to high-quality care, wherever they are being cared for. End of life care includes but is not only, palliative care and terminal care. If a patient has an illness that cannot be cured, end of life care aims to make patients as comfortable as possible, by managing pain and other distressing symptoms.

Key concepts

End of life care	Bereavement
Symptom assessment and	'Last offices'
management	Holistic care

Learning outcomes

By the end of this chapter you will be able to:

- Define end of life care
- Identify national initiatives related to end of life care
- List the conditions when patients may require end of life care
- Identify issues with symptom control and the interventions available to address these issues
- Identify interventions appropriate for a variety of patients in a diverse range of settings at the end of their life
- Explain and justify the procedures before and after the episode of death.

Introduction

Traditionally end of life care (EoLC) has been viewed as a specialist area of work. In reality, it incorporates all elements of the daily lives of people nearing the end of their lives. EoLC, palliative care and terminal care are terms that are often confused and used interchangeably but do have some differences (see later). Sensitive and patient-centred EoLC is a key skill for all nurses, as, in many areas of nursing, patients may receive life-limiting diagnoses. It also involves psychological, social and spiritual support for the patient and their family or carers. Practical skills are required and it ought to be remembered that any task or skills ought to be undertaken with the whole person in mind. 'You matter because you are you, and you matter to the end of your life' (Saunders, 1967).

In 2013, 506,790 people died in England (ONS, 2013), with cancer being the commonest cause of death (ibid.). Research by Gao *et al.* (2013) found that hospital was the commonest place of death for patients with cancer (48 per cent) with 24.5 per cent dying at home and a smaller per cent in a hospice. However, EoLC is also a feature in many areas: medical wards, emergency rooms and community settings, in fact, all the places people are cared for. These findings illustrate the need for nurses working in any area to be able to deliver high-quality EoLC. EoLC is provided by a range of organisations; within the NHS provision, patients may be admitted to general medical or oncology wards or receive care in the community from district nurses, health visitors or specialist community EoLC nurses.

Activity 6.1

Reflect on a patient you cared for who was dying.

- How did you feel planning care for this patient?
- In what way did any health professionals talk about death and dying?
- How much time did the patient spend with their family or carers during this period?

In nursing models, death is often identified as part of the life span, e.g., the Roper, Logan and Tierney Model of Care (2000). The rationale for the skill of EoLC is that it is an integral part of delivering a high standard of nursing care to 'treat people as individuals and uphold their dignity', specifically to 'recognise and respond compassionately to the needs of those who are in the last few days and hours of life' (NMC, 2015: 3.32).

Priorities in end of life care

There have been many studies considering what patients want from EoLC and during the phase of dying – the so-called 'good death'. The End of Life Care Strategy (DoH, 2008) proposes key priorities for approaching patient care:

- Being treated as an individual, with dignity and respect
- Being without pain and other symptoms
- Being in familiar surroundings
- Being in the company of close family and/or friends.

Activity 6.2

Find the NICE Quality Standard for End of Life Care: www.england.nhs.uk/wp-content/uploads/2014/11/actions-eolc.pdf

On the website are 16 statements about caring for people at the end of their life. Which of these statements apply to you as a student nurse? In what way? What might be issues arising in providing EoLC for the following patients?:

- Patients in their own home
- Homeless patients living in hostels or temporary accommodation
- Children and young persons and their families
- Patients with dementia or cognitive impairment.

It is possible to achieve these priorities in any area of care. The Liverpool Care Pathway for the Dying Patient (LCP) was developed as a partnership between Marie Curie Cancer Care and the Royal Liverpool University Hospital. The aim of the pathway was to translate best practice in EoLC from the hospice to the hospital setting. This approach was severely criticised and received poor media coverage as being 'misunderstood' despite the core principles being sound, and thus it closed in 2012. 'One Chance to Get it Right' (LACDP, 2014), replaced the LCP approach, citing five priorities for the care of the dying patient (ibid., p. 7):

- This possibility (death) is recognised and communicated clearly, decisions made and actions taken in accordance with the person's needs and wishes and these are regularly reviewed and decisions revised accordingly
- Sensitive communication takes place between staff and the dying person and those identified as important to them
- The dying person and those identified as important to them are involved in decisions about treatment and care to the extent that the dying person wants
- The needs of families and others identified as important to the dying person are actively explored, respected and met as far as possible
- An individual plan of care, which includes food and drink, symptom control and psychological, social and spiritual support, is agreed, co-ordinated and delivered with compassion.

Patients with learning disabilities and patients with existing mental health diagnosis also become physically ill and may require EoLC services; similarly, patients may develop a physical illness unrelated to their life-limiting diagnosis. It is important to recognise that these patients will have specific care requirements related to their other diagnosis which must be managed alongside their life-limiting diagnosis and EoLC requirements.

Distinguishing between palliative care, end of life care and terminal care

These three terms are often used interchangeably but have subtle differences. The term palliative derives from the Latin verb *palliare* 'to cloak'. The analogy is to cover as a protective mechanism, both the diagnosis and death, in the same way a cloak protects a person from the elements.

The World Health Organisation (2015) defined EoLC as 'palliative' in its approach which improves the quality of life of patients and their families facing the problems associated with life-threatening illness, through the prevention and relief of suffering by means of early identification and impeccable assessment and treatment of pain and other problems including physical, psychological and spiritual. Terminal care is care at the last days, hours or minutes of life but may be longer. Therefore, end of life or terminal care:

- Requires palliation
- Requires relief from pain and other distressing symptoms
- Regards dying as a normal process
- Intends neither to hasten nor postpone death
- Integrates the psychological and spiritual aspects of patient care
- Offers a support system to help patients live as actively as possible until death
- Offers a support system to help the family cope during the patient's illness and in their own bereavement
- Uses a team approach to address the needs of patients and their families, including bereavement counselling, if indicated
- Will enhance the quality of life
- Is applicable early in the course of illness, in conjunction with other therapies that are intended to prolong life, such as chemotherapy or radiation therapy, and includes those investigations needed to better understand and manage distressing clinical complications.

(WHO, 2015)

Palliative care for children represents a special, yet closely related field to adult palliative care. The WHO's definition of palliative care appropriate for children and their families is as follows however the principles apply to other paediatric chronic disorders (EAPC, 2009):

- Palliative care for children is the active total care of the child's body, mind and spirit, and also involves giving support to the family
- Effective palliative care requires a broad multi-disciplinary approach that includes the family and makes use of available community resources
- It can be provided in tertiary care facilities, in community health centres and even in children's homes.

Case study 6.1

Marcus is a 56-year-old man who was diagnosed with autism at the age of 7. Marcus has received care in a variety of settings during his life, having spent some time in a residential special school as a teenager, in residential care settings as an adult and at home with his parents as his full-time carers. Marcus has challenging behaviour as a result of his autism and can be violent at times. He finds verbal communication difficult and uses a combination of aids to assist in communication. Marcus has assistance with all his activities of daily living and has difficulty concentrating on tasks and can become frustrated and distressed at times. Marcus sometimes hits himself and screams for up to 5 minutes. He has been diagnosed with cancer of the prostate, with metastases in his bones. Marcus has pain which centres in his lower back and groin and has been nauseated and vomiting, affecting both his appetite and food intake. He has had intermittent retention of urine and has required catheterisation. At the time of referral to EoLC services, he is living at home with his parents who are both now in their eighties and who are finding it difficult to cope.

- What are Marcus' key problems?
- What specific challenges are there in practice for the nurses caring for Marcus?

Skills in end of life care: care before death

In a life-limiting illness patients are encouraged to plan ahead and make their wishes for the remainder of their life and their care preferences known (see the NHS National End of Life Care Programme). Sensitive person-centred care starts with the recognition of the dying stage. This can be very difficult to identify and recognise but Dougherty *et al.* (2015) indicate it is a progressive period of decline with the patient unable to undertake their activities of daily living (ADLs) they may be physically unable to drink, be rather sleepy or semi-comatose or unable to get out of bed. The core skills for delivering high quality EoLC nursing are both in the delivery of physical, psychosocial and spiritual care in a person centred way.

Top tip

The term 'psychosocial' care includes the psychological, social, spiritual, and practical needs of the patient and carers, all of which need to be assessed and addressed where possible.

Care of the dying child

Together for Short Lives (2011) is a care pathway approach for children with life-threatening and life-limiting conditions and their families, from diagnosis, throughout their care journey, at the time of death and beyond death. This includes EoLC, care of the child after death, and extends to the care of the body and the cultural and spiritual care of the family. This encompasses before, during and after death and addresses similar aspects to that of adults but with additional considerations of age and development. Caring for or facing the imminent death of a child has a significant impact on their physical, social, emotional and potentially the family's financial circumstances. This places an increasing demand on parents and carers. The need for meaningful, non-judgemental support at end of life is critical, and practical and emotional support is needed which can take a number of expressions.

Physical care

This is a key concern in patients who are dying. Physically patients will have a need for symptom control and management and assistance with ADLs. Patients may be admitted for periods of rehabilitation following treatment or surgery where life expectancy may be months or years and the overall goal of care is for the patient to return home. It is necessary for nurses to be able to assess each patient individually and establish the goal of the care episode. Anticipatory measures will aid comfort, e.g.:

- Pressure-relieving mattress if spending more time in bed
- Switching to continuous syringe pumps for medications in patients unable to swallow
- Frequent oral hygiene if unable to eat or drink as usual
- Observing for symptoms and initiating relief without alarming patients or relatives.

Spiritual and cultural care

Part of what makes people human is the need to make sense of life and death and find meaning and purpose in them. The RCN (2011) identified that spirituality is different from religion and is overwhelmingly difficult to define. Since the UK is a multicultural country, individual needs are complex and vary, and thus so do approaches to spiritual as well as physical care. Respect for the patient's cultural beliefs and needs at the end of life is essential, in order to assist the patient to live fully within their belief system until death. It is acknowledged that spiritual care can be provided by a variety of people, including healthcare professionals, patients and their families/carers. However, it is a particular speciality or expertise of the chaplain (or spiritual care coordinator) and patients may wish them to be involved. There is a wealth of resources to guide staff in providing spiritual and cultural care, and it is not the intention of this chapter to cover these in depth but merely to point to considerations for effective care. It is important to learn about the patients' culture through the assessment process and how they practise within it, so that interventions can be developed to facilitate the patient continuing to live within their chosen cultural frame. However, it would be dangerous to make assumptions about people, such as if they wish to align with a cultural or religious faith but not practise in a traditional sense, so this is best to determine on assessment by asking them. Practices around and after death vary according to cultural groups and local policies will address these to aid the nurse. The dying child may have specific religious or cultural interventions which differ from the adult profession or expression of their faith. The nurse or healthcare worker should follow this advice:

- Be guided by the family and ask if they are unsure
- Never assume the practices which will follow if a family have declared they are of a certain faith
- If a family are outside of their home or country, they may wish to be guided by their local community or embassy as to cultural and religious practices at the time of death.

Communication

Excellent communication is vital for patients receiving EoLC. On a daily basis there will be a need to communicate with patients about their activities for the day; physical care needs or management of symptoms such as pain and nausea and vomiting. Patients may also wish to discuss the future and there may be a need to have challenging discussion such as breaking bad news to both patients and family or carers. Patients who cannot communicate in English may need an interpreter. Dying patients may not be able to communicate honestly and openly through a member of their family or a friend acting as an interpreter, however this practice has implications for patient confidentiality.

The End of Life Care Strategy (DoH, 2008), the Gold Standards Framework Guide (GSF, 2006) and One Chance to Get it Right (LACDP, 2014) all emphasise the importance of good communication, both open and honest, as vital to the delivery of high quality EoLC. In a setting where patients are receiving EoLC, breaking bad news will be a regular activity. For communication to be achieved, the patient needs to feel they can trust the nurse or health professional, it is necessary to spend time with the patient to build a therapeutic relationship and it is important to actively listen to the patient. Health professionals need a careful skilled approach to assess and judge what the patient is saying and actually asking, e.g., a patient who says 'my pain seems to be getting worse' may actually be asking whether their condition is deteriorating.

For relatives and loved ones the way bad news is broken may impact on the bereavement process, particularly where a health professional is informing a relative or carer of the patient's death. Above all, it is necessary to plan as carefully as possible and to respect people at all stages and be responsive to their wishes and reactions, which will be diverse. For a dying child, there are additional issues and skills to consider:

- Age and development
- Awareness and understanding of illness and death
- Family connections – the values and beliefs of the family and how they make and process decisions
- Truth telling and confidentiality.

Furthermore, it is also important when talking to the dying child to do the following:

- Talk with them, not about them
- Speak in the child's language (recognise their body language and play language)
- Show them respect – don't rush them and don't interrupt
- Listen attentively.

Talking to young adults can be challenging and Together for Short Lives (2011) provides resources to support this and tackle the difficult conversations and approaches to care choices: www.togetherforshortlives.org.uk/assets/0001/0096/Difficult_Conversations_ for_Young_Adults_-_Final_PDF.pdf.

Case study 6.2

Read the following case study: have you encountered any similar situations or attitudes on placement?

Rosa and Christopher had been married for 10 years, with children aged 3 and 5, when Christopher was diagnosed with a brain tumour. He was admitted to an acute medical ward, as he was becoming confused at home. The following morning at 7.30 one of the wards nurses telephoned Rosa to inform her that Christopher's condition had deteriorated and she should come to the hospital. As Rosa's children had just got up and she was making their breakfast, Rosa decided to let her children have breakfast before going to the hospital. When Rosa arrived at the hospital, Christopher had recently died.

Rosa was very distressed that she had not been present when her husband died and said to the nurse: 'It's my fault, I stopped to give the children breakfast when I should have come straight here.' The nurse was upset by this and when discussing the case with the team during handover stated that Christopher was already dead when Rosa was telephoned but that she did not want to tell her over the telephone and had instead decided to tell Rosa Christopher had deteriorated.

What might the implications of such actions be for the therapeutic relationship and long-term grieving?

Clinical significance

Grieving may be affected by many influences, such as religious beliefs, previous experience, culture, relationship in life, presence at death and viewing of the body following death. In all communication situations, health professionals need to be aware that it is unlikely any actions can make the person 'feel better' as is often the stated desire remember, be genuine.

Symptoms and symptom management

Pain

Pain is not experienced by all patients at the end of life nor is it synonymous with cancer or other chronic disorders. The concept of 'total pain' was first articulated by Cicely Saunders in 1967 as a holistic definition of pain integrating the inseparability of physical pain from mental processes. The concept of total pain is of pain as a multi-faceted experience impacted by influences which are not all amenable to management by medications. The contribution of each component (see Figure 6.1) will be specific to each individual and his or her situation.

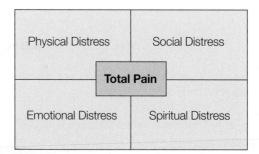

Figure 6.1 **Total pain**
Source: adapted from Saunders (1967).

Management of pain

Effective frequent pain assessment is imperative. This was addressed in Chapter 5. There are three key means of effective pain management in adults and in children and young people:

■ By mouth – the oral route ideally
■ By the clock – given regularly and not waiting for pain to appear
■ By the ladder (the WHO analgesic ladder) – increasing in strength as needed.

Patients may take medications bought over the counter alongside prescribed medications, complementary and alternative medicines (CAM) too and appropriate advice given for actions or interactions. Overall a holistic assessment of pain aids decisions about how best to manage the patient's pain.

The strategies available for pain management in EoLC are likely to be most effective if combinations of approaches are used. If the concept of 'total pain' is accepted, then it follows that different management strategies may be needed for each source of pain. There are some simple interventions the nurse can use which may help to reduce the patient's pain, e.g.:

■ Assisting the patient to reposition and find a comfortable resting position, perhaps supported by pillows

- Giving a warm bath or use of a heat pad
- Distraction may be effective and activities such as reading to the patient, chatting to the patient or watching television may be helpful
- Many hospice environments will offer other therapies such as massage, aromatherapy and hypnotherapy which may provide relief from pain.

In EoLC or terminal phase care, the patient may have regular medication, such as morphine sulphate or diamorphine, administered via slow release or syringe pump to achieve a consistent level of pain control. It would be really distressing for patients to experience pain and for family to witness this suffering. For effective analgesia, pain medication ought to be given even if the patient does not look to be in pain.

Nausea and vomiting

Patients receiving EoLC may have nausea and vomiting which can be quite distressing. This may be due to a number of causes, e.g. primary disease or a side effect of opiate analgesia.

If a patient is nauseated (retching) or vomiting, the care revolves around privacy and comfort and eliminating the cause if known. For example, patients with disease in their bones, may have hypercalcaemia (calcium); this condition is classified as an EoLC emergency causing nausea and vomiting, but also confusion, constipation and fatigue. Treatment of hypercalcaemia would include medication to reduce calcium levels.

The nursing interventions for the patient will range from appropriate assessment, hygiene and comfort measures; giving the patient a vomit bowl and tissues; providing privacy; giving mouth care and using touch appropriately; to administration of an appropriate antiemetic as prescribed and helping the patient to find a comfortable resting position. Avoidance of strong odours or food smells may also help.

Equipment needed at the bedside

- Non-sterile gloves and apron
- Vomit bowls
- Tissues
- Disposable wipe
- Water for personal hygiene.

Procedure for care of patient who is vomiting

1   Undertake an assessment of the patient's level of nausea and vomiting.
2   Ensure patient is safe, either in position or location to avoid injury or falling.
3   If they are in an open area, draw curtains/screens for privacy.
4   Provide vomit bowl and tissues to the patient.
5   Wash hands if able to.
6   Put on an apron and gloves.
7   When vomiting finishes, remove vomit container, offer water and hand towels to wash their face/hands. Comfort the patient throughout this.

8   Assist the patient into a comfortable position, not lying on their back.

9   Ensure patient has a clean vomit bowl and tissues.

10   Examine vomit for volume and presence of colour/consistency/smell/blood to determine cause and document this (NMC, 2015).

11   Discard the vomit bowl and contents according to the local policy.

12   Wash and dry hands.

13   Reassess the patient and record further incidents or changes. Remove any offending odours or irritants.

When assessing the patient, ask:

- When did you start to feel this way?
- Did anything precipitate it?
- Have you felt like this before?
- If so, did anything help last time?
- Do drinking and/or eating make you feel better or worse?
- Do you feel thirsty or hungry?

Also check:

- Are the patient's mucous membranes dry?
- What medication is the patient prescribed and taking?
- What is the location of the patient's disease and potential link to the nausea?

Patients may have antiemetic (nausea medication) prescribed regularly and this may be administered via a syringe driver with analgesia. If the patient has 'breakthrough' nausea, it may be necessary to give a combination of antiemetics regularly and as prescribed and planned with the care team.

Constipation

Constipation is a key nursing issue in EoLC settings. Defined as 'infrequent or difficult defecation' (Becker, 2010, p. 226), it may be complicated by patients taking prescribed opiate analgesia to manage pain or following reduced appetite, lack of mobility and low fluid intake. It is individual and holistic assessment guides decisions about this. This is further addressed in Chapter 4.

Common interventions for constipation include increased exercise and increased fluid and fibre intake, but these may not be effective for patients with an advanced disease. Many patients have reduced appetite and, therefore, increasing their fibre intake will be challenging; patients may be fatigued and, therefore, increasing mobility will be difficult, as a result, management may centre more on administration of laxatives and/ or rectal preparations.

Bowel care is best delivered in the morning and patients may appreciate this before personal hygiene. It is important that the patient feels relaxed and able to communicate with their nurse; it may be helpful for the patient to have a hot drink early in the morning

Don't forget!

Diarrhoea maybe overflow and therefore is a sign of constipation.

as this may help their bowels to start moving. As with other sensitive interventions, privacy and dignity are essential to good bowel assessment and care.

Fatigue and weight loss

Many patients with advanced disease experience fatigue and weight loss, the term 'terminal cachexia' may be used to describe significant loss of weight and 'wasting away' associated with the terminal phase of disease. There may be a range of causes for the feeling of fatigue; some, such as anaemia, insomnia and depression, may be improved by medication. Dehydration and anxiety may be improved by nursing interventions. As with all symptom control issues, the cause of the patient's feeling of fatigue should be identified through accurate assessment, so that appropriate interventions can be implemented.

Causes of feeling tired and fatigued include:

- Anaemia
- Weight loss
- Depression
- Anxiety and worry
- Insomnia
- Poor appetite and nutrition
- Dehydration.

Although the logical nursing intervention for fatigue may be to promote rest, some organisations, e.g. Macmillan Cancer, advocate gentle exercise to help to increase energy levels and improve appetite. The nurse may encourage and assist the patient to move around the bed area, the public or social spaces or at home. The physiotherapist or occupational therapist may give the patient some simple sitting exercises to do, which can also give the patient a focus and help the patient to feel they are 'helping themselves' while also improving their psychological well-being.

Confusion

Confusion and agitation, which can develop during the phase of dying, can be very distressing for both the patient and their loved ones, due to a range of possible causes and interventions. Appropriate interventions require accurate assessment of the patient. The patient may experience hallucinations and paranoia and this may be exhibited in a wide variety of ways: their behaviour may be aggressive and restless or they may speak in a way it is not possible to understand. This will be very distressing for the patient and their family or carers. Assessment of agitated patients can be very challenging, as the patient may not be able to answer questions or give any coherent information. Other sources of assessment, such as family or carers (maintaining confidentiality) and community practitioners, other members of staff who have been caring for the patient and the patient's medical and nursing notes may provide valuable assessment information as well as observation of the patient's non-verbal cues.

Don't forget!

Patients having EoLC may become confused as a result of infection or constipation, as well as issues related to their primary disease.

Creating a calm environment is recommended and although a relatively simple intervention, this may have a very positive effect and demonstrates nursing care with advocacy at its centre. Limiting noise and bright light, employing good communication by talking to the patient in a calm way, at their level, explaining interventions and offering simple choices with closed questions will be beneficial.

A number of medications may be administered to manage this symptom. Agitation caused by cerebral metastases may respond well to the administration of prescribed steroids, such as dexamethasone, or palliative radiotherapy treatment. Sedatives such as midazolam may be given as single one-off doses or via a syringe driver. For the nurse to select the appropriate 'as required' medication, it is necessary to have an understanding of the cause of the agitation and the action of the medications available. Prevention of delirium is better than management, however, this may be unexpected. A comprehensive assessment tool can be found on the NICE website (www.nice.org.uk/guidance/CG103) but general principles for this skill are as follows.

Assessment of confusion and agitation

If possible, ensure that patients at risk of delirium are cared for by a team of healthcare professionals who are familiar to the person at risk. Is the behaviour new or has it been experienced before?

1   If the patient has experienced this before, what helped last time?
2   Was the onset of behaviour sudden or gradual?
3   Does the patient have any lucid moments?
4   Does the patient seem able to respond to closed questions appropriately?
5   Can the patient follow simple instructions?
6   Is the patient a danger to themselves or other patients?
7   What medication is the patient prescribed?
8   Is the patient in pain?
9   Are there any signs of hypoxia (skin colour, breathlessness)?

10   Are there any signs of infection? The patient's urine will need to be tested.
11   Is the patient expectorating anything?
12   Is the patient poorly nourished?
13   When did the patient last open their bowels?
14   Are there any signs of dehydration? Is the patient passing urine or drinking orally?
15   Are the patient's mucous membranes dry?

This will form the baseline to develop an appropriate patient-centred care plan to address any issues which arise.

Mouth care

Oral hygiene is very important for patients in care situations and at end of life stages. This is especially important if they have difficulty taking food or fluids or are dehydrated. Causes vary but may be due to dry mouth, ulcers or oral fungal candidiasis (thrush), which, as well as being painful and unpleasant, further reduces oral intake. A number of factors can contribute to patients' oral hygiene being compromised. If the patient has advanced disease and their immunity is reduced, they may have poor appetite, reduced oral intake and poor nutritional status; the patient may physically be unable to perform their own oral hygiene and treatment with chemotherapy has the side effect of causing oral candida and ulcers.

It is part of the nurses' role to assess and manage the patient's oral hygiene (Chapter 3). Oral care is one of the areas of care the patient's family or carers can be actively involved with if this is desired by them and the patient. The patient's mouth will need frequent cleansing, their teeth and tongue should be regularly brushed and oral care kits can be used to clean around the gums. There is old yet useful evidence that pineapple juice is effective in reducing oral candidiasis, due to the action of proteolytic enzyme, ananase in pineapple juice that is cleansing to the mouth (ananase is still active despite the canning process of canned fruit) (Regnard and Tempest, 1998). A second line of approach may be to administer artificial saliva that buffers the acidity of the mouth and lubricates the mucous membranes but only provides transient relief (Twycross and Wilcock, 2007). For a sore or ulcerated mouth, topical analgesia may be needed too. It may also be appropriate to moisten the patient's lips, if they are dry, with lip salve or petroleum jelly. Oral candidiasis can still be a problem at times. They may be prescribed antifungal medications such as nystatin and fluconazole which will need to be given regularly.

Dyspnoea and upper airway secretions

Patients at the end of life may experience dyspnoea during their illness and the phase of dying, this may be related to their primary diagnosis, e.g.; a lung tumour or metastatic spread to the lungs, or it may be related to a pre-existing diagnosis such as emphysema or asthma. Accurate assessment such as outlined in Chapter 7 is needed. It may not be possible for the patient to give answers to open questions, and assessment may need to be focused on closed questions, non-verbal observation and pre-existing knowledge of the patient's medical history.

The nursing interventions for the management of dyspnoea are fundamental; the patient should be nursed in a supported upright position, in a calm, ventilated environment and encouraged to breathe regular, deep breaths (as much as they can). Essential oils, such as eucalyptus, may be helpful and if the care area has an aromatherapy massage practitioner, they can be consulted.

In addition, the patient may have excessive upper airway secretions, as a result of decreased mobility, coughing and swallowing, coupled with reducing consciousness. The symptom will be evident from the patient's breathing, which will be noisy, gurgled, rattling and laboured; this is sometimes referred to as a 'death rattle'. The symptom may be very distressing for family or carers to see; however, there is no evidence that the symptom is uncomfortable for the patient nor is there any medication to reduce it (Campbell and Yarandi, 2013). Changing the patient's position may alleviate the symptom temporarily. Suctioning as an intervention is not recommended in EoLC, as this is an unpleasant procedure and is generally done only as a last resort.

During the actual process of death, the body naturally dehydrates itself as a protective mechanism. Artificially hydrating the patient during the phase of dying, by subcutaneous or intravenous infusion or via a nasogastric tube, interrupts this process and may make the symptom of retained secretions worse.

Psychological care and coping

When patients have a diagnosis for which a cure cannot be achieved, this will affect patients in different ways and may be influenced by a range of factors: the age of the patient, the social support network the patient has, the patient's religious or spiritual beliefs, the patient's previous experience of illness and whether the patient has any pre-existing diagnosis or mental health condition, to name but a few.

As with any symptom, it is necessary to assess the patient. Communication with the patient on difficult and sensitive issues is a key skill in delivering care at the end of life (Box 6.1). When communicating with the patient, the patient will need time to express themselves, so adopting open questions and appropriate body language can facilitate this. It is important to spend time with the patient and for the patient not to feel rushed.

The patient may have practical concerns which are causing them distress, such as the need to make a will or worry about family members; it may be necessary to facilitate family discussions or to arrange this for the patient. The patient may need information

Box 6.1 The HOPE approach

Old and Swagerty (2007) outline the 'HOPE' approach:

H: Hope – sources of hope, meaning, comfort, strength, peace, love, connection
O: Organised religion
P: Personal practices
E: Effects of medical care and end of life issues.

about the process of dying and how this can be managed, as many patients are fearful of suffering pain and discomfort at the end of their life.

The patient's religious or spiritual beliefs will be an important influence on their care. Some patients may suffer a crisis of faith in the phase of dying, which will be distressing for them and which the nurse will need to support them through. It is important to ascertain what the patient wants; some patients may be comforted by seeing representatives from their faith and discussing issues with them, however, other patients may find this more distressing. Patients may be spiritual without believing in a religion and be religious without being spiritual. Many patients wish to find meaning and many will ask the 'why me?' question or become frustrated and angry.

When dealing with an angry patient, there are some key approaches to care and interventions which are effective. It is important not to be angry back to the patient or to argue with the patient, listening to the patient and allowing them time to express their anger are more effective, this may convey caring to show the patient you are listening, by validating their feelings. This may be achieved by acknowledging the patient's feelings (you have every right to feel angry) and showing the patient that their anger is a normal part of the process they are going through (it is normal to feel angry). Dying children can feel frustrated and their family and parents may be angry or upset, expressing their frustration as anger. It remains important to validate their feelings and give them space and opportunity to express themselves.

Care of the patient's family or carers

Caring for the patient's relatives, family or carers is a fundamental part of caring for patients at the end of life. The patient is not going through the process in isolation and their family or carers have needs which the nurse should address. They may need information, however, confidentiality of the patient still needs to be observed. This can be very challenging, the patient has the ultimate decision over what information is passed to whom and on admission.

Family or carers also have a need to be with the patient, if this is the patient's wish, to be helpful, involved in the patient's care and comfort (Campbell and Yarandi, 2013). Following the patient's death, it is important the family or carers are able to spend time with the patient and to view their body; there is also a need to give information about the registration of death, funeral arrangements and bereavement care and counselling.

Whatever the age of the patient, they may have family who are children, the patient may be a close relative, such as a parent, grandparent, aunt or uncle or friend of the family. Children who are well informed about the illness often have a better recovery from their relative's death. It is important to be honest and use the correct terminology: dying, death, died. Terms like 'going away with the angels' may be taken literally by a child depending on their age and create fear or unrealistic expectation.

Play and laughter remain important parts of a child's world, even where a parent is terminally ill. It can be therapeutic to encourage children and patients to play and laugh together. There is also evidence that children who are encouraged to help the patient and be involved in caring for them, develop more positive self-esteem and grief reactions. This can be encouraged in simple ways – helping the patient to have a drink, turning the pages of a magazine or newspaper, brushing the patient's hair or putting on their slippers.

It is suggested that an important part of preparing children for the death of a family member or carer is in the sharing and building of memories. Activities such as making memory boxes together (if the child is old enough) or a patient might be encouraged to write letters for the child maybe helpful for significant milestones such as birthdays, graduation, Building memories, by encouraging and facilitating the patient and child doing things they enjoy together, gives children positive memories. In the case of young children, it may be appropriate to video the patient and child, so the child has the memory in a different form for later life. For children of a terminally ill parent, this may be the surviving parent, who can be a constant in the child's life and offer support in the future (Box 6.2).

Box 6.2 Care requirements for children when a relative/parent/grandparent is terminally ill

- *Information*: honest, age-appropriate, with the opportunity to ask questions
- *Space*: a safe environment in which to share and express feelings, to be listened to and be heard
- *Routine*: normality and structure will help the child to develop a sense of safety
- *A key person*: someone chosen by the relative/parent to support and provide continuity for the child
- *Connection with the person they have lost*: memory boxes, photographs and video, a special present from the patient
- *Memory making*: memory boxes and activities to maintain memories
- *Support in bereavement*: time to talk and express feelings
- *Care from specialist bereavement services*: it is important to introduce the services before the patient dies if possible.

The assumption that young children are too young to understand bereavement and are not affected by it is misguided; children of any age are able to experience loss and may express this in different ways, even for a young baby, when their mother leaves the room, the baby may cry as an expression of her leaving, albeit temporarily. Although a child may not have the cognitive ability to understand bereavement, they still experience the loss.

Between the ages of 2 and 5, a child may not understand that death is permanent and may expect the patient to return at some point, although they may understand that the patient has gone at the moment. From around age 5, a child will begin to understand that death means the end of life and by age 7 most children will understand that death is a part of life which all people experience. By teenage years, children will have a greater understanding of death and the permanence of it. Reactions to grief, as with other emotions at this age, may be intense. Children may worry about who will perform the activities of the person who has died, such as taking them to school or making their meals. Support from professional bereavement services is recommended for all bereaved parties and if this can be introduced prior to the patient's death, this is optimal. Charities, such as Cruse and Winston's Wish, offer specialist care for children and families.

Ethical dilemmas

There are key ethical issues related to the present-day care of dying patients: do not resuscitate orders, withdrawal of feeding and hydration, advanced directives, assisted suicide and euthanasia being the significant ones. It is not possible to address these here in any depth in this chapter.

It is good practice to discuss issues openly, candidly and honestly as a team, with the patient and if appropriate, the family or carers. Shared decision-making is promoted by ethicists to minimise confusion and dilemma. One point worthy of mention is Advance Decision and Consent. The Mental Capacity Act (2005) sets out the conditions for consent with incapacitated adults, and for advance directives, the Act applies to patients over the age of 18. An Advance Decision (also known as a 'living will' colloquially or an Advance Decision to Refuse Treatment, ADRT), is generally an advanced refusal of consent to particular treatment and may set out how a patient wishes to be cared for when they have lost capacity. Advance Decisions are legally binding providing certain conditions are met (written, signed and witnessed) (Box 6.3). It is not the same as an Advance Statement which is a written statement that sets down a patient's preferences, wishes, beliefs and values regarding their future care which is not legally binding but informs everyone involved in the patient's care about these items if the patient is not able to tell them.

Box 6.3 Conditions for a legally binding Advance Decision

- The patient making the directive has mental capacity and competence to do so and is over 18 years old
- The patient was fully informed of the nature and consequences of the directive at the time it was made
- The patient states clearly the advance directive applies to all circumstances
- No one has influenced or pressurised the patient
- The directive has not been changed since it was established (verbally or in writing)
- In the present situation, the patient is mentally incapable of making a decision.

Adapted from Becker (2010)

Caring for a dying child can be challenging and involve complex decisions and advance care planning. Together for Short Lives (2011) identifies that Advance Care Planning (ACP) can ensure effective care and consideration of the wider dimensions of preparing for death and recognises the need for discussions on organ donation, preferred place of care and anticipatory symptom management planning.

Watch out

There is a presumption of capacity, and the test of competence is set out in the Mental Capacity Act (2005). The Act is based on a presumption of competence, the burden of proof rests with the nurse to demonstrate incompetence, not the patient to demonstrate competence.

When the patient dies

When the patient is in the final phase of dying, their family or carers may be present all the time and should be given the opportunity to fully participate in the patient's care, if they and the patient wish it. The family or carers may not realise when the patient dies and it will be important to communicate this to them sensitively; to avoid any confusion, the use of euphemisms for death should be avoided, the most appropriate words to use are died, dead and dying (Box 6.4).

Box 6.4 Colloquial terms used to describe death

- Passed away
- Passed over
- Gone to the other side
- With God
- Is gone
- No longer with us.

The RCN (2014) advocates asking the person (if this is possible and/or appropriate) who they would like to be present at the time of their death. If this is not possible, try to find out from the family/carers, as well as details of how they wish the news of the death to be communicated if they are not present. Then relevant contact details will need to be recorded and readily accessible by all appropriate staff. In any event, information should be honest and accurate, tailored to meet the family's needs and shared in an empathetic and caring way. Relatives may also wish practical advice on what to do next and this ought to be anticipated.

In care home and home settings where death is expected, it is crucial that the general practitioner reviews the person regularly and at least every 14 days, both from a care point of view and in order that a Medical Certificate of Cause of Death (MCCD) can be appropriately issued without involving the coroner.

Care of the body after death

Care of the patient after death is as much a part of EoLC nursing, as is care of the patient in the phase of dying. Each clinical area will have their own policy on how patients'

Activity 6.3

Homelessness is a big issue in some large urban areas. It is not confined to these areas. What are the considerations for EoLC for homeless persons or those in hostels?

St Mungo's and Marie Curie (2011) provides resources to address these: see the resource at: www.mungos.org/endoflifecare/resources_section and reflect on these questions:

1   What key people are involved in supporting people at the end stage of life?
2   An eco-map is proposed to help residents or clients to understand the different ways in which people in their life are important to them. To make the eco-map, put the resident under review in the centre of it (Figure 6.2). Then locate the people or organisations important to them and mark how strong, weak or stressful the connection is. The connection may relate to emotional or practical support that a person or organisation can offer to the individual. What do each have to offer (hint: physical, psychological, spiritual, emotional, etc. support)? Finally, consider what support hostel staff might need when a resident dies.

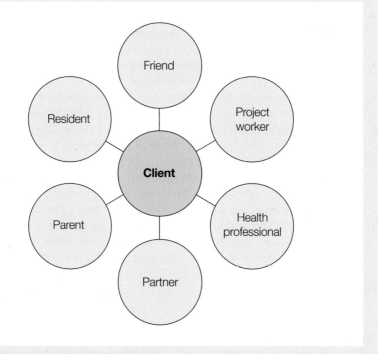

Figure 6.2 **An example of an eco-map**

bodies are treated following death, which has also been known as 'last offices'. The new terminology 'care after death' is recommended by the End of Life Care programme to reflect the differing nursing tasks involved, including ongoing support of the family and carers. The physical preparation of the body itself will be called 'personal care after death'. In all cases the patient needs to be shown dignity and respect, as do the family or carers who may have been present when the patient died.

In EoLC settings, as the philosophy of care is inclusive of family or carers, in the same way that they are encouraged to be part of the patient's care when alive, this is extended following death. For many close family or carers, being able to prepare the patient's body is an important part of the process and can positively assist with grieving, therefore, the family or carers will be able to take part in the last offices if they wish and the opportunity will be given. The following steps ought to be considered as key to this skill:

1   If present at the time of the death, the nurse records the time, who was present, the nature of the death, and details of any relevant devices (such as cardiac defibrillators), as well as their own name and contact details in the nursing, medical or ambulance documentation. If relatives have any concerns about the death, these should also be documented.

2   Inform the doctor or appropriately qualified nurse to provide verification of death. This is required before the body is transferred from the care setting. This person is also responsible for confirming the identity of the body. The responsible person may vary according to local policy.

3   If the relatives or carers are not present at the time of death, they need to be informed by a professional with appropriate communication skills and offered support, including access to a spiritual or religious person as they wish.

4   Check with the local policy about reporting to the local coroner (if unexpected death) or if a complicated death has occurred.

5   Tasks such as laying the deceased flat (while supporting the head with a pillow), and preparing them and the room for viewing, need to be completed as soon as possible.

6   Relatives, friends or significant others may wish to view the deceased and an appropriate location for this ought to be identified and prepared.

7   Family may wish to sit with their relative in the period immediately after death. They may need to be prepared for the changes which occur to bodies following death and any tubes, lines or other devices which may still be visible. Offer age-appropriate support, e.g., parents may wish a bereaved child to have a favourite toy.

8   Pack personal property showing consideration for the feelings of those receiving it and in line with local policy. Discuss the issue of soiled clothes sensitively with the family and ask whether they wish them to be disposed of or returned.

Personal care of the body after death

In some religions, last offices may be performed by a member of the religion. For example, for Jewish patients, this may be organised by the Jewish Funeral Service and performed by a Rabbi, with burial usually taking place on the same day if possible (see Table 6.1). These regulations are very broad and the nurse is advised to consult with the patient or family (or both) regarding specific rituals they wish to observe. It is important

Table 6.1 Common cultural and religious groups encountered and considerations for dying patients and families (NB this is a very broad guide do seek more details)

Religion	Cultural or religious routines	Preparing the body	Considerations after death	Further information
Buddhism	Buddhists believe the state of mind of the dying patient will influence their rebirth; they therefore place considerable importance on a state of conscious and focused peace. Monks or nuns may be present and chant or pray, maintaining a calm environment.	No specific rituals. It is traditional for the body to be left undisturbed for some time to allow any remaining consciousness to depart.	Buddhists believe in rebirth and that happens when they die. Cremation is preferred.	www.thebuddhistsociety.org/page/buddhist-funerals
Christian (Many: Catholic, Methodist, Church of England and many more)	Support is often sought from a minister or priest.	Nurses or healthcare workers can prepare the body.	Religious symbols may be requested, i.e. crucifix, rosary beads, relics or images of saints.	www.funeralwise.com/customs/christian_overview/
Islam/Muslim	Prayers from the Qu'ran may be read out to the dying person but not recited near the deceased.	Muslims prefer non-Muslims not to touch the body. Clothing removed and family ritually wash the body (same gender). The head is turned to the right or the body is pointed to Mecca (east). The body is then covered with a sheet.	If necessary, consent needs to be sought and gloves worn to touch the body. Burial is ideally performed within 24 hours.	www.islamreligion.com/articles/4946/viewall/funeral-rites-in-islam/
Hindus	It is preferred if the eldest son is present at the time of death. Care during dying involves holy water sprinkled over the dying person, and laying them on the floor to symbolise closeness to Mother Earth.	No problem for non-Hindus to touch the body but many prefer to wash the body at home as part of the funeral rites. If possible, the Hindu prefers to die at home. Do not remove any jewellery or religious objects.	The family may wish to stay with the patient all the time. Post-mortems are considered disrespectful but accepted if required by law.	www.hinduismtoday.com/modules/smartsection/item.php?itemid=1667

Table 6.1 Common cultural and religious groups encountered and considerations for dying patients and families (continued)

Religion	Cultural or religious routines	Preparing the body	Considerations after death	Further information
Sikh	Do not remove the five '5Ks', which are personal objects sacred to Sikhs and take care when touching these objects. Dying person may be given holy water to drink or be sprinkled with it.	No problem for non-Sikhs to touch the body but many prefer to wash the body at home as part of the funeral rites. Do not trim the hair or beard.	Cremation ideally within 24 hours of death. Access to a Sikh Granthi (a Sikh), who can recite Gurbani (writings of the Gurus) and perform Sikh prayers. Sikhs console themselves with the recitation of their sacred hymns.	www.sikhs.org/fest.htm
Judaism	It is considered immodest for men to touch women other than their wives. Contact the Rabbi as soon as possible after death if not present.	Eight minutes are required to elapse before the body is touched. Handle the body as little as possible. Straighten limbs with the hands open. The body would usually be washed by a nominated group.	Relatives may wish to keep vigil over the body. Burial is within 24 hours ideally. If death happens during the Sabbath (between sunset on Friday and sunset on Saturday), the body should be left.	www.jewishvirtuallibrary.org/jsource/Judaism/death.html

to be calm, respectful and treat the death of a person who was living until recently with dignity and respect. Care also ought to be seen with due regard to infection control and manual handling policies. The key personal care skills are outlined in the Guidance for staff responsible for care after death (NNCG, 2011) and address the following aspects:

Equipment that is needed at the bedside

- Sheets
- Shroud
- Basin
- Water
- Towel.

Procedure for preparing a deceased person

1   Deal with and speak to the deceased body respectfully.
2   Lay the deceased person on their back, straighten their limbs (if possible) with their arms lying by their sides. Leave one pillow under the head as it supports alignment and helps the mouth stay closed. It may be necessary to use a rolled towel to assist shutting the jaw – apply this without using pressure.
3   If possible, close the eyes by applying light pressure for 30 seconds.
4   Clean the mouth to remove debris and secretions. Clean and replace dentures as soon as possible after death if possible. If not, then ensure they stay with the deceased for the funeral directors.
5   Comb or tidy the deceased's hair if visible.
6   When the death is not being referred to the coroner, remove mechanical aids, such as syringe drivers, apply gauze and tape to syringe driver sites and document disposal of medication. Do check the local policy first.
7   Cover wounds, stomas, lines, which may leak.
8   Bladder or bowels may loosen and evacuate and so padding may be required.
9   Wash the deceased (unless requested or prohibited by faith or culture) maintaining dignity throughout.
10 Dress the deceased in the appropriate clothing – in hospital, this may be a shroud, in the community setting, it may be their own clothes. They are not to be left naked.
11 Check the deceased has an identity tag and this is securely fastened onto the body.
12 Gently wrap the deceased in a clean sheet and secure loosely.
13 Transfer the body to the mortuary (in hospital) or in community setting this may be to the undertakers.

Don't forget!

While it would be rare in an EoLC setting for a patient's death to be referred to the coroner, but if that is the case, their body must not be washed following death and medical devices must be left in place until the coroner releases the body.

Summary

Caring for and supporting people approaching the end of their life is considered the most challenging work any healthcare worker faces. It can also be the most rewarding – if they have the right knowledge, skills and attitude to provide the care and support needed. Individualised patient-centred care and frequent assessment will ensure patients are treated and cared for in the right way at the right point of their last stages of life. Open and frank communication is important and will enable the key priorities of care to be met.

References

ACT (2011) Basic symptom control in paediatric palliative care. Available at: www. togetherforshortlives.org.uk/assets/0000/1052/Basic_Symptom_Contro_in_Paediatric_ Palliative_Care_2011.pdf (accessed 1 February 2016).

Becker, R. (2010) Palliative nursing skills: what are they? In R. Becker, *Fundamental Skills for Palliative Care Nursing. An Evidence Based Handbook for Student Nurses*, 2nd edn. London: Quay Books.

Campbell, M.L. and Yarandi, H.N. (2013) Death rattle is not associated with patient respiratory distress: is pharmacologic treatment indicated? *Journal of Palliative Medicine.* 16(10):1255–9. doi: 10.1089/jpm.2013.0122

DoH (Department of Health) (2008) *End of Life Care Strategy*. Available at: www.gov.uk/ government/uploads/system/uploads/attachment_data/file/136431/End_of_life_strategy. pdf (accessed 25 November 2015).

DoH (Department of Health) (2015) *One Chance to Get it Right: One Year On Report*. Available at: www.gov.uk/government/uploads/system/uploads/attachment_data/ file/450391/One_chance_-_one_year_on_acc.pdf (accessed 1 February 2016).

Dougherty. L., Lister. S. and West-Oram. A. (2015) Patient comfort and end of life care. In L. Dougherty, S. Lister and A. West-Oram (eds) *The Royal Marsden Manual of Clinical Nursing Procedures*, Student Edition, 9th edn. London: Wiley.

EAPC (European Association for Palliative Care) (2009) *Report on Palliative Care for Infants, Children and Young People*. Available at: www.maruzza.org/maruzza_en/ Palliativecarcinchildren.html (accessed 1 February 2016).

Gao. W., Ho, Y., Verne. J., Glickman. M. and Higginson. I.J. (2013) Changing patterns in place of cancer death in England: a population-based study. *PLoS Med* 10(3); doi: 10.1371/journal.pmed.1001410.

Gold Standards Framework Guide (2006) *The National Gold Standards Framework (GSF) Centre in End of Life Care*. Available at: www.goldstandardsframework.org.uk/ (accessed 12 September 2015).

LACDP (Leadership Alliance for the Care of Dying People) (2014) *One Chance to Get it Right*. Available at: www.gov.uk/government/uploads/system/uploads/attachment_data/ file/323188/One_chance_to_get_it_right.pdf (accessed 5 January 2016).

Mental Capacity Act (2005) Available at: www.legislation.gov.uk/ukpga/2005/9/contents (accessed 20 January 2016).

NMC (Nursing and Midwifery Council) (2015) *The Code: Professional Standards of Practice and Behaviour for Nurses and Midwives*. London: NMC.

NNCG (National Nurse Consultant Group Palliative Care) (2011) Guidance for staff responsible for care after death (last offices). Available at: www.nhsiq.nhs.uk/media/2426968/ care_after_death___guidance.pdf (accessed 20 January 2016).

Old, J.L. and Swagerty, D.L. (2007) *A Practical Guide to Palliative Care*. Philadelphia, PA: Lippincott, Williams and Wilkins.

ONS (Office for National Statistics) (2013) What do we die from? Available at: www. ons.gov.uk/ons/rel/vsob1/mortality-statistics--deaths-registered-in-england-and-wales-- series-dr-/2014/sty-what-do-we-die-from.html (accessed 5 January 2016).

RCN (Royal College of Nursing) (2011) Spirituality: online resource. Available at: www2. rcn.org.uk/__data/assets/pdf_file/0008/395864/Sprituality_online_resource_Final.pdf (accessed 5 January 2016).

RCN (Royal College of Nursing) (2014) Getting it right every time: fundamentals of nursing at the end of life. Available at: http://rcnendoflife.org.uk/ (accessed 5 January 2016).

Regnard, C. and Tempest, S. (1998) *A Guide to Symptom Relief in Advanced Disease*, 4th edn. London: Hochland and Hochland Ltd.

Roper, N., Logan, W., Tierney A. (2000), *The Roper-Logan and Tierney Model of Nursing: Based on Activities of Living*. Churchill and Livingstone: London.

Saunders, C. (1967) *The Management of Terminal Illness*. London: Hospital Medicine Publications Ltd.

St Mungo's and Marie Curie (2011) End of life resources. Available at: www.mungos.org/endoflifecare/resources_section (accessed 25 May 2016).

Together for Short Lives (2011) A guide to end of life care. Available at: www.togetherforshortlives.org.uk/assets/0000/1855/TfSL_A_Guide_to_End_of_Life_Care_5_FINAL_VERSION.pdf (accessed 5 January 2016).

Twycross, R. and Wilcock, A. (2007) Palliative Care Formulary (PCF3). Available at: www.palliativedrugs.com.uk (accessed 5 January 2016).

Twycross, R.G., Wilcock, A. and Toller, C.S. (2009) *Symptom Management in Advanced Cancer*, 4th edn. Nottingham: Palliativecaredrugs.com

WHO (World Health Organisation) (2015) Palliative Care, Fact Sheet No. 402. Available at: www.who.int/mediacentre/factsheets/fs402/en/ (accessed 1 February 2016).

Part II

Essential and Advanced skills

Chapter 7

Observations and monitoring
Vital signs

Tina Moore

Vital signs are 'vital'.

A number of reports conclude that patients are not being assessed properly. Much of this assessment is in relation to vital signs. Nurses are failing to conduct a comprehensive assessment on the patient, nor are they interpreting the data gained from that assessment adequately.

(NCEPOD, 2007; NICE, 2007; DoH, 2009)

Key concepts

Recording/measuring respiration, pulse, blood pressure and temperature
Apex and radial pulses
Tachycardia
Bradycardia

Cardiac output
Stroke volume
Systemic vascular resistance
Hypertension
Hypotension

Learning outcomes

By the end of this chapter you will be able to:

- Revise anatomy and physiology in relation to pulse, blood pressure and temperature
- Demonstrate a comprehensive assessment of the pulse, respiration, blood pressure and temperature
- Select the correct equipment and use the correct technique in the assessment of a pulse (including apex and radial), respirations and blood pressure
- Analyse the significance of the assessment of respiration, pulse, blood pressure and temperature in relation to clinical practice
- Clearly identify factors influencing the assessment of the vital signs.

Introduction

Vital signs (also referred to as 'signs of life') are observations and measurements essentially of temperature, respiratory rate, pulse and blood pressure but may include other measurements, e.g. pulse oximetry. These measurements are considered to be vital for life and provide valuable information about the patient's physiological status. Normal ranges of measurements change with age, sex, weight, exercise tolerance and medical condition. Knowing these measurements also aids in the diagnosis and evaluation of medical problems. National Early Warning Scores (NEWS) exist in clinical practice which provide a quick overview of the patient's physiological status and identify areas of concern/deterioration. This is discussed further in Chapter 10. For information on the process of breathing and gas exchange, see Chapter 9.

This particular chapter will consider the skills in assessing four vital signs (respiration, pulse, blood pressure and temperature) and provide justification for these skills used in clinical practice.

Purpose of recording vital signs

Nurses have more contact with the patient than any other healthcare professional. Monitoring, interpreting and acting upon vital signs are a key part of the nurse's role, which places them in the best position to monitor the patient's progress, identify (or predict) problems early and make decisions about the best interventions required to resolve or minimise the problem. Vital signs are taken and recorded in a number of different situations, e.g. when the patient is admitted to the accident and emergency department; on admission to the practice setting; at regular intervals as part of the care package; prior to and following some procedures such as surgery (for investigation or treatment); and when the patient's condition is deteriorating.

After having taken the vital signs, nurses should compare the observation data to previous ones (analysing) and, in particular, look at any trends and patterns. Any abnormalities can then be identified and acted upon promptly. In identifying a patient's normal baseline, current measurements can be compared against what is considered normal for that particular patient. What needs to be considered when analysing observation data is the patient's normal baseline. Do remember that what is normal for one patient may be abnormal and potentially life-threatening to someone else, e.g. a patient with chronic obstructive pulmonary disease (COPD) may have a normally higher breathing rate. Where possible, knowledge of normal parameters for that patient, and their past medical history, is essential to enable an individualised assessment.

Nurses have a responsibility to take and record vital signs, i.e. using the correct (and fully functioning) equipment and following the correct technique. Documentation should reflect the findings and should be legible. Decisions regarding treatment are likely to be based upon the findings, any misrepresentation of the true findings could have detrimental effects on the patient's outcome or condition.

Any abnormalities in vital signs should be reported to the healthcare professional in charge of care, e.g. the nurse in charge or the doctor. The frequency of monitoring and recording vital signs varies and should reflect the severity of the patient's condition. Hence, for critically ill patients, vital signs should be recorded at least every 15 minutes to half an hour. If the patient has recovered from their illness uneventfully, this may then be every four hours. Senior staff will make a decision about the frequency of recordings.

Respiration

Changes in respiratory status are one of the early indicators of acute illness or deterioration and account for one of the main reasons for admission to critical care units and are a key predictor of cardiac arrest. Despite evidence from the NPSA (2007) and NCEPOD (2012) showing that patients have a clear recorded evidence of marked physiological deterioration before a cardiac arrest, anecdotal observations suggest that a comprehensive respiratory assessment continues to be neglected in general clinical practice.

An audit on observations concluded that respiratory rate was missing from many patients' charts, even when shortness of breath was identified as an actual problem (NPSA, 2007). This is in spite of the fact that recording respiratory rate is a simple, basic, bedside observation.

Rationale for respiratory assessment

There are many reasons why patients have dyspnoea (difficulty in breathing) or shortness of breath. Causes of dyspnoea may not necessarily originate from direct lung problems (e.g. asthma, chronic obstructive pulmonary disorder (COPD), and pulmonary embolism), but can also be cardiac (e.g. left ventricular failure); due to the central nervous system (e.g. head injury, opiate drugs, sedatives); circulatory (e.g. shock); or endocrine (e.g. diabetic ketoacidosis (DKA)). It is beyond the remit of this chapter to discuss these conditions. Dyspnoea has been identified as a significant preceding factor to adverse events and is the first early warning sign of patient deterioration. Therefore, this particular assessment should be performed at regular and appropriate intervals on most patients, i.e. those who may develop potential problems with their breathing as well as patients with identified respiratory problems.

The main purpose of respiratory assessment is to assess the efficiency of gas exchange, i.e. the adequate intake and transportation of oxygen into the body and the removal of waste products from the body. Therefore, a sound knowledge of normal anatomy and particularly the physiology of the respiratory system is crucial. A comprehensive and competent assessment enables the early recognition of a compromised respiratory status and allows the nurse to initiate early intervention to support and improve gas exchange. During the immediate assessment it is vital to recognise and treat immediately any life-threatening conditions that may be the underlying cause of respiratory dysfunction, e.g. severe asthma, pulmonary oedema (fluid accumulation in alveoli). Changes in the respiratory system affect every other system in the body, hence, a detailed respiratory assessment constitutes a critical component of a patient's physiological health status.

History taking is important as this will affect expectations from the assessment data in terms of normal parameters. This information also aids an individualised, contextualised assessment and the setting of expected outcomes. History taking also enables the assessment of mental status, establishing whether the patient is oriented to time and place.

Don't forget!

The mental health status of a person may have an effect on their breathing. Studies have found that an estimated 4.4 per cent of people in England experience a generalised anxiety disorder (McManus *et al.*, 2009) and that panic attacks affect 3–4 per cent of the population (Stein *et al.*, 2009). These disorders may give rise to phenomena such as feelings of shortness of breath, or hyperventilation. Other studies have found that people who have a serious mental illness are more likely than the general population to suffer respiratory diseases such as chronic bronchitis, emphysema and asthma (Robson and Gray, 2007) due to lifestyle behaviours, particularly smoking.

Top tip

- Those patients prone to feelings of anxiety or panic may experience an exacerbation of these symptoms during a physical assessment. Quiet reassurance by the nurse or carer, together with encouragement for the person to practise simple relaxation techniques, such as deep breathing, may help allay their feelings of anxiety.
- The patient's age and stage of development should be considered alongside the respiratory assessment, including children. The assessment should be performed as discreetly as possible, so as to avoid them being aware of the process and altering their breathing patterns.

Activity 7.1

Reflect on a patient that you have cared for.

- How did you assess their respiratory status?
- What clinical signs would indicate to you that they are struggling to breathe and required help? Consider the areas below;
  - Rate, pattern, depth, sounds, work of breathing, posture, skin colour, symmetry of chest movement, deformities of chest, pain, mental status, cough, secretions.

Case study (adult) 7.1

Read the following case studies, discuss what and how you would assess the patients' respiratory status. Compare your answers to the discussions in the text.

John Ross, 55 years old, is married, with two grown-up children who live away from home. Generally, he strives to live an active life but has smoked for most of his adult life. He has a history of depression and is finding it very difficult to give up smoking, although he has told the medical team that he has given up. Currently, he is smoking 25 cigarettes a day.

John has suffered from intermittent abdominal pain for the past two years. In the past, John has chosen to ignore the pain. Over the past three days his pain has become progressively worse. He has seen his General Practitioner, who referred him immediately to his local hospital for investigation and treatment.

This is John's first admission to hospital. A diagnosis of gastric ulceration was made which required surgery. Initially John was very nervous about being admitted to hospital and had numerous sleepless nights prior to admission. On admission to the ward he looks visibly anxious, his pulse rate and blood pressure are higher than normal.

John had his surgery as planned. He had a vagotomy (cutting of the vagus nerve to reduce hydrochloric acid secretion in the stomach). This was performed through a laparoscopy (a surgical procedure where a fibre optic instrument is inserted through abdominal wall). There were no immediate complications post-surgery. John returned to the ward to recover.

The first two post-operative days were uneventful. On the third day he looks unwell and is complaining of severe abdominal pain (his post-operative pain has never completely been under control). This pain is making it difficult for John to breathe properly (especially deep breathing) and he cannot get out of bed and move around as he should do, post operatively.

Findings

John is breathing spontaneously but is dyspnoeic (finding it difficult to breathe). His respiratory rate is 30 per minute, regular but shallow and he is using his accessory muscles (Sternocleidomastoid – passes obliquely across side of neck; Scalenus – side of neck; Trapezius – across neck, shoulders and vertebrae and abdominal). He has an unproductive cough (absence of coughing up sputum). He looks pale but has no other changes in skin colour.

John's heart rate is variable, with an average rate of 120 beats/minute. He looks pale and sweaty. His blood pressure is 160/110 mmHg and oxygen saturation levels are 87% on 40% inspired oxygen. John responds to verbal instructions but appears drowsy.

Case study (child) 7.2

Baby Charlie, aged 4 months, has been unwell for the past 24 hours. His mum, Jayne, is concerned as he has not been feeding well, taking only half of his normal milk feed. To mum, he appears lethargic. He has a temperature of 38.1°C, a runny nose and a dry cough. Over the past 6 hours, he has vomited his feed, appears to be breathing faster and is irritable.

Findings

Jayne has seen the GP who makes a diagnosis of Acute Bronchiolitis (inflammation of the bronchioles) and refers Charlie to the local paediatric unit at the hospital.

On admission, Charlie has a temperature of 38.5°C, respiratory rate of 66 (tachypnoea) and is using his accessory muscles for breathing. His pulse rate is 152 bpm (tachycardia), and blood pressure is 72/55 mmHg. He has a cough and is irritable. He looks pale with no other changes in colour.

Preparation of the patient

This is best conducted in a well-illuminated environment (which is not always easy to accomplish). The room should not be cold, as shivering distorts assessment findings.

When performing this skill, where possible, there needs to be minimal distraction to nurse and patient, if patients are anxious, it may cause false changes in their respiratory rate and pattern. If able, the patient should be sitting upright (supported by pillows) to facilitate lung expansion, allow access to the anterior and posterior thorax and provide an opportunity for a more accurate assessment. Document the position of the patient when the assessment was performed, as this could influence findings.

Try not to make it too obvious when assessing the patient as this may also be a cause of anxiety to them. Some aspects of the assessment will require consent. For example, if you are assessing for deformities of the chest, you will need access to patient's bare chest. You may also need to put your hand on the patient's chest to assess the depth of breathing.

Rate

■ Rate is considered the most useful sign in determining clinical signs of deterioration and is also viewed as antecedent to an adverse event.

Consider what the patient was doing before the assessment and allow them to rest (where possible) for 5 minutes before counting. Count the patient's breathing (inhalation-exhalation) for 1 full minute. This allows assessment of any irregular patterns of breathing. In some practice settings, if the patient's respiratory pattern is regular, the practice is to count the rate for 30 seconds and then multiply the answer by two. This is not viewed as good practice as the patient's respiratory rate can change from one reading to the next very quickly.

In children, it is important to count the breathing for one full minute, observing the movement of the chest. Children have a limited ability to increase their pulmonary functional residual capacity, hence, they increase their ventilation primarily by an increased respiratory rate rather than taking deeper breaths.

Clinical significance

The patient's level of activity immediately prior to assessing their rate of breathing may influence results. If the patient is aware that their breathing is being counted, it may prompt them to breathe faster.

Box 7.1 Normal respiratory rate

What is considered normal respiratory rate is age-related (Table 7.1). Common alterations to rate include tachypnoea and bradypnoea:

- *Tachypnoea* – higher than the normal rate. This is the most common abnormality of rate and represents the first indicators of respiratory distress (for both adults and children). It can also be seen as a result of pain, hyperventilation/anxiety, sepsis (severe infection), and pulmonary embolism.
- *Bradypnoea* – lower than the normal rate. This includes disorders that cause central nervous system depression, e.g. opiates, fatigue, severe hypoxia, hypothermia.

Table 7.1 Normal respiratory rate and age

Age	Rate (breaths per minute)
Newborn–1 year	30–60
1–3 years	24–40
4–5 years	22–34
6–12 years	18–30
Adolescent	12–16
Adult	12–20

Source: Dieckmann *et al.* (2000).

Pattern

- The normal breathing pattern has regular intervals with expiration lasting slightly longer than inspiration. The ratio of breaths per heart rate usually 1:4 (Ball *et al.*, 2015).

Altered patterns of breathing may indicate underlying disorders, e.g. Kussmaul's respiration (referred to as 'air hunger'). This is seen in diabetic ketoacidosis as deep and rapid breathing. It is the body's attempt to correct acidosis. Cheyne-Stokes respiration is an irregular pattern with periods of apnoea, and generally indicates marked hypoxaemia.

Depth

■   Depth of respiration gives an indication of the adequacy of the tidal volume.

Measuring the depth of respiration (volume normally inspired or expired during one breath) can be subjective if you are relying on looking at the chest. A spirometer (Figure 7.1) should be used if available, as this is the most accurate way of measurement (through tidal volume). The normal tidal volume for an 'average' adult is 500 mls and for a school-aged child is 8–10 mls/kg. For the infant and small child, who is self-ventilating, this measurement is not always accurate.

Note whether the patient is breathing deeply or in a shallow manner. If unsure, put your hand on their chest and gauge how far it rises and falls. If little movement is felt under your hand, then respirations are assessed as being 'shallow'. Shallow breathing is cause for concern as this is a characteristic of respiratory distress (see 'Work of breathing' section). It is highly likely that patients with tachypnoea will have a low tidal volume (shallow breathing).

Chest movements may be difficult to view in a patient with quiet shallow breathing, particularly when unconscious. Sometimes, if patients feel that they are being watched, it may lead them to automatically breathe deeply.

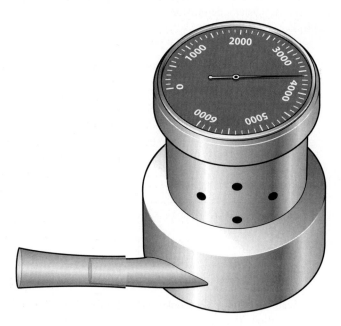

Figure 7.1 **Spirometer**

Procedure for measuring tidal volume using a spirometer

1 Explain the procedure to the patient and where possible gain consent.
2 Wash and dry hands before and after procedure.
3 Instruct the patient to breathe normally into the tube and then read the dial.
4 Do not instruct the patient to take a deep breath as you want to measure their true tidal volume at that time. A deep breath will falsely increase the results.
5 Take the best result out of three readings.

Sounds of breathing

Normal respiration is quiet but unusual sounds such as grunting, snoring, gurgling may indicate respiratory distress and this is a medical emergency, see Chapter 10. For breath sounds, see Chapter 9.

Work of breathing

■ This is an indication that the patient is finding it difficult to breathe, i.e. there is an increase in the 'work of breathing'.

If an intervention does not occur quickly, or the patient/child does not respond to treatment, they will become exhausted and require help with their breathing (non-invasive or invasive ventilation). The patient will use their accessory muscles (sternocleidomastoid, scalene and trapezius) (Figure 7.2) to help them increase their lung expansion. They will also feel sweaty and slightly cool (unless they have a high temperature) and in this instance would be hot to touch.

The patient's difficulty in breathing may be relieved by sitting upright (orthopnea) or may not (platypnoea is difficulty in breathing when sitting upright).

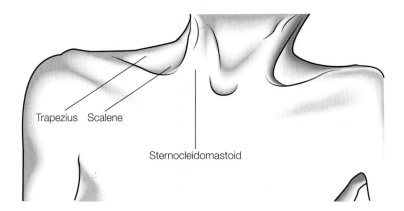

Figure 7.2 **Active accessory muscles of respiration**

Clinical significance

An inability to talk in complete sentences, known as 'staccato speech', indicates that the patient's main effort is focused on trying to breathe adequately and this is a sign of severe respiratory distress. In addition, patients feeling sweaty or clammy may indicate increased work of breathing.

Children can deteriorate very quickly. Nasal flaring (nostrils move in and out during breathing – like an angry bull) and mouth breathing are more common in children with difficulty in breathing. Increased respiratory rate, shoulders rising on inspiration, head bobbing (movement of the head) with intercostal retractions (an inward movement of the intercostal muscles between the ribs, resulting from reduced pressure in the chest cavity), the abdomen and chest will look like they are being sucked in with every breath, indicate respiratory distress.

A baby normally uses their abdominal muscles to breathe and a school-aged child uses their costal muscles for breathing. Respiratory distress should be suspected in a baby who uses its costal muscles and a child using its abdominal muscles to breathe.

Posture

- Description of the patient's posture is often omitted in the assessment.

Those with impaired respiratory function often adopt a 'tripod' position. The patient leans forward with hands on knees or a table, it is a technique to 'splint' the lungs to allow maximum expansion (Figure 7.3). This is a sign of impending decline in respiratory function. The patient sits in the Fowler's (upright) position. Splinting is a technique used to help minimise pain on coughing and moving and enable the expulsion of sputum and secretions. This allows increased diaphragmatic movement as the internal organs gravitate downwards.

Skin colour

- This can be difficult to detect and is subject to observer variability, particularly in dark-skinned patients, although it may be observed by looking at the oral mucosa.

Changes in skin/mucous membrane colour (nail beds, fingertips, nose and under the tongue) provide information regarding the adequate or insufficient removal of carbon dioxide. Central cyanosis (a bluish discoloration) is a late clinical sign of respiratory problems and so other assessment information should be noted and acted upon before changes in skin colour become apparent.

There are two levels of cyanosis:

1   *Peripheral cyanosis* occurs when there is adequate oxygenation of the circulating blood, but abnormalities of local circulation are present (sluggish peripheral circulation) as seen in shock. This is visible in nail beds, fingertips and toes.
2   *Central cyanosis* represents gross hypoxaemia, indicating that the patient is very ill.

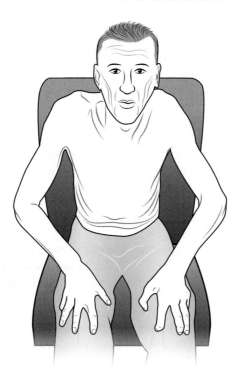

Figure 7.3 **Tripod position**

It is usually detectable when the arterial oxygen saturation is less than 85 per cent (BTS, 2008). Central cyanosis can be seen in any disorder that can cause hypoventilation (shallow breaths), e.g. pneumonia, severe asthma, pulmonary oedema, pulmonary embolism, COPD, polycythaemia (increased amount of red blood cells). Clinical signs include blue discoloration of lips, nose, mucous membrane of the mouth and tongue.

Watch out

Cyanosis is a late sign and should not be relied upon entirely. Extreme caution should be exercised with patients who are anaemic as they will rarely appear cyanosed due to insufficient haemoglobin to produce the blue colour of the mucous membranes, characteristic of cyanosis (Moore, 2007).

Symmetry of chest movement

■ Chest should be moving bilateral and equal, expanding on inspiration and expiration (see Chapter 9).

This includes assessing both sides of the chest wall which should normally expand equally during breathing (i.e. both sides are rising and falling together). If this cannot be seen clearly, stand in front of the patient with both hands firmly placed on the anterior thorax so that equal expansion of the chest wall can be assessed. The depth of each breath and equality of chest movement should also be noted. It may be necessary for both hands to be placed on each side of the anterior chest wall on the lower ribcage to simultaneously feel the chest movement.

Failure of the chest wall to rise adequately may indicate lung fibrosis, collapse of upper lobes or bronchial obstruction. If one side demonstrates less movement, this may be indicative of pneumothorax. Delayed chest movement may suggest congestion or consolidation of the underlying lung tissue.

Deformities of chest

■ Any deformity of the chest can influence lung expansion and reduce the gas exchange.

Look at the chest – it may appear as a 'barrel' shape (anterior and posterior diameter is approximately double the measurement of the side-to-side diameter (Figure 7.4)). This is associated with emphysema, affecting lung expansion. Look at the spine for deformities: kyphosis or scoliosis (abnormal curvature of the spine) (Figures 7.5 and 7.6). Spinal deformities can compromise tidal volume and the capacity to breathe normally.

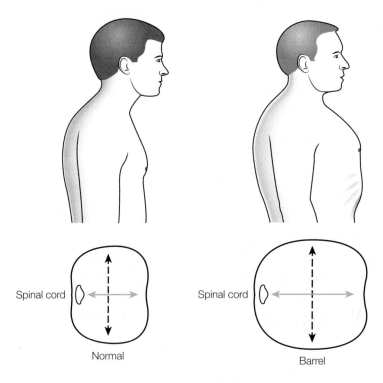

Figure 7.4 **Barrel-shaped chest**

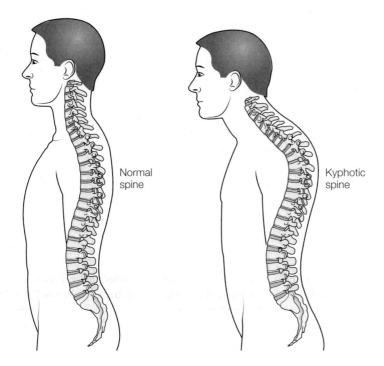

Normal
spine

Kyphotic
spine

Figure 7.5 **Kyphosis of the spine**

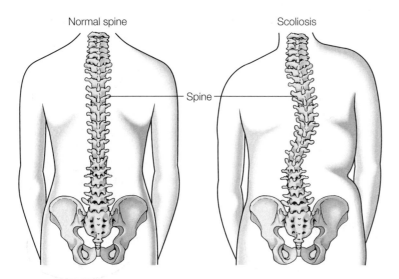

Normal spine

Scoliosis

Spine

Figure 7.6 **Scoliosis of the spine**

Other deformities such as clubbing (abnormal curvature of the nail and swelling of the terminal part of the digit of fingertips/toes), nail thinning and an abnormal alteration in the angle of the finger and toes may be present (indicative of pulmonary or cardio-vascular disease).

Pain

▨   The pain experienced may not necessarily be from the lung in origin but could still influence the patient's ability to breathe properly.

Note the type of pain – central stabbing chest pain with or without radiation down left arm and up left side of face or chest tightness – may indicate myocardial ischaemia. Pleuritic chest pain is characterised by sharp/stabbing/localised pain which is worse when breathing or coughing and may indicate pulmonary embolism or pneumothorax.

Pain often causes a reduction in tidal volume, this may also be complicated by retention of sputum in the alveoli, resulting in possible alveoli collapse (atelectasis). Assessment of pain in a child should be performed using an appropriate assessment pain tool, depending on the child's age and stage of development together with the use of play. Their family or carer may also help with this if required.

Remember to ask the patient to describe (if able to) the location, type, frequency, severity of pain in their own words (see chapter 5).

Mental status

▨   The findings of the assessment may demonstrate that the patient has developed hypoxaemia.

Answering the following questions will help you in this assessment.

▨   Does the patient look alert?
▨   Is the patient orientated to time and place? Speak to them, ask simple questions (in relation to time; where they are; who they are).
▨   Do consider age, stage of development cultural differences that may affect interpre-tation/understating of questions.

In babies, assessment could include recognition of a familiar voice, carer's face, favourite toy. Young children who can vocalise can be asked the above questions, using simple, age-appropriate language. Ask parents/carer for their conclusions of the child's mental status.

Clinical significance

A reduced level of consciousness or confusion often presents with hypoxaemia, and aggression or agitation are seen with hypercapnia. Patients may also experience a feeling of suffocation and panic. In addition, language barriers/cultural influences must be considered with the assessment process as the patient may simply not understand instructions or questions.

Cough

- Inflammation or infection almost anywhere in the upper or lower respiratory tract may produce a cough
- A cough is a defence mechanism to protect the airway from inhaled foreign material as well as clearing secretions. It can be a voluntary action but most are involuntary responses to an irritant, e.g. dust, smoke, upper/lower respiratory tract infections.

If the patient has a cough, the assessment should include observing the following characteristics:

- Regularity
- Presence or absence of pain
- Distinctive sounds (e.g. whoop or bark, bubbling)
- Strength of cough
- Is the cough unproductive (dry and or 'tickly') or productive (producing sputum)?
- Secretions – listen to their breathing, there may be a 'rattling' sound heard which could indicate fluid or sputum in the lungs. If a spontaneous cough is not present and you suspect that there is some retention, ask the patient to cough in order to try and expectorate it
- Degree of breathlessness after coughing
- Change of colour to face during coughing (may become blue, red, very pale).

Sputum can be a useful indicator of lung pathology:

- White, frothy, pink (bloodstained) – may indicate pulmonary oedema
- Frank blood (haemoptysis) – possible pulmonary embolism or active tuberculosis (TB)
- Bloodstained (streaks) – could imply pneumonia, abscess, aspiration (stomach contents)
- Purulent green and copious – usually suggests infection
- Black (tar) – usually old blood from very heavy smoking or industrial job, e.g. mining
- Rusty/brown – may be a sign of tuberculosis (TB), lung cancer.

This is an important assessment to perform as it can indicate if the patient has difficulty in clearing the lungs of sputum or fluid. If the patient is unable to cough and expectorate, the sputum can build up and their condition will deteriorate very quickly.

Don't forget!

The respiratory system's function is to exchange oxygen and carbon dioxide in the lungs and tissues and the regulation of the acid-base balance. The elimination of carbon dioxide relies upon adequate total ventilation (minute volume) of the lung and adequate blood supply of oxygen.

Top tip

Ideally, during one shift, the same nurse is required to conduct the complete assessment, reducing the risk of observer variations, particularly in terms of depth of breathing and skin colour.

Pulse

Assessing the pulse is a quick and non-invasive way of examining the patient's cardiovascular status. Change in the pulse is another early warning sign of clinical deterioration.

The main purpose of pulse assessment is to assess the efficiency with which the heart acts as a pump – distributing adequate blood to the organs of the body. Therefore, a sound level of knowledge of normal anatomy and physiology of the cardiovascular system is vital. A comprehensive and competent assessment enables the early recognition of a compromised cardiovascular status and will help in the initiation of early intervention (to support and improve cardiac output). During the immediate assessment it is vital to diagnose and treat immediately any life-threatening conditions, e.g. shock.

Rationale for assessing pulse

Assessing the pulse is an integral part of clinical assessment of a patient. All patients at some point would have had this assessment performed, on admission or initial contact to establish a baseline for comparison of future measurements.

Essentially, the rationale is the same for both adult and child. All clinical conditions will affect the pulse in some way, so knowledge and understanding of the role of the pulse are essential. Changes in the pulse will inevitably affect the blood pressure (normally lowering it), potentially impacting on every bodily system. Hence, assessment of the pulse constitutes an essential component of a patient's physiological health status.

This particular assessment should be performed at regular and appropriate intervals and should not be restricted to patients with identified cardiovascular problems as some patients may develop potential problems with their cardiovascular status (e.g. complications post operatively).

Other reasons for assessing the pulse include:

- Assessment/evaluation of treatment, e.g. digoxin which slows and regulates the heart. Note: this medication must not be administered if the pulse rate is below 60 beats per minute (bpm)
- Monitoring for signs of reaction to blood transfusion/pharmacological intervention
- Assess for signs of clinical deterioration, e.g. early warning sign of shock.

The pulse is a wave of pressure representing the expansion of arteries during the systolic phase (blood ejected into the aorta), initiating a wave of pressure through the arterial system and recoil during the diastolic phase of each cardiac cycle.

The pulse can be felt as pulsations wherever an artery passes near the skin and over a firm or bony surface of the body. The pulse is strongest in arteries closest to the heart (central pulses, e.g. carotid, femoral) (Figure 7.7) and becomes progressively weaker as it passes through the arterial system (peripheral pulses, e.g. radial), disappearing in the capillaries as each pulse wave corresponds to a heartbeat.

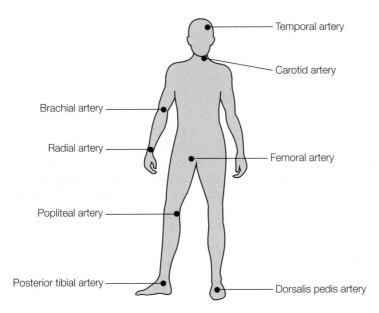

Figure 7.7 Arterial Pulse sites

Activity 7.2

Think about the challenges that you have encountered when assessing the patient's pulse.

■   How did you overcome these challenges?
■   Describe how you assessed the patient's pulse.

Pulse taking

Ideally, the patient should be resting for a period of ten minutes prior to this assessment. If the patient shows signs of emotional worries, this should be documented, as this may influence the pulse rate. If possible, wait until the emotion has minimised.

Assessment of the pulse involves the rate, rhythm and depth (the latter is sometimes referred to as pulse volume). Normally the radial pulse is assessed, however, if this is very weak or it cannot be felt (as in the case of shock when the blood pressure is severely low), then the central pulses should be assessed. Privacy and dignity should be maintained when measuring the femoral pulse. In this situation the patient is usually very ill and requires immediate medical attention.

Don't forget!

Care should be exercised when feeling the carotid pulse. This is because oxygenated blood is delivered to the brain via the carotid artery. Applying too much pressure too long, could reduce (or even stop) the blood flow to the brain, possibly causing a reduction in the level of consciousness.

Procedure for taking a pulse

1 Wash and dry hands before and after procedure.
2 Explain the procedure and where possible obtain consent.
3 Make sure the limb (normally the forearm and hand) is supported on a table, bed or your hand.
4 Hold the patient's hand and turn the palm of the hand upward.
5 Use the tips of your first two fingers (index and middle) from your other hand to locate the pulse. The radial artery is on the thumb's side (or outside) of the wrist.
6 Locate the thumb and slide your fingers down the 'groove' (half-way between the tendons that run down the centre of your forearm and the edge of the patient's arm).
7 Make sure your fingers are vertical (side by side) and not one finger 'stacked' on top of each other (Figure 7.8).
8 Press firmly (not too hard or you may occlude the artery and reduce/stop the blood flow). You should be able to palpate (feel) a pulse here. You will feel a pulsating motion under your fingers.
9 Count the number of beats for a whole minute. Also note the strength and rhythm of the pulse.
10 Document your findings (NMC, 2015).

For the newborn, babies and infants, use a stethoscope to hear the sound of the heartbeat. Place the stethoscope on the infant's chest, between the sternum and left nipple. The heartbeat has a double sound. Listen for a whole minute to establish the rate of the heart (apex beat).

For the child, assess the heart rate by palpating the brachial arterial pulse. Place your index and middle fingers on the pulse point to establish the pulse. Count the pulse for one full minute. The literature is variable in what is considered to be 'normal' parameters for the child (Table 7.2). Local policies should offer direction in terms of local policies and expectations.

A slow heart rate is called bradycardia (Box 7.2) and a fast heart rate is called tachycardia (Box 7.3).

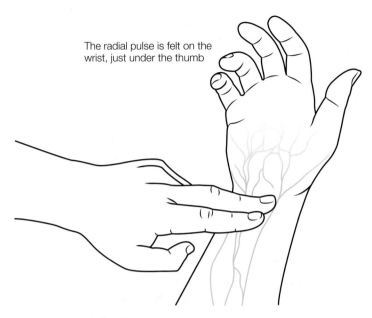

The radial pulse is felt on the wrist, just under the thumb

Figure 7.8 Taking a radial pulse

Table 7.2 Normal pulse rates at rest

Age	bpm
Newborn	120–160
1–12 months	80–140
1–2 years	80–130
2–6 years	75–120
6–12 years	75–110
Adolescent and adult	60–100
Well-trained athletes	40–60

Box 7.2 Causes of bradycardia, slow heart rhythm

- *Cardiac dysrhythmias* – due to problems with the sinoatrial or atrial ventricular node (see Chapter 10)
- *Hypothermia* (temperature less than 35 degrees Celsius) – due to decreased impulses from the sinoatrial node
- *Disorders of the nervous system/neurological insult* – due to impaired control of autonomic nervous system (sympathetic and parasympathetic nerves)
- *Drugs* e.g. beta-blockers – reducing the effects of epinephrine.

Box 7.3 Causes of tachycardia, fast heart rhythm

- *Emotion* (anger or excitability) – e.g. if a patient is very anxious, the sympathetic nerve would be stimulated and there would also be a surge of adrenaline into the circulation (blood) increasing the heart rate
- *Exercise* – due to release of epinephrine and lactic acid into the bloodstream
- *Drugs* – e.g. bronchodilators (to relax the smooth muscle in the bronchi); thyroid hormone replacement, anti-depressants, amphetamines (to stimulate the sympathetic nerves)
- *Temperature* – due to increased metabolic rate
- *Shock* – due to increased sympathetic nervous activity and release of adrenaline, vasoconstriction
- *Hypoxaemia* – due to increased sympathetic activity to distribute oxygen around the body.

Rate

- Electrical impulses are generated from the heart itself, this creates muscular contraction to eject blood from the ventricles. The sympathetic and parasympathetic nerves; hormones (epinephrine or norephinephrine) influence the pulse rate.

If the pulse rate is either too fast (greater than the highest parameter) or too slow (less than the lowest parameter), the filling of the heart (with blood) during each cardiac cycle may be reduced. In turn, cardiac output may be reduced, causing a lowering of blood pressure.

Rhythm

- Normal rhythm should be regular but some patients may have long-term arrhythmias, e.g. atrial fibrillation. Any changes to their 'normal' rhythm should be noted and reported immediately.

Note if the pulse has a regular, irregular or regular irregular pattern. Irregular patterns feel erratic, unsteady and uneven. Regular irregular patterns are regular patterns overall with 'skipped' (missed) beats (see Chapter 8).

Volume

Volume is indicative of the patient's circulatory blood volume. So, if the blood volume is low (e.g. bleeding, loss of bodily fluids), the pulse volume will also be low (weak and thready). If the pulse is slow, it may indicate a high stroke volume and, as there is a long time between each ejection of blood, the pulse pressure (the difference between systolic and diastolic pressure) will be high.

When counting the rate of the pulse, also note whether the pulse is weak, normal, or too strong (bounding). This is a subjective observation that should become more accurate with experience.

Apex and radial assessment

There is a cardiac condition known as atrial fibrillation (see Chapter 8), and this creates a difference between the heart rate and the pulse rate. This is known as the 'pulse deficit'. Two measurements are required to assess a pulse deficit: apex and radial.

Procedure for assessing a pulse deficit

1   Wash and dry hands before and after procedure.
2   Explain the procedure and its purpose (this will help reduce any anxieties that will influence the heart rate) and where possible gain consent.
3   This procedure requires two people – one to assess the apex pulse rate and the other to assess the radial pulse rate. This assessment also requires effective coordination.
4   The apex pulse is listened to through a stethoscope.
5   Locate the pulse site on the left side of the chest (apex of the heart) below the left nipple. Put the diaphragm of the stethoscope over the apex pulse and listen for heart sounds, which sound like 'lub dub'.
6   At the same time, the second person should locate the radial pulse.
7   A watch with a second hand should be visible to both people undertaking the assessment.
8   At the same time both the apex pulse and radial pulse are counted for one full minute. Hence, starting and finishing times should be the same.
9   One person should take responsibility to indicate when to start counting and when to finish. Apart from the rate, rhythm and depth (radial pulse volume) should also be noted.

Ensure that the apex pulse rate, the radial pulse rate and the difference between the two (pulse deficit) are recorded (NMC, 2015). In good health, the pulse deficit should be zero. A pulse deficit occurs when some of the chaotic impulses from the sinoatrial node do not filter through the atrioventricular node.

If a patient has atrial fibrillation, the recording could be as follows:

Apex pulse rate is 124, radial pulse rate 96, making the pulse deficit = 28 bpm.

The apex pulse will ALWAYS be higher or equal to the radial pulse, never lower.

Top tip

In clinical practice, machines (pulse oximeters) are frequently used to record the pulse. However, the pulse should always be assessed manually (apart from critical care areas), these only record the rate and not the volume or rhythm of the pulse.

Don't forget!

For patients who have a tachycardia, you should always feel the depth of the pulse and this is likely to be weak. Do not rely on the machines only when observing the pulse.

Blood pressure

In addition to assessing the pulse, blood pressure monitoring is one of the most frequently observed vital signs and provides valuable information about the integrity of the cardiovascular system. It is another marker for clinical deterioration in patients but is viewed as a later sign.

Blood pressure represents the pressure exerted on the walls of the arteries during ventricular systole and diastole. Systole is the highest pressure of ventricular contraction and represents the pressure of the surge of blood going into the arteries. Diastole is the lowest pressure in the ventricles and occurs during relaxation of the heart.

Blood pressure is measured in millimetres of mercury (mmHg) and is written as a fraction – with systolic on the top and diastolic on the bottom – e.g. 120/80. It is dependent upon cardiac output (CO) and systemic vascular resistance (SVR) (Figure 7.9):

$$BP = CO \times SVR$$

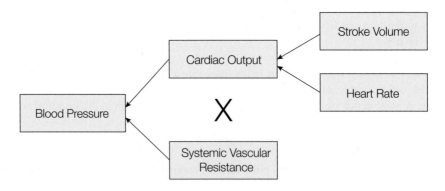

Figure 7.9 **Measuring blood pressure**

Cardiac output (CO) is the amount of blood ejected from the left ventricle during each minute and is influenced by the heart rate (HR) and stroke volume (SV) (Figure 7.10). Stroke volume is the amount of blood ejected from the ventricle during each beat:

$$CO = HR \times SV$$

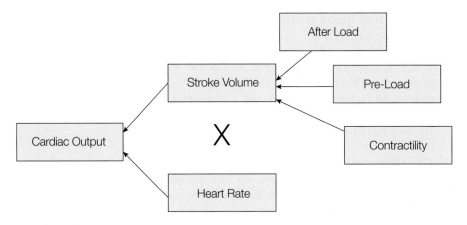

Figure 7.10 Measuring cardiac output

Stroke volume is dependent upon factors such as circulatory blood volume, vascular tone, vascular resistance, and contractility of the myocardium.

Neural and hormonal systems also play a role in the regulation of blood pressure. Baroreceptors (found mainly in the aorta and internal carotid arteries) detect the pressure within the vessels. Compensatory mechanisms to maintain adequate blood occur, a reduction in pressure would stimulate vasoconstriction (narrowing of the arteries and arterioles) in an attempt to maintain blood pressure.

Hormonal influences include production of angiotensin 2, causing vasoconstriction and stimulating the release of aldosterone (which reabsorbs water and increases blood pressure). Vasoconstriction is also caused by the production of epinephrine and norepinephrine, ensuring the blood flow to the organs is reduced.

Antidiuretic hormone (ADH) is released as a response to the reduced osmotic pressure. This stimulates the release of ADH, causing vasoconstriction and a decrease in cardiac output.

Watch out

Due to the body's compensatory mechanisms, blood pressure may be the last sign to indicate deterioration. Therefore, other clinical signs should be closely monitored.

Changes in the blood pressure (particularly compensatory) will affect the pulse (normally tachycardia). As the blood pressure controls the perfusion to the organs, potentially every organ in the body is affected by changes in the blood pressure.

Rationale for assessing blood pressure

Assessing the blood pressure provides information relating to cardiac output, the ability of the heart as a pump and the integrity of the blood vessels in order to maintain adequate tissue perfusion. This assessment is an integral part of clinical practice. Like the pulse assessment, all patients would have had a blood pressure assessment performed on admission or initial contact.

The purpose of recording blood pressure is:

- To enable baseline comparisons
- To monitor post procedures/operations for complications (hypo- or hypertension)
- To monitor alterations caused by the disease processes, e.g. cardiovascular disease, renal disease
- To provide an assessment/evaluation of treatment, e.g. antihypertensive drugs, which lower the blood pressure
- To monitor for signs of reaction to blood transfusion or pharmacological intervention
- So that undetected hypertension may be diagnosed.

Essentially, all clinical conditions may affect the blood pressure, hence knowledge and understanding of the role of the blood pressure are essential. A comprehensive and competent assessment enables the early recognition of a compromised cardiovascular status and the initiation of early intervention to support and improve cardiac output.

Factors affecting blood pressure

These factors can be a combination or physiological, social, psychological origins and include the following:

- *Contraction (pumping action) of the heart* – a weak myocardium (heart muscle) will result in a reduced stroke volume and consequently cardiac output and a low blood pressure (hypotension). Alterations to the apex pulse (increased rate) will reduce the filling time of the heart and therefore a reduced cardiac output
- *Systemic vascular resistance* – vasoconstriction can occur, e.g. shock and hypothermia. This results in a temporary increase in blood pressure. Vasodilatation (widening of the arteries/arterioles) occurs, resulting in reduction in the amount of blood to the heart, thus lowering blood pressure
- *Disease process* – e.g. arteriosclerosis (hardening of the inner layer of the artery)
- *Blood volume* – hypovolaemia, a decrease in circulating blood volume from fluid loss, haemorrhage or dehydration will reduce the amount of blood returning to the heart (pre-load). Thus, affecting the amount of blood (cardiac output) leaving the heart, lowering the blood pressure. Equally, if there is an increase in blood volume by the patient retaining fluid or being overloaded with too much fluid from infusions, the blood pressure will increase (hypertension)
- *Anxiety/stress/emotions/pain* – increases the heart rate, reduces the filling time of the ventricles and hence causes a reduction in blood pressure

- *Diet* – too much salt (causes fluid retention), alcohol and caffeine increase blood pressure
- *Ethnicity* – people of Afro-Caribbean and Asian origin have a higher incidence of hypertension, due to their diet
- *Drugs* – normally as part of treatment. There are many medications available to either increase or decrease blood pressure, e.g. ibuprofen can increase blood pressure and diuretics can decrease blood pressure
- *Gender* – women who are premenopausal have lower blood pressure than men of the same age. Those who are postmenopausal have higher blood pressure
- *Age* – blood pressure gradually increases with age due to atherosclerotic changes in the arteries
- *Diurnal variations* – blood pressure peaks in the late afternoon or evening and is at its lowest in the early hours of the morning during deep sleep.

A child's blood pressure varies with age and is closely related to the child's height and weight. Emotional states, including pain, may result in a rise in actual blood pressure.

Factors affecting blood pressure recording

- *Poor technique*: This includes the incorrect procedure for measuring blood pressure; failing to use equipment as recommended by the manufacturer's guidance; using incorrect size cuff; or if there are leaks, kinks and twists in the stethoscope
- *Faulty equipment*: Equipment should be regularly maintained and calibrated (particularly automated devices). The bladder and cuff should not be worn or torn. There should be no leaks in the outlet valve and tubing.

Watch out

It is imperative that this procedure is performed using the correct technique. Failure to do so will lead to the wrong blood pressure measurement being recorded and a possible wrong diagnosis that could result in unnecessary or inappropriate management for the patient.

If the patient has a problem with their blood pressure, ALWAYS use a manual device.

Normal blood pressure

Blood pressure increases throughout the ageing process. In the literature there are inconsistencies as to what constitutes a 'normal' range of blood pressure for children (Table 7.3).

Table 7.3 **Normal blood pressure and age**

Age	Systolic (mmHg)	Diastolic (mmHg)
0–3 months	65–85	45–55
3–6 months	70–90	50–65
6–12 months	80–100	55–65
1–3 years	90–105	55–70
3–6 years	95–110	60–75
6–12 years	100–120	60–75
12 years +	110–135	65–85
Adult	120–140	80–90

Source: Dieckmann *et al.* (2000).

Procedure for taking blood pressure

Prepare the patient:

1 Ideally, the patient should be resting for a period of five minutes prior to this assessment. This may prove difficult to achieve and is not always appropriate, particularly in the instance when the patient's physiological condition is deteriorating.

2 Note if the patient is showing any emotions, has pain, has ingested caffeine, a meal, alcohol or smoked 30 minutes prior (these may cause an increase in blood pressure). In children, sucking, crying and eating can also influence results and should be documented. If possible, give the patient time to calm down, and administer analgesia for pain.

3 Explain the procedure to the patient in accordance with their level of knowledge and understanding, including why it is important for them to keep their limb still.

4 Gain their consent especially in relation to applying cuff pressure, which can cause discomfort and pain. Caution is required for the child as this may cause more distress than the actual procedure.

5 When taking this assessment for the first time, it is necessary to record the blood pressure on both limbs (patient's general condition allowing). If there is a difference of more than 10 mmHg, this should be reported and further assessment undertaken (usually by the doctor).

6 The limb should be free from any clothing as this will influence the measurement, providing false results.

7 Maintain patient privacy and dignity.

8 The patient's legs should not be crossed as this elevates the blood pressure.

The devices used to measure the blood pressure are:

■ Aneroid sphygmomanometer (Figure 7.11)
■ Digital sphygmomanometer (Figure 7.12)

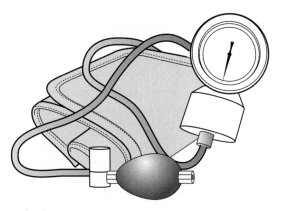

Figure 7.11 **Aneroid sphygmomanometer**

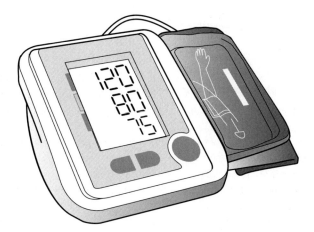

Figure 7.12 **Digital sphygmomanometer**

- Automated device (Figure 7.13)
- Generally the mercury sphygmomanometer has been phased out of use in clinical practice (MHRA, 2005) due to its danger (if the column containing the mercury was broken) but these may still be seen in some GP practices (Figure 7.14).

The manufacturer's guidance should be followed when using any of the devices. The use of the automated device is very popular in clinical practice. It is advisable that all students should practise manual blood pressure measurements as often as possible.

Normally, the upper arm is selected for this procedure. The upper arm should not be used if a patient has the following affecting both arms:

- Burns
- Amputation
- Trauma or fractures

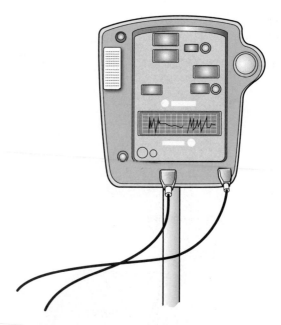

Figure 7.13 Automated device to measure blood pressure

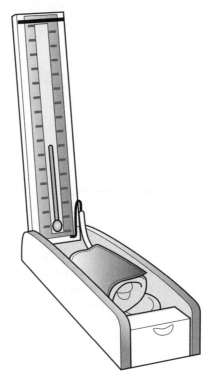

Figure 7.14 Mercury sphygmomanometer

■ Intravenous infusions
■ Diseased or injured shoulder.

The thigh should be used in these instances, using the popliteal artery (Figure 7.15).

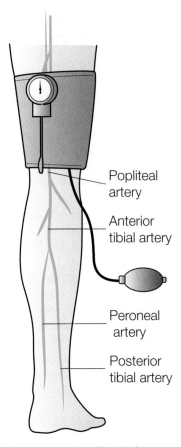

Popliteal
artery

Anterior
tibial artery

Peroneal
artery

Posterior
tibial artery

Figure 7.15 Taking blood pressure using the thigh

However, it is inappropriate to use the thigh if:

■ Any of the problems for the upper arm stated above affect the thigh
■ There is occlusion by large dressings or bandages
■ The patient is receiving renal dialysis (creation of arteriovenous fistula).

Alternatively, a cannula may be inserted into the femoral artery and attached to a monitor. The blood pressure will then be continuously recorded on the monitor (wave-like forms). This is known as direct (invasive) blood pressure monitoring. The radial artery is selected and usually performed in critical care areas.

For children under 3 years of age, the palpation method should be used. Use play to explain this procedure, e.g. demonstrate it on a doll. This measurement may need to be done first as other uncomfortable procedures will cause emotional disturbances and hence affect blood pressure.

1   The patient should be in a sitting position, unless their condition contradicts this; for example, low blood pressure and spinal injury.

2   Ensure that the device is working properly with no leaks or kinks in the rubber tubing.

3   Select an appropriate size blood pressure cuff. Size is considered in relation to the width of the cuff. The circumference of the patient's limb (normally upper arm) is used to determine this. The cuff width should be 40 per cent of the limb circumference, and the length should be 80 per cent of the circumference of the patient's limb. Hence, limb circumference and not age determines the size of the cuff.

4   Cuff sizes are infant, child/paediatric, small adult, adult, and large adult (i.e. 14–45 cm). The right size is important. If the cuff is too small, it will over-inflate, over-constrict and be very uncomfortable for the patient. In addition, the recording will be falsely high. If the cuff is too large, it will move around the arm and the recording will be falsely low. A variety of different size cuffs should be readily available.

5   Wash and dry hands before and after the procedure. Ideally, the patient's same arm should be used for the pulse assessment. Avoid using the arm with intravenous fluids administered or pulse oximetry readings.

6   Feel the patient's pulse – if the pulse is irregular, use a manual device NOT an automated device (NICE, 2011) as recordings may be inaccurate.

7   The arm should be slightly flexed and with the palm of the hand facing upwards and supported (on a table if possible). The position should be at the same level as the heart. If the arm is below the level of the heart, the blood pressure will be decreased, if the arm is above the level of the heart, blood pressure will be increased.

8   Completely deflate the cuff (Figure 7.16) and ensure it is free from any trapped air (this can be achieved by opening the valve fully (turning it counter-clockwise) and squeezing the cuff).

9   Apply the cuff over the brachial artery (Figure 7.17). There is an arrow on the cuff to indicate its correct position. Place the cuff approximately 2.5 cm above the antecubital fossa (the crease of the arm, anterior to the elbow, this is the position of the brachial pulse).

10   Place the device at the same level as the limb.

11   The systolic pressure should be identified to prevent over-inflation of the cuff. This is achieved by closing the valve (turning it clockwise), with the other hand, palpate the brachial pulse (see section on pulse above) and inflate the cuff until the pulse disappears. Quickly inflate for a further 20 mmHg with the bulb (NICE, 2011) and then release the valve slowly, paying close attention to the dial. The systolic pressure will be indicated when the pulse is felt again.

12   Deflate the cuff quickly and fully. Now, locate the brachial pulse (located on the inner side of the antecubital fossa), place and hold the diaphragm side of the stethoscope over this position on the skin, and inflate the cuff to 20–30 mmHg (NICE, 2006) above the previous systolic reading, release the pressure slowly and at a

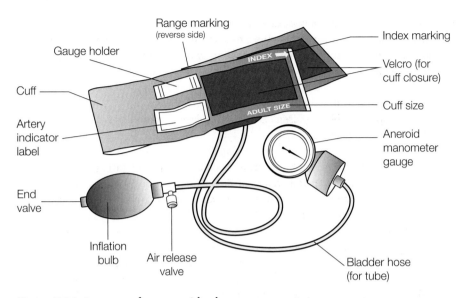

Figure 7.16 **Anatomy of an aneroid sphygmomanometer**

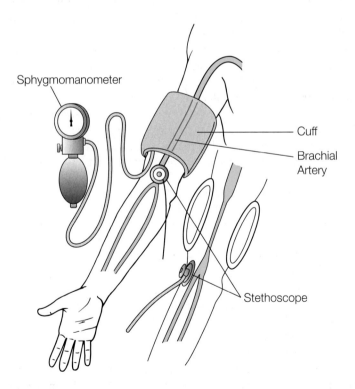

Figure 7.17 **Taking blood pressure using the brachial artery**

controlled rate (a deflation rate of 2–3 mmHg per second, NICE, 2011), otherwise the sound will be missed, watching the dial at all times (accuracy of recording is imperative). The sound phases you need to identify are the first (systolic) and last (diastolic) sounds. These are called the Korotkoff sounds (Table 7.4).

13 Once the very last sound is heard, continue to deflate quickly, ensuring all air has been removed from the cuff.

14 Document your findings (NMC, 2015). Normally the systolic and diastolic pressures are recorded.

15 Follow local policy in relation to cleaning the cuff. This is a source of infection and should be cleaned after each use (unless one is used per patient).

16 If there is a significant difference in blood pressure from the last reading, it is necessary to recheck it. Report any significant changes to the person in charge.

Table 7.4 **Korotkoff sounds**

Phase	Sound
1	A faint, sharp 'thudding' sound
2	Softer, swishing sound
3	Return to a sharp thudding sound but softer than phase 1
4	Fading, muffling that is softer in quality
5	Sound has completely disappeared.

Top tip

Try not to let the patients see the rise and fall of mercury, it could lead to unnecessary anxiety and cause an increase in blood pressure.

Clinical significance

Clinical signs of hypotension (generally more acute, sudden) include: increased pulse, dizziness, skin looks pale and is clammy (sweaty) to touch, urine output is decreased.

Signs of hypertension (generally more chronic) include: headache, warm flushed face, nose bleeds without injury.

Don't forget!

DO NOT round up or down to the nearest 5 mmHg or 10 mmHg of the reading. Record the exact measurements. The wrong recordings will initiate the wrong treatment, or worse, the seriousness of the patient's physiological condition may not be realised. Report immediately any changes in the patient's blood pressure.

Don't forget!

There is a difference of approximately 20–30 mmHg (adult) and approximately 10 mmHg (child) in the systolic pressures of the posterior popliteal artery and the brachial artery. The diastolic is generally the same (Frese *et al.*, 2011).

Automated devices

An automated device is non-invasive, and quick and easy to use, reducing the need to listen. As a result, its use has become more popular in clinical practice, particularly in acute settings.

However, this device has been proven to be unreliable in patients with existing alterations to their blood pressure (Bern *et al.*, 2007). A sensor in the cuff detects pulsations from the patient, therefore it is unreliable when pulse pressures are low, or when arrhythmias or hypertension are present. Where the accuracy of blood pressure monitoring is essential, or pulse pressures are low, manual recordings should be taken. Some machines over-inflate the cuff causing gross discomfort and bruising.

Procedure for taking a lying and standing blood pressure

Sometimes it is necessary to assess the patient's blood pressure in a lying and standing position. This is to assess a clinical condition known as postural hypotension, where the patient stands up from a lying position and their blood pressure drops considerably. As a result, they feel dizzy or may even faint (syncope). Caution needs to be exercised during this procedure in order to maintain patient safety.

1   Wash and dry hands before and after procedure.
2   Explain the procedure to the patient and where possible gain consent.
3   Lying blood pressure should be recorded first.
4   Ensure that the patient has been lying supine (on their back) for approximately ten minutes.
5   Take and record the blood pressure as described earlier.
6   Allow sufficient time for the position change to standing (patient should be standing for one minute (NICE, 2011)) before measuring the blood pressure. If the patient cannot stand at the side of the bed, record the blood pressure in the sitting position with the legs hanging down over the edge of the bed.
7   If the patient complains of feeling dizzy, put them in the supine position immediately then take the blood pressure.
8   Report to the nurse in charge.
9   Clearly document findings (NMC, 2015).

Alternative interventions

If the Korotkoff sounds cannot be heard, it will be necessary to palpate the brachial artery instead. It is important that this information is documented as it may indicate that the patient's cardiac output is low. Korotkoff sounds may not be reliably heard in children under the age of three. When measured in the legs, the blood pressure reading might be slightly higher than that recorded in the arms.

Using the thigh to measure the blood pressure will involve the patient lying supine with their knee slightly flexed as the posterior popliteal artery (see Figure 7.15) is used. If the prone position cannot be tolerated by the patient, then the supine position should be adopted.

Follow the same procedure as highlighted, the cuff selected will need to be larger (as the circumference of the thigh is larger). Ensure that the bladder of the cuff is placed directly over the posterior popliteal artery.

Temperature

Body temperature is not assessed as often as pulse, breathing, pulse and blood pressure unless the patient has an identified problem with temperature regulation. Nonetheless, it is an important observation and should be performed at regular and appropriate intervals.

Rationale for assessing temperature

Assessing temperature can provide information regarding the body's ability to successfully maintain homeostasis. Maintaining a constant temperature is vital for a suitable environment to support body cell function. By measuring body temperature, the core temperature is estimated.

Reasons for assessing temperature include:

- To establish baseline data and to determine if the core temperature is within normal range
- To identify changes which could indicate clinical problems, e.g. post-operative hypothermia, sepsis
- To evaluate patients who are at risk of temperature alterations, e.g. hypothermia in the elderly, very young, the homeless, unconscious patients, or hyperthermia due to infection
- To evaluate treatment, e.g. antipyretic medication, antibiotics
- To monitor for signs of an allergic reaction, e.g. reaction to blood transfusion
- To monitor patients who have diseases affecting the metabolic rate, e.g. thyroid (hypothyroidism/hyperthyroidism).

As well as recording the temperature with a thermometer, additional observations should also be performed. For example, note if the patient's skin feels cold, warm, hot or sweaty to touch; is the patient complaining of feeling hot or cold?; is the patient shivering or huddled in a ball to try and keep warm?

Thermoregulation

In order to understand the significance of taking a temperature, it is important to understand normal temperature regulation (Box 7.4). Despite variations in extreme heat (hot and cold), the body is remarkably good at maintaining a constant temperature. Regulation of temperature is a homeostatic process that ensures a balance between heat production and heat loss. This is due to a negative feedback mechanism – any changes start a physiological response in order to maintain a constant body temperature. The hypothalamus, the body's thermostat, is located in the brain and controls the body temperature.

Box 7.4 Factors affecting body temperature

The following factors should be taken into consideration when assessing the patient's temperature:

Exercise	Body metabolism is increased, therefore increasing body temperature
Stress	Metabolic activity is again increased
Age	The very young and very old are sensitive to environmental changes in temperature. Due to the ageing process, older people have a decreased thermoregulatory control, making them susceptible in extreme weathers (i.e. extreme heat/ extreme cold)
Environment	If the body's homeostatic control cannot regulate changes in the environmental temperature, the body will not adjust
Circadian rhythms	Fluctuations in body temperature can be as much as 1°C and it is at its highest point normally between (20.00 and 24.00 hours) and lowest during deep sleep.

If the skin temperature is hot, the hypothalamus sends signals to the parasympathetic nervous system causing vasodilation of the arterioles in the skin, directing warm blood from the core organs (e.g. liver, heart) to the skin. Heat loss through radiation and conduction is increased. The patient will feel sweaty as the sweat glands in the skin produce more sweat.

If the skin temperature is cold, a variety of responses are initiated to conserve the heat in the body and to increase heat production. Peripheral temperature receptors in the skin stimulate the hypothalamus to send signals to the sympathetic nervous system, causing vasoconstriction, decreasing the flow of blood and thus heat to the skin, preventing heat loss. Shivering, which is the involuntary constriction and relaxation of the skeletal muscle, occurs in an attempt to increase heat production in the muscles by increasing the metabolic rate. To maintain an adequate core temperature, blood is also redirected to the vital organs (e.g. heart, brain, kidneys). This causes the skin to feel cool.

Heat is produced as a by-product of cellular metabolism and is lost through the mechanisms of:

- *Radiation* – transfer of heat without contact between the surfaces of both objects, mainly in the form of infrared rays, e.g. the sun transfers heat to the Earth through radiation
- *Convection* – the process of losing heat through the movement of air or water molecules across the skin, e.g. the use of a fan to cool the body
- *Conduction* – is the transfer of heat through physical contact with another object or body of a lower temperature, e.g. if touching someone who is very cold, the heat from one person would transfer to the colder person
- *Vaporisation* – this is the evaporation moisture from the skin, mouth and respiratory tract. Heat is lost through the conversion of water to gas (respiration).

Activity 7.3

Reflect on the ways in which you have measured a patient's temperature.

- Did the patient have problems with maintaining a normal body temperature? What were the causes?
- How did you measure the patient's temperature?

Watch out

Alterations in body temperature such as hypothermia include severe shivering, pale cool skin, hypotension (low blood pressure), tachycardia, and confusion. Coma can occur in severe cases. Causes of hypothermia are usually accidental (exposure to cold) or could reflect problems with the thermoregulatory system.

Causes of pyrexia usually represent infection somewhere in the body. Clinical signs include warm/hot skin, sweating and tachycardia.

Different areas of the body have different temperatures. The core temperature (inside the body) is higher than the 'shell' temperature (skin). Generally, temperature is measured in degrees Celsius. Normal body temperature is considered to be:

Oral	36.5 °C–37.5 °C (NICE, 2008)
Axillary	36.0 °C–36.7 °C
Tympanic	37.5 °C
Rectal	36.2 °C–37.7 °C

Top tip

Whenever a child feels warm to touch, measure their temperature immediately, even if it was previously normal a short period of time prior (NICE, 2013). Children under 3 are vulnerable to seizures (febrile convulsion) as a result of a high temperature.

It is important that nurses choose the most appropriate device/route to assess the patient's temperature. In order to achieve this, advantages and limitations of each should be noted. There are four main routes for taking a temperature – oral, axillary, rectal and tympanic. The same route should be used to assess the temperature at regular intervals and the route should be recorded.

There are various types of thermometers in use, e.g. alcohol (disposable or non-disposable) (Figure 7.18); digital (Figure 7.19), single use (Figure 7.20), and tympanic.

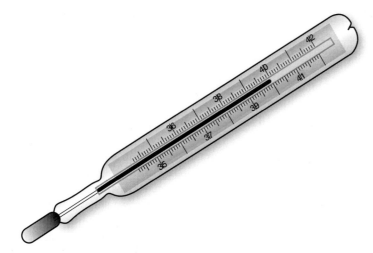

Figure 7.18 Alcohol thermometer

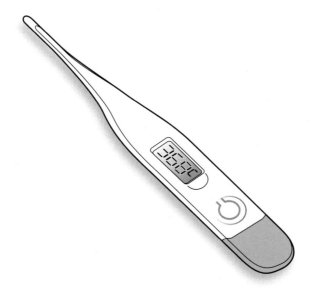

Figure 7.19 Digital thermometer

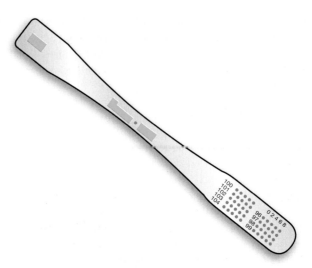

Figure 7.20 Single use clinical thermometer

■ *Alcohol thermometers*: Alcohol thermometers are either disposable or reusable. If reusable, it may have a sheath (plastic covering). The use of mercury thermometers should now be obsolete as mercury is a dangerous substance when ingested
■ *Digital thermometers*: These have a digital display and are usually for the oral or axillary route. They have a disposable plastic cover (for the silver end)
■ *Single use clinical thermometers*. This is a single use disposable thermometer. There are markings on the paddle side of the thermometer. A chemical mixture contained in each dot will turn blue when it gets to a certain temperature. Each dot represents half a degree.

Procedure for taking an oral temperature

The sublingual area (under the tongue) has a rich blood supply derived from the carotid arteries, which are close to the hypothalamus and the heart. Therefore, this allows changes in temperature to be quickly detected. The temperature taken by this route is also close to the core temperature.

Do not perform this procedure on the patients who are:

■ Confused
■ Mentally unpredictable
■ Semi-conscious or unconscious
■ Recovering from facial/oral surgery
■ Experiencing damage to the mouth, teeth and face (including sores)
■ Having difficulty in breathing
■ Receiving oxygen therapy.

NICE guidelines (NICE, 2013) suggest that this method should not be used with infants or very young children (0–5 years of age), as they have difficulty holding oral thermometers under their tongues long enough for their temperatures to be accurately measured. In addition, the child may accidentally bite or break the thermometer! For infants under the age of 4 weeks, an electronic thermometer should be used in the axilla and for infants and children who are 4 weeks to 5 years old, electronic or the single use clinical thermometers should be used instead either tympanic or axillary.

1 When taking an oral temperature, the patient should not have ingested orally hot or cold fluids, or have been smoking for at least 30 minutes prior to the measurement.
2 Wash and dry hands before and after procedure.
3 Explain procedure to the patient and where possible gain consent.
4 With the silver end of the alcohol thermometer pointing downwards, hold firmly at the clear end, use the wrist movement to flick it quickly a few times. This will move the fluid (silver line in the middle) down to the bottom.
5 There is no need to shake the digital thermometers. The result is displayed on the liquid crystal display (LCD) screen. It is important to ensure that it is switched on and that the screen is clear from old readings.
6 Ask the patient to open their mouth and curl up their tongue (Figure 7.21).
7 Place the thermometer (the silver tip end) under the tongue (posterior sublingual pocket of tissue).
8 Leave the thermometer in place as guided by the manufacturers – (alcohol thermometer, a minimum of 3 minutes; single use, 1 minute minimum). The digital thermometers will give a 'beeping' sound when ready. Look at the thermometer, where the silver line has stopped (on the graduated line), that is the temperature.
9 Clean the thermometer with an antiseptic (follow the manufacturer's guidance) and store in an appropriate container (usually plastic) to prevent breakage, or discard the covering sheath, this reduces the risk of infection.
10 Document findings (NMC, 2015).

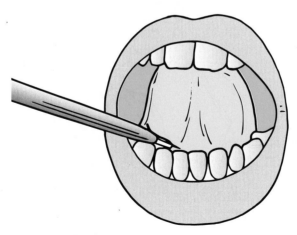

Figure 7.21 Thermometer under the tongue

Don't forget!

Oral temperature assessment should never be performed on a patient who is confused, mentally unpredictable, semi-conscious or unconscious as they may risk ingesting/swallowing the device.

Procedure for taking an axillary temperature

Taking the temperature under the axilla (under the armpit) is an alternative to oral temperature recording where the oral temperature cannot be taken. Do not perform this procedure on patients who are emaciated as there will be a large gap between the folds of skin in the axilla and the chest wall, allowing air to get through. It is also not suitable for those who are obese as the excessive fat layer may prevent the thermometer from being close to the axillary artery.

1   Wash hands before and after the procedure.
2   Explain procedure and where possible gain consent.
3   Maintain patient's privacy and dignity.
4   Ask the patient to elevate their elbow to expose the axilla. If they cannot do this, gently manually elevate this arm (taking care to support the elbow).
5   Ensure the axilla is clean and dry.
6   The silver tip of the thermometer should be placed vertically under the right armpit (Figure 7.22).

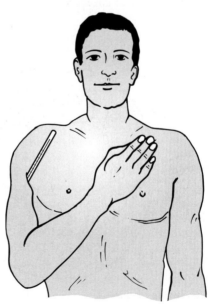

Figure 7.22 **Taking an axillary temperature**

7   Close the arm over the thermometer so that it is firmly against the chest, making it secure.

8   Follow the manufacturer's guidance for how long the thermometer should stay in place (a minimum of 7 minutes, (alcohol thermometer); 3 minutes for single use).

9   Remove and read the thermometer.

10   Wash hands and document findings (NMC, 2015).

Don't forget!

The axillary method provides the least accurate results, so another method should be used if accuracy of the temperature is important.

Procedure for taking a tympanic temperature (ear drum)

Blood flowing through the tympanic membrane is measured via a tympanic thermometer (Figure 7.23). The thermometer is placed in the external auditory canal. It is recommended for use with children under 5 years (NICE, 2013). Do not use this type of thermometer on patients following aural (ear) surgery or those with excessive ear wax/ear discharge.

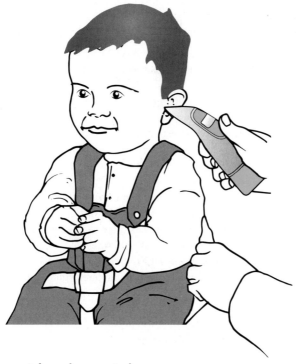

Figure 7.23 Using an infra-red tympanic thermometer

1   Wash hands before and after procedure.
2   Explain procedure and where possible gain consent.
3   Use play techniques with children to gain cooperation.
4   Place the disposable cover over the probe.
5   Instruct the patient to keep their head still, gently pull the earlobe up then back and insert the probe into the ear canal. DO NOT FORCE THE PROBE. This is a quick procedure, normally 1–2 seconds. A beeping sound will indicate when the results are ready.
6   Remove the thermometer and discard the disposable cover.
7   Record the findings (NMC, 2015).

Procedure for taking a rectal temperature

This route is considered to be closest to the core body temperature and is therefore more accurate than the other routes. Except in the instance of critical illness or hypothermia, this method should not be routinely performed on children (NICE, 2013), and never on babies younger than 6 months. Student nurses should always be supervised when taking a rectal temperature because of the risk of perforating the rectum.

For the same reasons, this procedure should not be performed on patients who have irritations to their large bowel (e.g. bowel perforation), have recently undergone rectal surgery, those who have diarrhoea or haemorrhoids and those with clotting disorders, as they can haemorrhage very easily.

1   Wash hands before and after procedure.
2   Explain the procedure and where possible gain consent.
3   Maintain the patient's privacy and dignity.
4   Ask the patient to lie on their side with knees flexed (left lateral position is best) (Figure 7.24).
5   Expose the buttocks only (taking great care to ensure privacy and dignity), exposing as little of the buttocks as possible.
6   Ensure that the rectal area is clean and dry.
7   Use thermometers designed solely for the use in the rectum. Some may have a sheath.
8   With a non-sterile gloved hand hold the thermometer and lubricate the first third (helps minimise trauma).
9   Insert up to 1.5 cm of the thermometer very gently inside the rectum. DO NOT FORCE THE THERMOMETER IN PLACE.
10 The patient may contract their buttocks – try to reassure them and distract them if possible. Maintain patient's dignity at all times.
11 Hold the thermometer in place until the end of the procedure, which should take approximately 3 minutes (follow the manufacturer's guidance in terms of the length of time). Remove carefully.
12 Wipe lubrication from the rectal area and thermometer.
13 Allow patient to get dressed.
14 Clean the thermometer with an antiseptic (follow manufacturer's guidance) and store in an appropriate container. If the thermometer has a sheath, discard it.
15 Document findings (NMC, 2015).

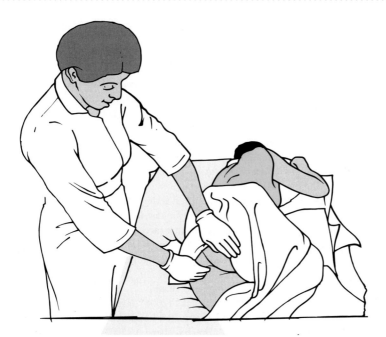

Figure 7.24 Inserting a rectal thermometer

Top tip

Do not take a rectal temperature on a patient who has a cardiac condition. The thermometer/probe could stimulate the vagus nerve in the rectum and cause cardiac arrhythmias (abnormal heart rhythm).

Summary

Monitoring and interpreting vital signs – temperature, pulse, respiration and blood pressure are a fundamental part of the nurse's role. A comprehensive assessment of vital signs in addition to using the correct assessment methods will reduce errors. From this information an evaluation of the patient's responses to intervention, i.e. improvement or deterioration in their physiological status can then be identified.

References

Ball, J.W., Danis, J.E., Flynn, J.A., Solomon, B.S. and Stewart, R.W (2015) *Seidels Guide to Physical Examination*, 8th edn. St Louis, MO: Elsevier.

Bern, L., Brandt, M., Mbelu, N., Asonye, U., Fisher, T., Shaver, Y. and Serrill C. (2007) Differences in blood pressure values obtained with automated and manual methods in medical inpatients. *MEDSURG Nursing*, 16(6): 356–361.

British Thoracic Society (2008) Guideline for emergency oxygen use in adult patients, *Thorax*, 63 (supplement V1): vi–68.

Dieckmann, R., Brownstein, D.R. and Gausche-Hill, M. (eds) (2000) *Pediatric Education for Pre-hospital Professionals.* Sudbury, MA: Jones & Bartlett.

DoH (Department of Health) (2009) *Competencies for Recognising and Responding to Acutely Ill Patients in Hospital.* London: Department of Health.

Frese, E.M., Fick, A. and Sadowsky, H. (2011) Pressure measurement guidelines for physical therapists. *Cardiopulmonary Physical Therapy Journal*, 22(2): 5–12.

McManus, S., Meltzer, H., Brugha, T., *et al.* (2009) *Adult Psychiatric Morbidity in England, 2007.* Leeds: The NHS Information Centre for Health and Social Care.

MHRA (2005) *Report of the Independent Advisory Group on Blood Pressure Monitoring in Clinical Practice.* London: MHRA.

Moore, T. (2007) Respiratory assessment in adults, *Nursing Standard* 21 (49): 48–59

National Patient Safety Agency (2007) *Safer Care for the Acutely Ill Patient; Learning from Serious Incidents.* HYPERLINK www.npsa.nhs.uk (accessed 9 September 2011)

NCEPOD (2007) *Emergency Admissions: A Journey in the Right Direction?* London: National Confidential Enquiry into Patient Outcome and Death.

NCEPOD (2012) *Cardiac Arrest Procedures: Time to Intervene?* London: National Confidential Enquiry into Patient Outcome and Death.

NICE (National Institute for Clinical Excellence) (2006) *Hypertension: Management of Hypertension in Adults in Primary Care.* CG no. 34. London: NICE.

NICE (National Institute for Health and Care Excellence) (2007) *Acutely Ill Patients in Hospital: Recognition of and Response to Acute Illness in Adults in Hospital.* CG no. 50. London: NICE.

NICE (National Institute for Health and Care Excellence) (2008) *Hypothermia: Prevention and Management in Adults Having Surgery.* CG no. 65. London: NICE.

NICE (National Institute for Health and Care Excellence) (2011) *Hypertension: Management of Hypertension in Adults in Primary Care.* CG no. 127. London: NICE.

NICE (National Institute for Health and Care Excellence) (2013) *Fever in Under 5s: Assessment and Initial Management*, CG no. 160. London: NICE.

NMC (Nursing and Midwifery Council) (2010) *Record Keeping: Guidance for Nurses & Midwives*, London: NMC.

NMC (Nursing and Midwifery Council) (2015) *The Code: Professional Standards of Practice and Behaviour for Nurses and Midwives.* London: NMC.

NPSA (National Patient Safety Agency) (2007) *Safer Care for the Acutely Ill Patient: Learning from Serious Incidents.* Available at: www.npsa.nhs.uk (accessed 9 Sept. 2011).

Robson, D. and Gray, R. (2007) Serious mental illness and physical health problems: a discussion paper. *International Journal of Nursing Studies*, 44: 457–466.

Stein, D., Hollander, E. and Rothbaum, B. (2009) *Textbook of Anxiety Disorders*, 2nd edn. Arlington, VA: American Psychiatric Publishing Inc.

Chapter 8

Monitoring and interpreting

Tina Moore

Any patient admitted into hospital is at risk of deterioration in their clinical condition due to their altered physiological state. For most of these patients, the monitoring of fundamental vital signs alone will be insufficient to detect significant physiological changes. Most patients will require more complex monitoring.

Key concepts

Central venous pressure (CVP) measurement

Mean arterial pressure (MAP) measurement

Lung auscultation

Arterial blood gas (ABG) measurement

Electrocardiography (ECG) interpretation

Reticular activating system (RAS)

Glasgow coma scale (GCS)

Arrhythmias

Neurological assessment

Learning outcomes

By the end of this chapter you will be able to:

- Demonstrate knowledge and understanding of how to assess and accurately measure a CVP, MAP, and GCS
- Select and correctly use appropriate equipment when measuring
- Discuss the complications associated with central lines and arterial stabs
- Understand the significance of measurement (CVP/MAP/ABG) in relation to the patient's cardiovascular (CVS) status
- Describe and interpret normal and abnormal lung sounds
- Recognise common arrhythmias.

Introduction

Often, when the patient's physiological condition deteriorates and they become acutely ill, the use of more complex equipment is necessary to monitor them safely. As a result, there will be occasions where student nurses will be allocated (under supervision) to care for such patients requiring more complex methods of assessment, making it necessary to use more specialised devices.

Normal ranges should be known and should act as comparative data. Any abnormalities in the patient's observations should be reported immediately to the nurse in charge of the patient's care. Generally, for acutely or critically ill patients, adults or children vital signs should be recorded at least every 15 minutes to half-hourly initially. If the patient's condition becomes stable or improves, this may be decreased to every 2–4 hours. But remember, the frequency of monitoring and recording observations will vary and reflect the severity of the patient's condition.

Central venous pressure measurement (CVP)

Central venous pressure measurements are often used to provide more in-depth knowledge of the patient's cardiovascular (CVS) status. Central venous pressure is the measurement of the blood pressure in the right atrium of the heart.

Rationale for CVP monitoring

While blood pressure measurements provide some essential information, they do not give information about intravascular blood volume, vascular tone, the effectiveness of the right ventricular function, the pulmonary vascular resistance and intra-thoracic pressure. Although the CVP does not measure blood volume directly, it can offer some information about intravascular volume, venous return, venous tone and intra-thoracic pressure. The use of CVP monitoring can provide early recognition of fluid imbalances and cardiac dysfunction – remember, this is crucial for the acutely or critically ill patient. Indications for central venous access would be for those patients who require the following:

- Continuous haemodynamic monitoring, e.g. if in shock
- Rapid administration of intravenous fluids, e.g. if in hypovolaemic shock
- Secure venous access for the infusion of drugs that cause irritation of the veins or that are administered directly into the heart, e.g. inotropic drugs. These drugs also require a very precise rate of delivery into the circulation
- Evaluation response to treatment, e.g. fluid resuscitation, inotropic support
- Frequent blood sampling (particularly in children)
- Venous access that cannot be obtained by other venous routes, e.g. the femoral vein.

Insertion routes

A central venous catheter (CVC) is an indwelling intravenous device that is inserted into a vein of the central vasculature and provides venous access into the right atrium of the heart. Common insertion sites include internal jugular vein (Figure 8.1) and the subclavian vein (Figure 8.2). The femoral vein (Figure 8.3) may also be used, particularly if there is no other option or in an emergency. However, this route has a higher risk of infection, haemorrhage and thrombosis, due to the length of the catheter – the distance from the femoral vein to the right atrium. Alternately, the basilic, cephalic or brachial vein just above or below the antecubital space (the area on the opposite side of the elbow) of the right arm may be used, this is known as a peripherally inserted central catheter (PICC). Using a PICC (Figure 8.4) route reduces the risk of pneumothorax that is associated with the subclavian access. PICC can be used for a range of treatments such as chemotherapy, blood transfusion, antibiotic therapy, IV therapy and withdrawal of blood. The line is a long, thin, flexible catheter that has a longer shelf life, and as a result, can be used in the community setting as well as hospital.

In children, the subclavian veins should not be used, particularly for those having

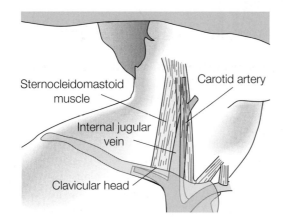

Figure 8.1 Internal jugular approach

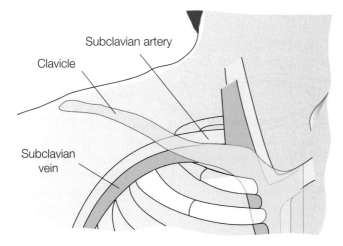

Figure 8.2 Subclavian approach

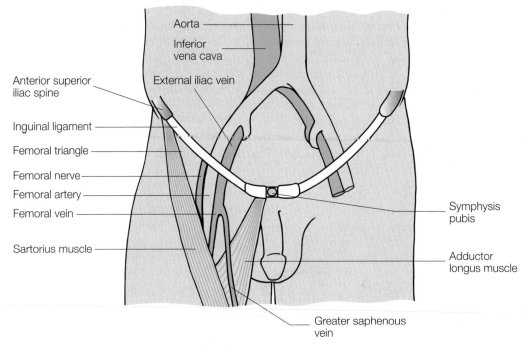

Figure 8.3 **Femoral approach**

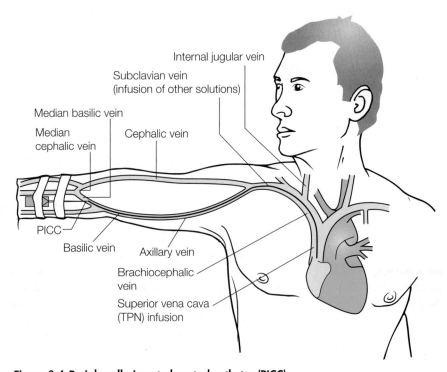

Figure 8.4 **Peripherally inserted central catheter (PICC)**

renal replacement therapy, as this can jeopardise future vascular access management if the child needs long-term therapy (BAPN, 2008). This is because cannulation of the subclavian vein has a high risk of stenosis or occlusion.

Types of central venous catheter are:

- single lumen (one line);
- double lumen (two lines);
- triple lumen (three lines) (Figure 8.5).

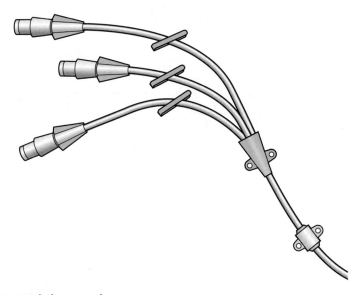

Figure 8.5 **Triple lumen catheter**

It is likely that more than one infusion will be prescribed, therefore a triple lumen should be used.

Ready-made CVP packs (Figure 8.6) are available, and consultation with local policies relating to equipment and procedure is advised.

Insertion of the CVC

Occasionally, in emergency situations, insertion of a CVC will be performed in non-critical care areas. As this is a sterile procedure and the risk of infection high, for non-emergencies, the patient may be transferred to the theatre department for this procedure. Ideally, two nurses should be available for this procedure – one to reassure the patient/parents and the other to assist in the procedure itself. Reassurance should include holding the patient's hand. Holding the patient's hand not only offers reassurance, but allows for detection of signs of deterioration (clinical signs of shock, i.e. pulse rate/ volume, warmth and colour of hand).

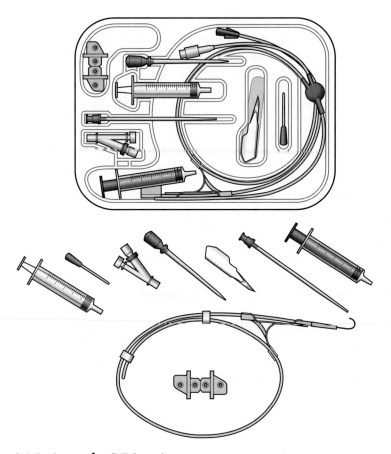

Figure 8.6 Equipment for CVP insertion

It is likely that the patient's face will be covered with the sterile drapes. Children and patients with mental health issues are less tolerant of their faces being covered, so the decision may be made to remove the drapes from the face. In this instance, it is important to ensure that the insertion area should be free from sources of infection (such as hair).

The insertion of the catheter should be performed by an experienced clinician. To reduce the risk of septicaemia, a strict sterile procedure has to be adhered to. Both the doctor inserting the line and the person assisting should wear sterile gowns, caps, gloves, and masks. The patient should be within a 'sterile field' with sterile drapes.

Ultrasound equipment may be used to aid with the location of the veins (NICE, 2002), making it a quicker and arguably safer procedure for the patient. For insertion, the patient should be in the supine (lying flat on the back) position. This enables the veins to become 'engorged' with blood, thus reducing the risk of air embolism on insertion. For easier access and to make the anatomical landmarks more visible, a pillow or rolled blanket (length-wise) may be placed under the shoulders for subclavian insertion (Figure 8.7).

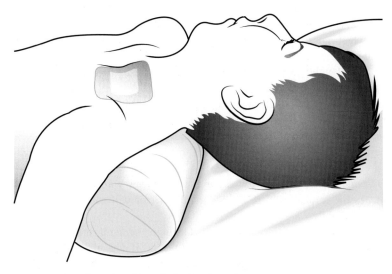

Figure 8.7 **Position of patient for subclavian insertion**

For jugular veins, place the pillow or back under the opposite shoulder. Some patients will have breathing difficulties and find lying flat impossible. If this position is not possible, then sitting slightly upright may have to be adopted but it will pose some risks.

Top tip

The use of play may be effective in gaining a child's cooperation. They may understand better if they are able to see a similar catheter in another child or in an adapted teddy bear or doll.

Once the catheter is inserted, an intravenous line is attached (usually 0.9 per cent sodium chloride) and infused very slowly until a chest x-ray has been performed to confirm the position of the catheter and rule out pneumothorax.

Problems which may occur during insertion

Some of these problems are now minimised with the use of ultrasound. However, during and after this procedure, an essential role of the nurse is to assess and monitor the patient's signs and symptoms for any problems. These could include:

■ *Arterial puncture* – positioned beside a large vein is often a larger artery (e.g. carotid, femoral, and subclavian). Therefore, there is a risk of accidentally puncturing the artery instead. Clinical signs may be missed in patients who are already hypoxic or hypotensive. If puncture of the artery is suspected, a senior healthcare professional may connect a length of manometer tubing to the needle/catheter and look for blood flow which goes higher than 30cm vertically or is strongly pulsatile. Remember, blood flow through the arteries pulsates, not in veins. If haemorrhage is evident, the doctor will withdraw the needle. Pressure should be applied to the puncture site for at least 5 minutes until the bleeding has stopped

■ *Pneumothorax* (subclavian access) – this occurs when the catheter punctures the chest wall and air enters the pleural space, causing collapse of a lung/segment of lung. Symptoms include breathlessness, chest pain, hypotension and tachycardia. A chest X-ray should always be performed post procedure to check if a pneumothorax is present

■ *Ventricular arrhythmias* – can occur if the catheter wire is inserted too far and touches the cardiac wall. If this occurs, the doctor will withdraw the wire of the catheter slightly

■ *Air embolus* – this can occur in hypovolaemia or wrong positioning, if the needle or cannula is left in the vein while open to the air. If possible, during insertion, the patient should be flat with the head slightly tilted down, this encourages venous engorgement and reduces risk of air entering the vein. All lines should be primed prior to connection

■ *Persistent bleeding at the point of entry* – apply firm pressure with a sterile dressing (as for arterial puncture). Any coagulation (blood clotting) abnormalities should be noted. Equally, any persistent severe bleeding may require surgical exploration and intervention

■ *Infection* – possibly resulting in septicaemia. Strict asepsis is critical.

Transducers

There may be times when it is essential to continually monitor the patient's CVP. In these instances, transducers (Figure 8.8) will be used. Transducers are used in critical care areas where the readings are displayed electronically on a monitor and are more accurate than manual recordings. To maintain patency of the line, the transducer tubing is kept under continuous pressure of 300 mmHg which causes a continuous flush of 3 ml/hr sodium chloride 0.9%.

The procedure to measure CVP

1   Explain the procedure to the patient/parents and where possible gain consent.
2   Wash and dry hands before and after procedure.
3   Position the patient – if possible, supine, although measurements can be taken in the semi-recumbent position (sitting up a 45 degree angle). Consistency is the key to whatever position is used to ensure accuracy for comparable readings. Clearly document the position selected.
4   Measurements can be taken at two points, i.e. sternal notch (Figure 8.9) and mid-axilla point (most common) (Figure 8.10).
5   Place the manometer arm (Figure 8.11) at the level of the right atrium (where the forth intercostal space and mid-axillary lines cross each other (phlebostatic

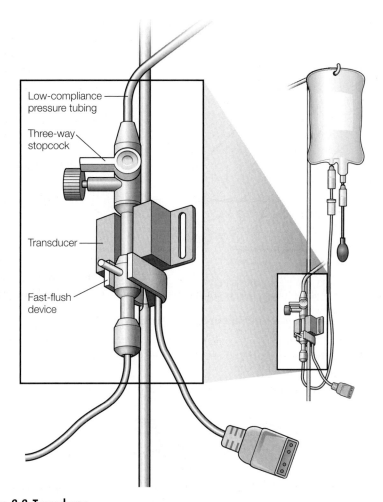

Low-compliance pressure tubing

Three-way stopcock

Transducer

Fast-flush device

Figure 8.8 **Transducer**

axis). Normally the area is documented and an 'x' placed on the patient's skin. For consistency of positioning and critical for accuracy of results, it is good practice for the nurse to locate the landmark for the first reading.

6   See Figure 8.12, for the direction of flow in the manometer. The white arrows on the three-way tap indicate the direction of fluid flow. Check the patency of the line (flush with 3–5 mls of fluid). Initially the white arrow (on the three-way tap) is turned straight up towards the manometer, allowing the fluid to flow from the fluid bag to the patient's CVC. If fluid does not flow freely into the patient's catheter, a valid CVP reading will not be obtained and the line has to be 'unblocked' before proceeding. Any fluid from this line infused into the patient should be recorded on the fluid balance chart. This is crucial in patients with problems associated with fluid balance and for children.

7   Position the manometer at the level of the right atrium (Figure 8.11).

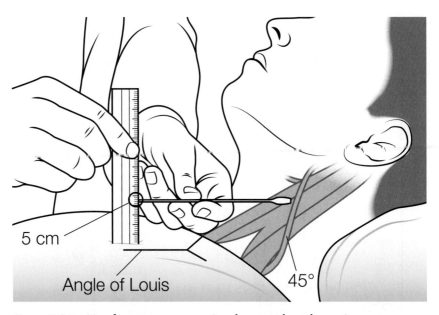

5 cm

Angle of Louis · 45°

Figure 8.9 Position for measurement using the sternal notch

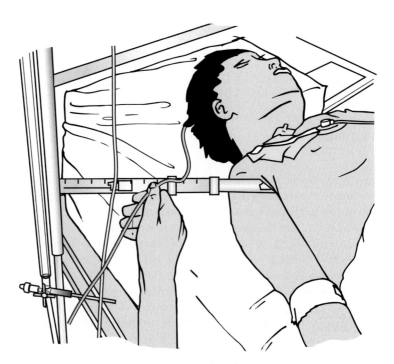

Figure 8.10 Position for measurement using mid-axilla point

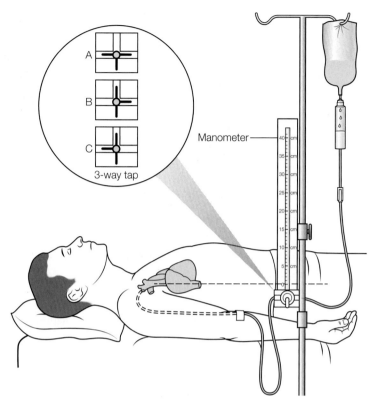

Figure 8.11 **Position of patient and manometer**

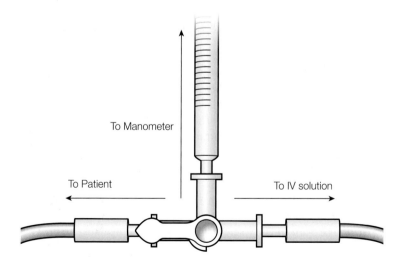

Figure 8.12 **Direction of flow in a manometer**

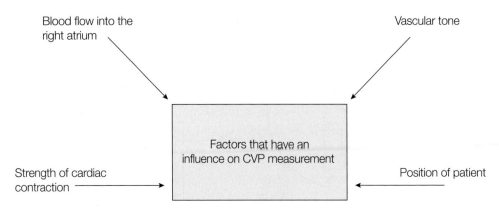

Figure 8.13 **Factors affecting CVP measurement**

8   Zero the manometer by moving the manometer scale up or down to allow the bubble (Figure 8.10) to be aligned with zero.

9   Turn the arrow toward the patient so that the fluid line is open to the manometer and the fluid will fill the manometer, taking care not to fill it right to the top. Some manometers have filters, if this gets wet, the readings will be inaccurate. The manometer should not contain any air bubbles or it will produce a false high reading.

10 If air is present in the manometer or fluid line going to the manometer, turn the clamps on luer lock connection, otherwise blood will flow out of the catheter. Disconnect the line and let the fluids run, overfilling the manometer until all air is purged from the system. Re-open the luer lock connection. Strict asepsis should be adhered to.

11 Turn the arrow toward the fluid line, closing this and opening the connection between the patient and manometer.

12 Observe the falling level in the manometer, fluid will run into the patient's catheter until the height of the fluid column exerts a pressure equivalent to the patient's central venous pressure.

13 The top of the fluid column will slightly oscillate up and down as the patient breathes. Record the mean level (where the fluid in the spirit level hovers).

14 Reposition and make patient comfortable.

15 Document findings (NMC, 2015). The trend of readings should be noted in conjunction with blood pressure, heart rate and urine output.

Significance of readings

A manual recording of CVP is measured in cmH_2o (centimetres of water), whereas those recorded via a monitor is in mmHg (millimetre of mercury). Generally, 'normal' values are considered to be 5–10 cmH_2o (manual) and 2–6 mmHg (monitor) for both adult and child.

Factors that affect CVP measurements (see Figure 8.13) are pre-load (amount of blood entering) into the right atrium, vascular tone, strength of cardiac contractions and patient's position. CVP may provide an inaccurate result if the patient has left ventricular dysfunction but the right ventricular function is unaffected. All observations of the patient (i.e. clinical signs, vital signs) need to be considered when interpreting results.

Causes of an *elevated* CVP (Figure 8.14) include: hypervolaemia – over-hydration (too much fluid intake); cardiac incompetence; heart failure (right- or left-sided); increased intra-thoracic pressure (tension pneumothorax, pulmonary embolism); obstructed or displaced catheter tip; or incorrect measuring technique. Additional assessment would include rate and depth of breathing (expecting tachypnoea and shallow breaths) and signs of pulmonary oedema (crackles on auscultation, dyspnoea, pink frothy sputum).

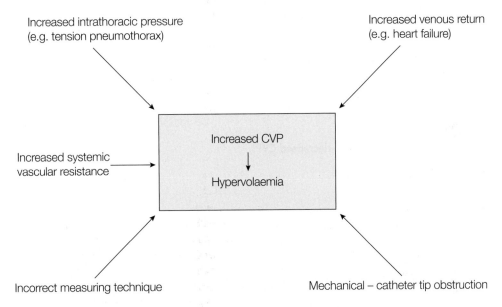

***Figure 8.14* Causes of increased CVP**

Decreased CVP (Figure 8.15) can be caused by: hypovolaemia/dehydration or excessive vasodilatation. Clinical signs include hypotension, tachycardia and oliguria. Intervention includes fluid challenge/replacement for hypovolaemia, possible inotropic support, or vasoconstrictive drugs.

Nursing care

To minimise the risk of infection, handling of the line should be kept to a minimum. The wound site should be covered by a non-occlusive dressing and wound management (see Chapter 12) performed in accordance to the local policy. Temperature should be monitored at least every 4 hours for signs of infection. It is necessary to inspect the wound site at least daily for signs of infection: swelling, redness or discharge (pus or blood).

Ensure lines are patent with no kinks or air bubbles. In the event of multiple drugs being administered, seek advice from the pharmacist regarding their compatibility and possible interaction.

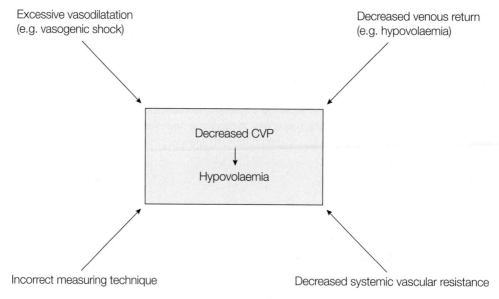

Figure 8.15 **Causes of decreased CVP**

Top tip

Patients are prone to neck stiffness and many are reluctant to move their head and neck as they may feel that they cannot do this, thinking they may dislodge the cannula. They should be encouraged to do gentle passive neck exercises and be reassured. Note – if the cannula is secure enough, it will not be dislodged by neck and head movements.

You should monitor for potential complications. These are shown in Box 8.1.

Removal of the CVC

Removal of the CVC requires the use of an aseptic technique. This procedure is performed by suitable qualified practitioners. Where possible, the patient should either be supine or slightly in the head-down position (the Trendelenberg position). The patient should be instructed to take a deep breath and hold or blow into a straw (the Valsalva manoeuvre). The catheter should then be gently removed.

Clinical significance

The Trendelenberg position and holding of the breath during expiration increase the intra-thoracic pressure, thus reducing the risk of air embolism.

Box 8.1 Potential complications of CVP

▪ *Haemorrhage* – from the catheter site or disconnection of the line. Patients who are particularly at risk are those with coagulation disorders.

▪ *Occlusion of the catheter* – from a thrombus or kinked tube. Keeping the line patent by a slow infusion if other infusions are not running through will reduce this occurrence.

▪ *Infection* – note any redness, pain, swelling around the catheter site. Send swabs for culture and sensitivity (C & S) if indicated.

▪ *Air embolus* – if the lines become disconnected, they should be checked before undertaking the measuring.

▪ *Catheter displacement* – demonstrated through arrhythmias and should be reported immediately.

▪ *Jugular access* – may be irritating for the patient and are more prone to blockage if the patient is mobile. Positioning may prove difficult in the unconscious patient, due to the possibility of dislodgment. In addition, keeping a dressing on may prove problematic.

Once the catheter has been removed, pressure should be applied for at least 5 minutes or longer (until bleeding has stopped). An airtight dressing should be placed on the wound site, which should be undisturbed for the first 48 hours, unless bleeding is present. The catheter tip should be sent for microbiological examination. This is achieved by cutting the catheter tip with sterile scissors and putting it in a sterile specimen pot. The catheter tip should NOT be contaminated.

Again, monitor the patient closely for bleeding/swelling around the insertion site and for general signs of shock, i.e. reduction in blood pressure, increased pulse rate, increased breathing rate, and cool, pale skin.

Mean arterial pressure (MAP)

Traditional observations of vital signs include respiratory rate, heart rate, blood pressure and temperature. Sometimes during acute/critical illness, mean arterial pressure (MAP) measurements are relied upon as a marker for cardiovascular deterioration or improvement. These measurements are used to evaluate the perfusion of vital body organs and are used for the goal and evaluation criteria in the physiological responses to interventions increasing blood pressure.

The MAP is determined by the cardiac output (flow), systemic vascular resistance (resistance) and central venous pressure (pressure), therefore:

$$MAP = (CO \times SVR) + CVP$$

The MAP provides an average blood pressure across the cardiac cycle and offers a better indication than either systolic or diastolic pressures as to whether the patient's brain and other vital organs are receiving sufficient oxygen. Measurements provide more in-depth knowledge relating to the patient's cardiovascular status, giving information about approximate perfusion pressures at the organ and cellular levels.

The MAP measures the average blood pressure over the entire cardiac cycle of systole and diastole. Because the heart spends twice as much time in diastole, while the atria and ventricles fill with blood, diastole counts twice as much as systole, when the chambers contract, i.e. the systole usually requires one-third and diastole two-thirds of the cardiac cycle time. This is reflected in the formulae of calculating the MAP:

Systolic + (diastolic × 2) ÷ 3.

For example:

B/P of 120 (systolic)/90 (diastolic) = MAP 100 mmHg
120 + (90 × 2 = 180) = 120 + 180 = 300. 300 divided by 3 = 100

B/P of 66 (systolic)/40 (diastolic) = 49 mmHg (rounded up)
66 + (40 × 2 = 80) = 66 + 80 = 146. 146 divided by 3 = 48.66 (49 rounded up).

This is an example of one formula. The principle is important. The average MAP is 70–100 mmHg. A MAP below 65 mmHg results in hypotension, poor perfusion, poor oxygenation to vital organs and peripheries; below 60 mmHg is considered incompatible with life. A high reading of above 110 mmHg indicates hypertension.

In clinical practice (other than critical care areas), automated blood pressure machines and most monitors at the bedside will automatically calculate the MAP. Where such devices are not available, the MAP should be calculated manually. It is good practice to calculate the MAP manually when using an automated device at least once per shift and of course when there are discrepancies between patient's condition, blood pressure readings and automated MAP readings.

Lung auscultation

Lung auscultation is a non-invasive method of listening to the internal sounds of the lungs. Assessment of breath sounds (with and without a stethoscope) should form part of the respiratory assessment. Indirect auscultation with a stethoscope is a procedure under-taken by experienced practitioners who should have undergone appropriate training and education. In general care areas, nurses may struggle to provide diagnostic names for what they hear and rely on description in communicating these sounds to other healthcare professionals. It is a subjective procedure, in that there are no measurements just descriptive information.

The procedure for lung auscultation

1   Wash and dry hands before and after the procedure.
2   Patient should be informed and, where possible, gain consent. If possible, the patient should be placed in an upright, leaning forward position (to facilitate

maximum lung expansion). Privacy must be ensured as the stethoscope should be placed on the bare skin. As a result, the chest should be exposed and free from clothing and dressings (these interfere with the transmission of sounds). In some instances shaving of the chest may be necessary as too much hair may also interfere with the sound transmission (remember to gain consent).

3   For children – in order to gain cooperation play will likely to be required. Use the stethoscope to listen to the lungs of the doll/teddy bear – let the child also listen.

4   Ensure the environment is warm as you may have to take off the patient's top layer(s) of clothing.

5   The flat diaphragm of the stethoscope (Figure 8.16) is normally used to identify high-pitched respiratory sounds and the bell for low and medium frequency sounds.

6   The tubing should be as short as possible, preferably around 48 cm. Conducting sound through a shorter distance of tubing reduces further background noise.

7   Teach the patient to take slow deep breaths and listen in an ordered sequence (Figures 8.17 and 8.18) listening to the main areas – i.e. apex, midzone, base of right and left lung, anterior and posterior.

8   It may be necessary to have someone else play a game with the child to distract them.

9   Check that there are no kinks in the tubing.

10   Check it is audible by tapping the diaphragm (a sound should be heard). Ensure that it is not too cold (as it should be placed directly on the patient's skin).

11   The room should be as quiet as possible, try and block visual senses by closing your eyes (helps with concentration of one sense).

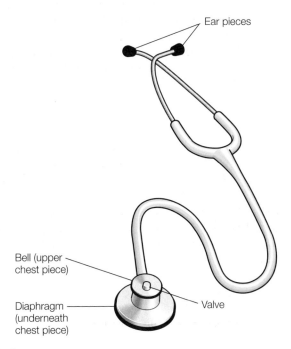

Ear pieces

Bell (upper chest piece)

Diaphragm (underneath chest piece)

Valve

Figure 8.16 **Stethoscope**

12   Listen to inspiration and expiration separately on the anterior wall of the chest. Do the same for the posterior wall (see Figures 8.17 and 8.18) – describe what is heard. Description of sounds are best, i.e. frequency, pitch, intensity, duration and quality, are breath sounds clear, decreased or absent?, and location of any adventitious (extra) sounds.

13   Document whether the sound is direct (heard without stethoscope) or indirect (heard with stethoscope), compare each side to the other, when and where sounds are heard, inspiratory or expiratory, cleared on coughing (NMC, 2015). These sounds can either be direct (sounds audible without a stethoscope) or indirect (use of stethoscope). Normally breathing should not be heard without the use of a stethoscope.

14   Clean the stethoscope between uses (infection control) with different patients or by different members of staff (ideally all staff should have their own stethoscope).

Lung sounds

The following website provides lung sounds for you to listen to: www.practicalclinicalskills. com/heart-lung-sounds-reference-guide-details.aspx?caseID=146&title=Crackles%20 -%20High%20Pitched%20(Rales).

Knowledge of the different types of lung sounds is important to aid description and diagnosis. Without a stethoscope, normal breathing should be quiet. Normal lung sounds are known as vesicular, broncho-vesicular and bronchial.

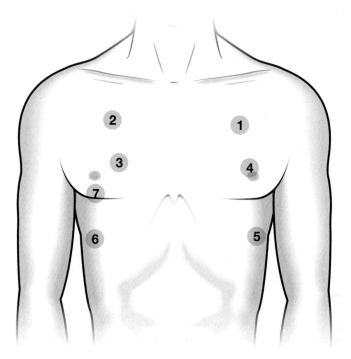

Figure 8.17 Main auscultation landmarks (anterior)

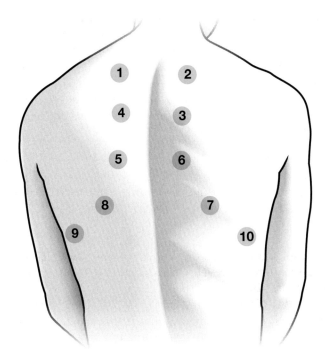

Figure 8.18 Main auscultation landmarks (posterior)

- Normally, *vesicular* sounds (low-pitched, low intensity – described as 'soft and breezy') can be heard over most of the lung fields. In normal breathing, air moves into the airway during inspiration, branching into progressively smaller and smaller airways as it moves to the alveoli. Turbulence of the airway occurs and it is this turbulence that produces the sound. It sounds like wind rushing through trees (a gentle 'swishing' sound)

  During expiration, the air is flowing from small airways to much larger ones, and while the air does contact some surfaces, it takes place in larger, less confining tubes. So there is much less turbulence created, therefore less sound. Sounds can be described as a smooth, swishing sound
- *Harsh vesicular breath sound.* Much louder sounds occurring in conditions where breathing is rapid, producing deep breaths that are longer and louder, i.e. patient is breathing faster and deeper
- *Diminished vesicular breath sound.* Softer, more distant in sound and can occur in the chest of someone who doesn't move as much air, (i.e. the patient's breathing is shallow). You may also hear this sound in the very obese patient (too much tissue mass that muffles the sound)
- *Broncho-vesicular* sounds should be heard in the anterior region, near the mainstem bronchi and posterior only between the scapulae; sounds are more moderate in pitch and intensity. It is heard equally throughout inspiration and expiration. There is no silent gap

■ *Bronchial* sounds are high-pitched, loud and hollow-sounding. These sounds are normally heard over the larger airways, and the trachea. They are coarse, loud, harsh sounds in which expiration is the predominant phase, usually heard throughout the whole of expiration and through only part of inspiration. If bronchial sounds are heard in other areas, this could indicate consolidation of lung tissue, e.g. in pneumonia (consolidated lung tissue transmits sounds better than air, making them louder). There is also a silent gap between inspiration and expiration.

Abnormal breath sounds

Absent breath sounds

Absent breath sounds may be localised, while the rest of the lung is normal or generalised, indicating:

■ Pneumothorax
■ Pneumonectomy (removed lung)
■ Pleural effusion
■ Massive atelectasis (collapsed alveoli)
■ Complete airway obstruction.

Adventitious (additional) sounds

Crackles

■ *Crackles* (also known as rales) are discontinuous, non-musical, breath sounds heard more commonly on inspiration and are indicative of small airway disease (alveoli) as can be found in pulmonary oedema. Here, small airways open during inspiration and collapse during expiration, causing the crackling (popping) sounds. This sound is often heard in the acutely, critically ill patient. They can be classified as fine (high-pitched, soft, very brief) or coarse (low-pitched, louder, less brief). When listening to crackles, pay special attention to their loudness, pitch, duration, number, timing in the respiratory cycle, location, pattern from breath to breath, change after a cough or shift in position
■ *Fine crackles* are high-pitched and are heard at the base of the lungs near the end of inspiration and normally represent the opening of the alveoli
■ *Medium crackles* are lower in pitch and are heard during the middle/latter part of inspiration
■ *Coarse crackles* are loud, bubbling sounds that are heard on both inspiration and expiration and are usually associated with mucous which may clear after the patient has coughed. If the sound is still present, it may be necessary to suction the patient.

Rhonchi

Rhonchi are described as musical, continuous, bubbling, gurgling sounds which indicate large airway disease. There are three categories of rhonchi:

- *Bubbling rhonchi*: due to secretions that are moving through the large bronchioles and bronchi. This type can occur in the patient following surgery, in someone with pneumonia, suffering from an overdose or on prolonged bed rest
- *Gurgling rhonchi*: sounds can be heard throughout inspiration and expiration
- *Sonorous rhonchi*: sounds similar to wheezing, but produces a low-pitched sound and is more musical and is heard most frequently during expiration.

Wheezes

Wheezes are high-pitched, squeaking, musical, continuous noises that are mainly heard during expiration, but can also be heard during inspiration. This sound is indicative of constriction of the larger airways. Wheezes are classified in accordance to the severity:

- *Mild wheeze*: seen in patients with some secretions
- *Moderate wheeze*: sounds for most of the expiratory phase
- *Severe wheeze*: occurs throughout the whole of inspiration and expiration.

Arterial blood gas (ABG) measurement

As more acutely ill patients are being cared for outside of critical care areas, analysing arterial blood gas (ABG) is becoming increasingly common. It is an established method of assessing the patient's respiratory and metabolic status and is indicative of clinical deterioration. Nurses are often the first to receive the blood results from the laboratory. Accurate interpretation is vital as results will dictate the course of intervention.

Rationale for ABG analysis

While pulse oximetry monitoring is effective in providing quick and non-invasive results on the oxygen saturation status of the patient (see Chapter 9), ABG analysis is more accurate in assessing the efficiency of the gas exchange, providing information about oxygenation (PaO_2) and elimination (carbon dioxide, $PaCO_2$). However, this investigation should not be performed as the first option. A clinical assessment and consideration of oxygen saturation levels would be undertaken first. However, the patient's condition may be severe enough to warrant this investigation immediately. The procedure for obtaining arterial blood is not only risky (bleeding, infection) but also extremely painful. Reasons for ABG analysis are seen in Box 8.2. Once the results are understood, there is an urgent need for the doctor to assess the problem.

Obtaining a sample of arterial blood

Arterial blood can be obtained through two routes – an arterial line (a cannula is inserted into the radial artery and a line established to a pressurised intravenous fluid bag containing sodium chloride 0.9%) (Figure 8.19). Normally, arterial lines are attached to a monitor via a transducer for continuous monitoring of arterial pressure (blood pressure and mean arterial pressure). Therefore, arterial lines are usually used in Critical Care Units and general High Dependency Units.

Box 8.2 Reasons for ABG analysis

- Diagnosis and severity of respiratory failure
- Evaluate interventions (e.g. fluid resuscitation)
- Managing the acutely/critically ill (assessment of respiratory or metabolic disorders e.g. diabetic ketoacidosis, respiratory failure)
- Assess patient's condition immediately following cardio-pulmonary resuscitation
- Establish baseline for surgery
- Some clinical guidelines advocate this investigation after 20 minutes of altering supplementary oxygen therapy
- Determine prognosis in the critically ill.

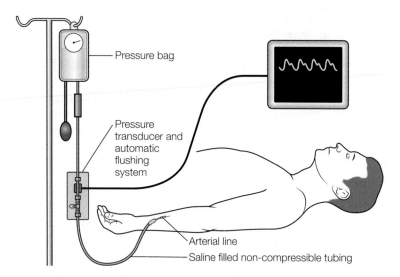

Figure 8.19 Arterial line

More commonly, the second route is via an arterial stab. Puncture sites are indicated in Figure 8.20. This procedure is performed by experienced practitioners who have undergone relevant training. Typically, the radial artery is selected as it is superficial, and therefore easier to palpate, stabilise and puncture. The radial artery also has a collateral blood flow, so if damage or obstruction occurs, the ulnar artery will maintain the blood flow to the tissues. Collateral blood flow is confirmed by the Allen test (performed by elevating the hand, occluding both ulnar and radial arteries and releasing compression of the ulnar artery) (Figure 8.21). If adequate collateral circulation is present, the hand should flush pink/warm within 5–7 seconds. However, this is difficult to determine in dark-skinned people, so warmth of skin should then be noted.

In the event of peripheral shutdown or if the radial artery cannot be palpated, the femoral artery may be selected (this is a larger artery) but the risk of bleeding is greater. If regular ABG analysis is required, an arterial line should be inserted.

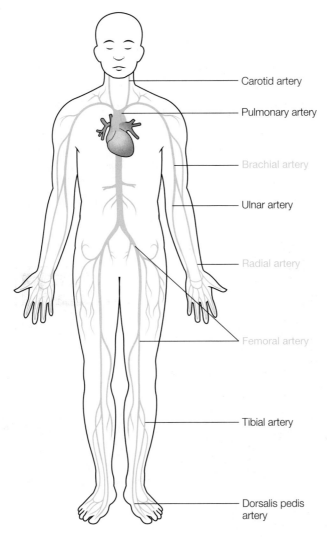

Carotid artery

Pulmonary artery

Brachial artery

Ulnar artery

Radial artery

Femoral artery

Tibial artery

Dorsalis pedis
artery

Figure 8.20 **Arterial puncture sites (in colour)**

Watch out

The puncture site for patients with haematological disorders should be monitored very closely for signs of bleeding. Once the needle has been removed, pressure should be applied for longer than the suggested five minutes.

Like any procedure, if possible, consent should be obtained. The pain induced by this procedure must never be underestimated – the needle has to be inserted very slowly through the skin into the artery (Figure 8.22). Precision is paramount. Local anaesthesia

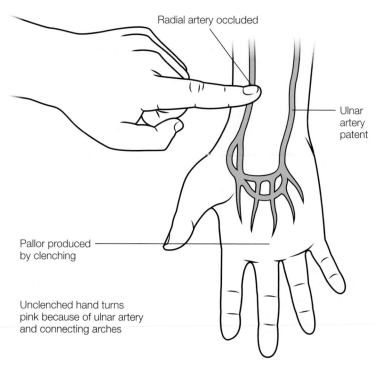

Figure 8.21 **The Allen test**

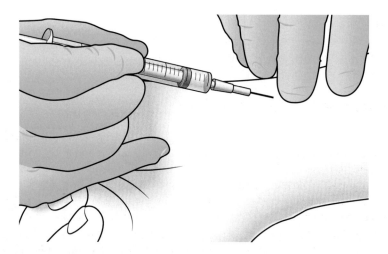

Figure 8.22 **Arterial stab**

should be given, but this is not common in adult practice. Anaesthetic cream must be used with children.

The arterial stab is performed by someone who is trained and assessed and competent in this procedure. There are pre-prepared syringes to use: 0.5–1 ml for aspirating blood is sufficient for adults and 0.1–0.2 ml for the child. The amount of blood taken each time should be noted and recorded. This is particularly important for children as the child's circulatory blood volume can become depleted very quickly. Ensure no air bubbles are in the syringe, as large air bubbles falsely increase the PaO_2 content and reduce the $PaCO_2$. The position of the patient should be noted, as the supine position can cause a false reduction in PaO_2 (as the rate and pattern of breathing are usually compromised). Where possible, an upright position is best for this procedure.

There is a high risk of bleeding with this procedure. Once the needle has been withdrawn from the artery, continuous pressure should be applied for at least 5 minutes (longer if the patient has haematological problems or high risk of bleeding). Observe closely for signs of ischaemia, obstruction and nerve trauma (pins and needles, numbness, loss of wrist/hand movement).

Don't forget!

Once blood has been taken, the syringe should NOT be shaken vigorously, as this leads to haemolysis, gentle rolling is sufficient. Results should be analysed within 15 minutes at room temperature or the cells will start to metabolise in the syringe (using oxygen), thus increasing $PaCO_2$ and reducing PaO_2.

Four main groups are analysed:

1 pH
2 Respiratory function (oxygen, carbon dioxide, saturation)
3 Metabolic measures (bicarbonate, base excess)
4 Electrolytes and metabolites.

For the purpose of this chapter, only the first three will be discussed.

Acid base balance: pH

The potential hydrogen (pH) concentration of ions measures acidity or alkalinity in the blood and provides information regarding the acid base balance. In absolute chemical terms, pH is on a scale (logarithmic) between 0 (absolute acid) to 14 (absolute alkaline). In human blood, the normal range of pH is 7.35–7.45 (Figure 8.23), making it alkaline. It is measured in moles per litre. Even small changes in pH are life-threatening.

An acid is a substance capable of providing hydrogen (H+) and a base (alkali) is capable of accepting H+. Two major organs involved in maintaining the balance are the lungs (respiratory) and the kidneys (metabolic). H+ is released by acids in the blood.

The normal by-product of cellular metabolism is carbon dioxide (CO_2). CO_2 is carried to the lungs and excreted, any excess combines with water (H_2O) to form carbonic acid (H_2CO_3) (a weak acid) via carbonic anhydrase. The pH changes in accordance to the amount of H_2CO_3 present. So, pH is inversely proportional to the number of hydrogen

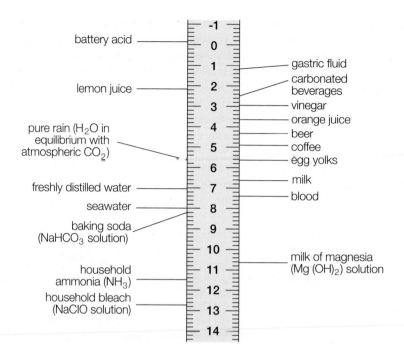

Figure 8.23 The pH scale

ions in the blood – as H+ accumulates, so pH reduces. The kidneys reabsorb bicarbonate (to increase pH) and excrete hydrogen ions (to decrease pH).

During homeostasis, acids and alkalines are physiologically balanced, any deviation can be potentially life-threatening. Changes will trigger a response from the respiratory centre either by increasing or decreasing the rate/depth of breathing.

Alkalis are chemicals that absorb hydrogen, so if the hydrogen levels decrease, the pH level increases. Blood pH below 7.35 is termed acidotic. pH above 7.45 is termed alkalotic. Note, pH does NOT tell us if the problem is respiratory or metabolic.

Respiratory acidosis

Respiratory acidosis (pH less than 7.35 mmol/L; $PaCO_2$ greater than 6.0 kPa) occurs as a result of ventilation failure (hypoventilation), i.e. the inability of the alveoli to sufficiently excrete CO_2 (leading to CO_2 retention). Causes include any condition causing the patient's breathing to become slower and shallow, e.g. central nervous system depression (head injury), excessive use of sedatives, massive pulmonary embolism, pulmonary oedema, or pneumonia.

Respiratory alkalosis

Respiratory alkalosis (pH greater than 7.45 mmol/L; $PaCO_2$ less than 4.5 kPa) can occur when the patient is hyperventilating. It is impossible to give a measurement in terms of breaths per minute as hyperventilation refers to an increase in the rate of alveolar ventilation that is disproportionate to the rate of carbon dioxide production. Therefore, inadequate alveolar ventilation will be different in each patient. Panic attacks, sepsis, over-use of respiratory stimulants can result in hyperventilation. The patient may complain of light-headedness, numbness, tingling, confusion, inability to concentrate, dry mouth, or diaphoresis (sweating).

Metabolic acidosis

Metabolic acidosis (pH less than 7.35 mmol/L; bicarbonate (HCO_3) less than 22 mmol/L) represents the failure to remove/buffer sufficient H+ which is caused by excessive production or accumulation of renal acids (renal failure); lactic acids (circulatory failure); ketoacids (diabetic ketoacidosis); ingestion of acids, e.g. salicylates and loss of base (associated with diarrhoea), causing metabolic acidosis.

Clinical signs include headache, confusion, lethargy, reduced levels of consciousness, cardiac arrhythmias, or Kussmaul respiration (deep, rapid breathing). The acidosis causes hyperventilation which is the body's attempt to 'blow off' CO_2 and compensate for acidosis.

Metabolic alkalosis

Metabolic alkalosis(pH greater than 7.45 mmol/L; HCO_3 greater than 26 mmol/L) is a disorder caused by a loss of acids – due to excessive vomiting/gastric drainage; potassium depletion through diuretic therapy; burns, and by an excess of base acids (from ingestion of acids/excessive use of bicarbonate). Symptoms include dizziness, muscle twitching/cramps, nausea, vomiting, and respiratory depression.

Bicarbonate (HCO_3)

Bicarbonate (normal 22–26 mmol/L) is the main chemical buffer in plasma, mainly produced in the liver and kidneys. It provides information regarding how much alkali there is in the blood. It indicates how well the metabolic system is functioning and relates closely to kidney function, i.e. excretion.

In an attempt to maintain the pH within its normal range, the kidneys excrete or retain bicarbonate (HCO_3). In the event of acidosis, HCO_3 is retained, increasing levels. With alkalosis, excretion of HCO_3 reduces levels.

Base excess

Base excess (normal −2 to +2 mmol/L) indicates the amount of excess or insufficient level of bicarbonate in the system, i.e. it represents the amount of acid or base required to store 1 litre of blood to its normal pH. It reflects only the metabolic component of any disturbance of acid base balance. In the case of metabolic acidosis, acid needs to be added to return the pH to normal, therefore the base excess is negative. For metabolic alkalosis, the acid needs to be removed, hence the base excess is positive. Zero is a neutral score.

Oxygen (PaO$_2$)

In the UK, gases are almost always measured in kilopascals (kPa). While oxygen (normal 11.5–13.5 kPa) is not associated with or influences the acid base balance or analysis, it does, however, provide vital information regarding respiratory function. PaO$_2$ represents the measurement of partial pressure of oxygen dissolved in arterial blood and is dependent upon the effectiveness of gas exchange (see Chapter 9). It is vital for the survival of cells. Prolonged used of high concentrations, resulting in hyperoxia (PaO$_2$ greater than 13.5), is usually iatrogenic and can cause toxic damage. O$_2$ is less soluble that CO$_2$ and therefore more likely to be altered first when the patient's condition deteriorates

Hypoxaemia (PaO$_2$ less than 8.0 kPa) (BTS, 2002) can occur as a result of type 1 respiratory failure and is usually caused by hypoventilation. Hypoxaemia will stimulate the respiratory centre to increase the rate and depth of breathing (see Chapter 9).

Carbon dioxide (PaCO$_2$)

Carbon dioxide (CO$_2$) (normal 4.5–6.0 kPa) is produced by body cells as a waste product of metabolism and is transported to the lungs in plasma in the form of carbonic acid (H$_2$CO$_3$). It provides information concerning ventilation (adequacy of gas exchange). PaCO$_2$ is used as a guide to measure CO$_2$ in the blood and is referred to as the respiratory parameter.

The respiratory centre in the brainstem (the medulla oblongata) responds primarily to the level of arterial carbon dioxide to stimulate breathing. When PaCO$_2$ levels rise, the respiratory centre is stimulated to increase the rate and depth of breathing, resulting in increased excretion of CO$_2$ (Figure 8.24).

People with chronic obstructive pulmonary disorders (COPD) develop alterations in the gas exchange as a result of adjusting and becoming used to a high PaCO$_2$. The central chemoreceptors become tolerant to high CO$_2$ levels. If given too much oxygen (O$_2$), this drive will be inhibited, causing respiratory failure. The respiratory stimulant becomes hypoxia (known as the hypoxic drive). Low PaCO$_2$ levels will eventually inhibit respiratory stimulation, resulting in an initial increase in the respiratory rate but eventually becoming slower and more shallow (leading to type II respiratory failure). Hypercapnia (PaCO$_2$ greater than 6.0 kPa) (BTS, 2002) stimulates the respiratory centre to increase the rate and depth of breathing.

Compensation

The aim of compensation is to maintain the normal acid base balance (homeostasis). Buffers, carbonic acid and bicarbonate are combined in a 1:20 ratio, i.e. 1 carbonic acid to 20 bicarbonate molecules. In order to maintain the 1:20 ratio, when carbonic acid levels increase, so do bicarbonate levels and when the carbonic acid levels decrease, so do the bicarbonate levels. If the pH becomes abnormal, the body will attempt to return it to normal through compensation. In compensation, the system that is NOT experiencing problems (i.e. respiratory or renal) but will attempt to correct the 1:20 ratio, to return the pH to normal.

This means that one system will compensate for the other. Therefore, blood values will not be as we expect them to be, i.e. movement in the opposite direction. For example,

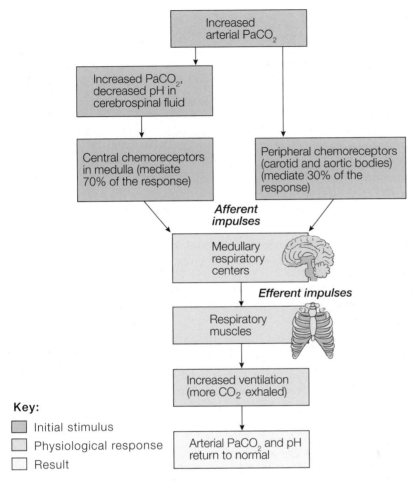

Figure 8.24 Increased CO_2 in the blood

respiratory disturbances are compensated for by the renal system and metabolic distur-bances by the respiratory system. Respiratory compensatory response is not fully activated until 24–48 hours after initial activation. Respiratory compensation occurs at a faster rate than renal. Any acute respiratory problem will always be uncompensated as the kidneys will not have time to compensate.

Interpreting ABGs

Interpreting ABGs is a learnt skill and requires perseverance. Student nurses are not expected to interpret results, but they are expected to do so post qualifying. By examining each variable in turn, it is possible to monitor the condition of a patient's clinical condition and any response to treatment. Box 8.3 is a checklist of questions to ask on pH.

Box 8.3

Questions to ask:

- Look at the pH– is there acidaemia or alkalaemia?
- Look at the $PaCO_2$ – is it high, low or normal?
- Look at the PaO_2 – is the patient hypoxaemic?
- Look at the HCO_3 – is it high, low or normal?
- Is compensation occurring?

Case studies

Test your knowledge and understanding, work out the acid base imbalance in the following case studies. The answers are also given.

Case study 8.1

Jack, a 42-year-old man, has recently returned to the ward following the removal of his large bowel and the creation of a colostomy. He is very sleepy following the effects of the anaesthetic and is finding it difficult to keep his eyes opened. His respiratory rate is 10 breaths per minute and shallow.

ABG profile:

pH	7.30 mmo/L
PaO_2	9.5 kPa
$PaCO_2$	6.4 kPa
HCO_3	25 mmol/L

Problem: respiratory acidosis. Primarily treatment should be focused upon the underlying cause and increasing ventilation, through enhancing lung expansion and increasing the amount of inspired air, e.g. wake patient up, encourage deep breaths, pain control, position should be upright if possible. Give supplementary oxygen.

Case study 8.2

Mabinda has recently been readmitted to hospital with a severe wound infection, pyrexia and her condition is deteriorating. She has developed sepsis as a result of her wound infection. Respiratory rate is 30 breaths per minute (normal = 12–20).

ABG profile:

pH	7.51 mmol/L
PaO_2	10.2 kPa

| PaCO$_2$ | 3.4 kPa |
| HCO$_3$ | 24 mmol/L |

Problem: respiratory alkalosis. The aim is to monitor closely for signs of exhaustion or respiratory muscle fatigue as respiratory failure can follow. In this case, aggressive antibiotic therapy and fluid resuscitation in line with clinical guidelines will be initiated.

Case study 8.3

Parvis is a 15-year-old youth, who has type 1 diabetes mellitus. He is non-compliant with his regime and as a result his condition is poorly controlled or managed. He has been admitted to the ward, with blood sugar levels 30 mmol/L (normal = 4–7 mmol/l) and diagnosed with diabetic ketoacidosis (DKA).

ABG profile:

pH	7.24 mmol/L
PaO$_2$	10.7 kPa
PaCO$_2$	4.0 kPa
HCO$_3$	12.5 mmol/L

Problem: metabolic acidosis. The aim of treatment is to control or treat the underlying cause; in this case, controlling the hyperglycaemia and addressing his non-compliance.

Case study 8.4

Erika, a 73-year-old, has heart failure requiring diuretic therapy. There have been problems in monitoring her urine output/fluid balance, this has resulted in over-administration of diuretics. Erika is clinically dehydrated.

ABG profile:

pH	7.59 mmol/L
PaO$_2$	9.8 kPa
PaCO$_2$	4.6 kPa
HCO$_3$	39 mmol/L
K+	2.9 mmol/L

Problem: metabolic alkalosis. This is the most difficult disorder to identify and in treating the underlying cause. This disorder is almost always a secondary problem to a primary complaint. Therefore, careful monitoring of the patient's responses to interventions is essential. In severe cases, IV administration of acids may be used.

Electrocardiography (ECG) interpretation

Irregularities of the rhythm will indicate the need for an ECG (12-lead) assessment. Note if the pulse has a regular, regular irregular or irregular irregular pattern. Irregular irregular rhythms feel erratic, unsteady, uneven and have no pattern.

During acute/critical illness the patient may develop a cardiac arrhythmia known as atrial fibrillation, resulting in an irregularly irregular pulse pattern. Cardiac arrhythmias are relatively common in the peri-arrest period. For the purpose of this chapter, only the most common arrhythmias are discussed.

Normal conducting pathway

An impulse is generated at the sino-atrial (SA) node and spreads across both atria, causing them to contract (atrial depolarisation) (this correlates with the P wave of the ECG). The fibro-fatty atrioventricular (AV) groove insulates the ventricles from the atrial impulse. The AV node is the only normal gateway of conduction to the ventricles. The impulse is delayed at the AV node and then travels down the AV bundle and its branches onto the Purkinje fibres. The ventricles are then stimulated to contract (ventricular depolarisation – the QRS complex). The T wave correlates with ventricular repolarisation. Figure 8.25 shows the conducting pathway for an ECG.

Sometimes a 'U' wave may occur when the ECG machine picks up repolarisation of the Purkinje fibres. A 'U' wave may also occur with hypokalaemia (low potassium).

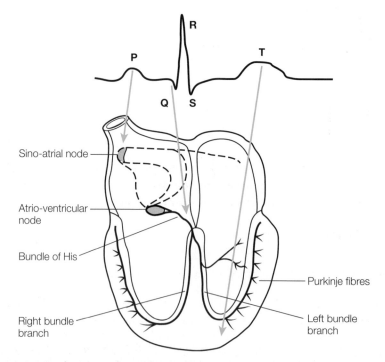

Figure 8.25 Conducting pathway for an ECG

For all patients, a 12-lead ECG should be taken. Taking a 12-lead ECG is beyond the remit of this particular section. Healthcare professionals who have undertaken the appropriate training should interpret a 12-lead ECG. The focus here is on 3-lead ECG reading and interpretation. It may be possible to take a trace (on paper) for the purpose of reading, documenting and filing (in patient's notes) (Figures 8.26 and 8.27).

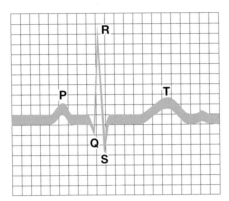

Figure 8.26 Normal ECG complex

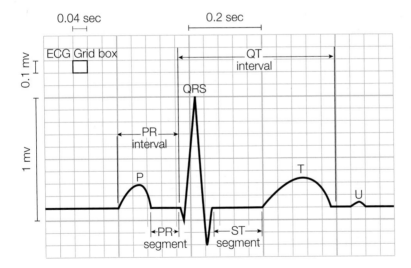

Figure 8.27 ECG trace on paper

Analysing an ECG means that you need to note the following:

- *Rate*: one small square = 0.04 seconds and one large square = 0.2 seconds. For manual rate calculations – count the number of QRS complex with six strip (30 seconds) times this by ten – will give you the heart rate per minute
- *Rhythm:* place plain paper over the rhythm strip and mark off three QRS complexes, marking the R wave, move the paper along to match and compare the distance with

the next three peaks (R–R interval). If they match, then the rhythm is regular. Note whether regular irregular or irregular irregular

- *QRS complex:* the QRS complex should be no wider that 0.11 seconds (i.e. three small squares), a widened complex may indicate a ventricular arrhythmia
- *P waves:* indicates atrial activity
- *Relationships and measurements:* P–R interval should be 0.12–0.20 seconds (3–4 small squares) greater than 0.2 seconds indicates first degree heart block.

When assessing an ECG, always note blood pressure (signs of shock), chest pain (resulting in cardiac ischaemia), pulmonary oedema (heart failure), or syncope (due to reduced blood flow to the brain), as this will indicate whether the patient is 'compensating' and therefore their condition is stable or unstable. Other influencing factors affecting the rhythm are blood potassium (K +), magnesium (Mg2+) and calcium (Ca+), therefore, blood levels should be checked and monitored closely.

Rhythm interpretation

Sinus rhythm (normal rhythm)

Key factors in sinus rhythm (Figure 8.28):

- P wave present
- QRS complex follows P wave
- P–R interval regular normal (0.12–0.20 seconds)
- QRS complex normal (less than 0.12 seconds)
- R–R interval regular
- Rate 60–100 beats per minute (bpm).

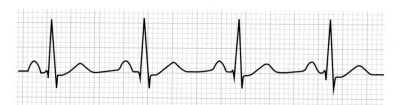

Figure 8.28 Sinus rhythm

Box 8.4 presents the criteria for a sinus rhythm.

Box 8.4 Criteria for sinus rhythm

- P wave always present and rounded in shape
- Each P wave followed by a QRS complex
- T wave present
- P–R interval should be regular and constant
- Rhythm should be regular R–R interval constant and regular.

Sinus tachycardia

This is not viewed as an arrhythmia as it is seen as a normal response to pain or, anxiety (Resuscitation Council, 2010). It may also occur in complications such as infection or blood loss.

Key factors in sinus tachycardia (Figure 8.29):

■ P wave present
■ QRS complex follows P wave
■ R–R interval regular
■ Rate (at rest) – greater than 100 bpm (not usually more than 140 bpm).

The underlying cause should be treated.

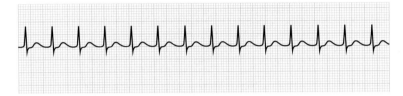

Figure 8.29 Sinus tachycardia

Arrhythmias

Arrhythmias include tachycardias (atrial fibrillation, atrial flutter, premature ventricular contraction (PVC), supra ventricular tachycardia, ventricular tachycardia, ventricular fibrillation).

For patients who are unstable and deteriorating, the treatment of choice is cardioversion. If this fails, amoiderone may be administered. If the patient is stable, then drug therapy is recommended. It is also recommended that oxygen should only be administered if the patient is hypoxaemic (Resuscitation Council UK, 2015). Vital signs should be monitored very closely.

Problems with atrial conduction (AV node) include atrial fibrillation and atrial flutter.

Atrial fibrillation

Atrial fibrillation is the most common arrhythmia in acutely/critically ill patients. Here, there are a large number of disorganised electrical impulses from the SA node. Some will transmit to the AV node and then follow the normal conducting pathway. This results in apex pulse beats being greater than radial pulse beats.

Key factors in atrial fibrillation (Figures 8.30 and 8.31):

■ Visible P wave is absent (SA node not functioning)
■ Normal QRS complex
■ R–R interval irregular irregular
■ Rate (ventricular/pulse) 110–200 bpm (atrial rate greater than 300 bpm).

Treatment – assessment (see Chapter 7), treat cause. Drugs such as beta blockers, amiodarone or digoxin may be prescribed. These patients are at high risk of developing thrombo-emboli and will require anticoagulation therapy.

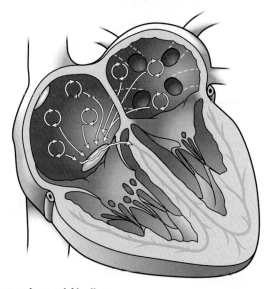

Figure 8.30 **Heart with atrial fibrillation**

Atrial fibrillation

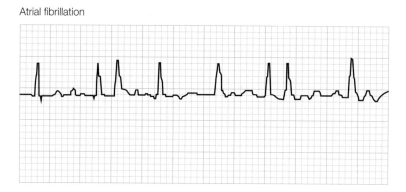

Figure 8.31 **Atrial fibrillation rhythm**

Atrial flutter

The SA node sends a premature electrical signal that moves in an organized circular motion, or 'circuit' (normally alternate signals (beats) (Figure 8.32). This causes the atria only to beat. The second impulse will follow the normal conducting pathway (known as 2:1 block). This arrhythmia can be caused by myocardial infarction.

Key factors in atrial flutter:

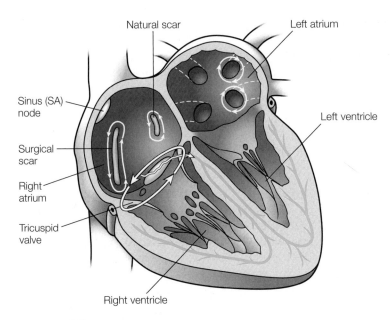

Figure 8.32 **Atrial flutter**

- P wave is replaced with 'sawtooth' pattern (SA node not functioning) (Figure 8.33)
- Normal QRS complex and T wave
- R–R interval irregular irrregular (usually 2:1 block)
- Rate (ventricular/pulse) 125–150 bpm (atrial rate greater than 300 bpm).

Treatment – assessment (see Chapter 7), vagal manoeuvres, i.e. carotid sinus massage or the Valsalva manoeuvre. If this fails, then adenosine IV may be prescribed.

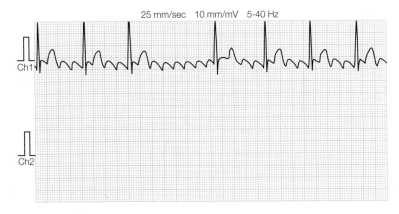

Figure 8.33 **Atrial flutter rhythm**

Supra-ventricular tachycardia (SVT)

Rapid abnormal heart rhythm that may occur in thyrotoxicosis, ischaemic heart disease. Key factors in supra-ventricular tachycardia (Figure 8.34):

- P wave is not easily identifiable
- QRS complex is narrow
- R–R interval irregular when premature beat occurs
- Rate – greater than 140 bpm.

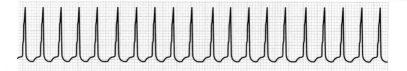

Figure 8.34 Supra ventricular tachycardia

Treatment – start with vagal manoeuvres. Carotid sinus massage (this HAS to be performed by a healthcare professional trained in this technique) or the Valsalva manoeuvre. If this fails, then adenosine IV may be prescribed. Electrical cardioversion is the last resort if patient does not respond to the other modes of treatment.

Premature ventricular contraction (PVC)

PVCs indicate the 'irritability' of the heart. They are premature beats initiated from the ventricles. Complexes are very wide and bizarre-looking.

Key factors in premature ventricular contraction (Figure 8.35):

- P wave absent (impulses originate in the ventricles)
- QRS complex is wide and looks bizarre (greater than 0.1 second). T wave absent
- R–R interval irregular when premature beat occurs

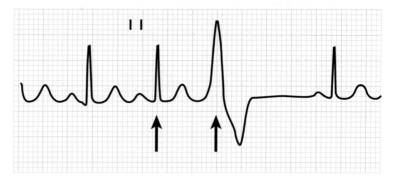

Figure 8.35 PVC

Note:

▦ *Count* how many per minute (the more per minute, the more dangerous the arrhythmia is, initiating ventricular tachycardia (VT))

▦ *Pattern* i.e. occurring every second beat (bigeminy) or third beat (trigeminy)

▦ *Shape* note there maybe different PVC shapes

▦ *Position* to previous complex (particularly T wave). An ectopic beat occurring repolarisation (T wave) is known as 'R on T' phenomenon and it can deteriorate to VT very quickly.

If the patient is symptomatic, then beta blockers or calcium channel blockers may be prescribed. Amiodarone may also be considered.

Ventricular tachycardia (VT)

Impulses from the SA node fail to reach the ventricles. As a result, the impulses are activated by the ventricles.

Key factors in ventricular tachycardia (Figures 8.36 and 8.37):

▦ P wave usually buried in QRS complex

▦ QRS complex is wide and bizarre

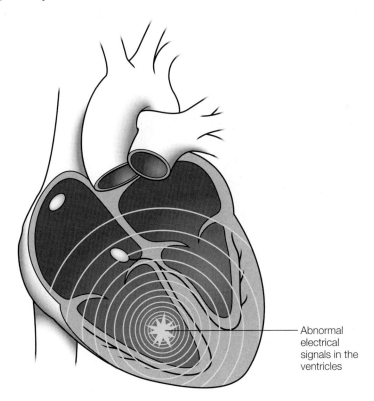

Abnormal electrical signals in the ventricles

Figure 8.36 Ventricular tachycardia

Ventricular tachycardia ECG

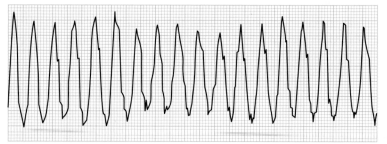

Figure 8.37 **ECG trace for VT**

- R–R interval usually regular
- Rate – ventricular 150–250 bpm
- Cardiac output may be maintained – no loss of consciousness. BUT THIS WILL NOT LAST FOR LONG PERIODS OF TIME.

Treatment – this is an emergency (Chapter 10).

Ventricular fibrillation (VF)

VF is an abnormal irregular heart rhythm caused by rapid, uncoordinated quivering (like a bag of worms) contractions of the ventricles.

Key factors in ventricular fibrillation (Figures 8.38 and 8.39):

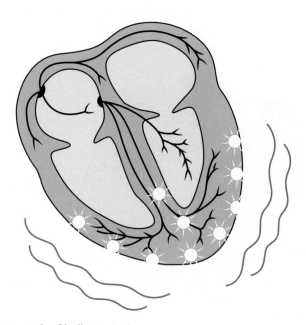

Figure 8.38 **Ventricular fibrillation (VF)**

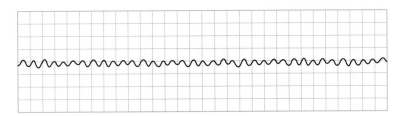

Figure 8.39 **ECG trace VF**

- Rate – ventricular 150–250 bpm
- No audible heart beat or palpable pulse
- Cardiac arrest situation (Chapter 10).

Bradycardia

Sinus bradycardia is a slow heart beat (less than 60 bpm) and can be caused by hypothermia, hypothyroidism, drug-induced state (beta blockers/digoxin), ischemia, hypoxaemia. Bradycardia may be a natural physiological response, i.e in athletes.

Key factors in bradycardia (Figure 8.40):

- All wave forms present with one P wave to each QRS complex
- R–R interval regular
- Rate – less than 60 bpm (not usually less than 40 bpm).

Treatment – atropine, oxygen, possible cardiac pacing (if unresponsive to drug therapy).

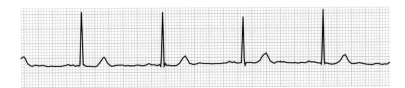

Figure 8.40 **Sinus bradycardia**

Conduction abnormalities

First degree AV block

Key factors in first degree AV block (Figure 8.41):

- P wave present but P–R interval is prolonged (greater than 0.2 seconds) (due to impulse delay in the AV node)
- QRS complex is normal
- R–R interval usually regular

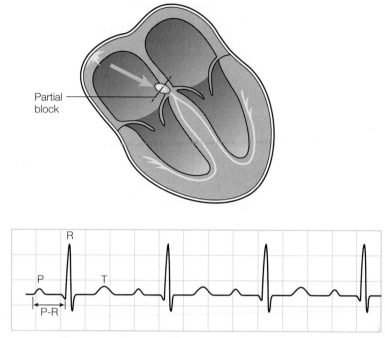

Partial block

R

P T

P-R

P-wave precedes each QRS-complex but interval is > 0.2 s

Figure 8.41 **First degree AV block**

- Rate – 60–100 bpm (patient is asymptomatic)
- Cardiac output may be maintained – no loss of consciousness.

Treatment – none – careful monitoring as may lead to more serious forms of heart block.

Second degree AV block (Mobitz type 1/Wenckebach)

Key factors in second degree AV block (Figure 8.42):

- P wave present but P–R interval is progressively prolonged (until P wave is not conducted (i.e. until a drop beat is seen)
- P–R interval is not constant
- QRS complex is normal
- Rate – 60–80 bpm
- R–R interval shortens as the P–R interval prolongs
- After each dropped beat, the P–R interval is normal and the cycle starts again.

Treatment – none – careful monitoring as may lead to more serious forms of heart block. Can progress to third degree heart block.

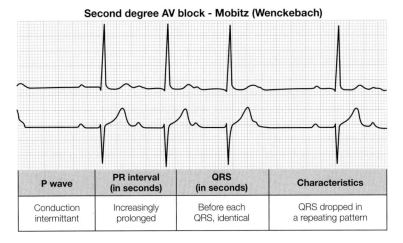

Second degree AV block - Mobitz (Wenckebach)

P wave	PR interval (in seconds)	QRS (in seconds)	Characteristics
Conduction intermittant	Increasingly prolonged	Before each QRS, identical	QRS dropped in a repeating pattern

Figure 8.42 **Second degree AV block (Mobitz type 1/Wenckebach)**

Second degree AV block (2:1)

Key factors in second degree AV block (2:1) (Figure 8.43):

- Ratio of two P waves to one QRS
- P–R interval is constant
- QRS complex is normal
- Rate – 60–80 bpm
- R–R interval is regular.

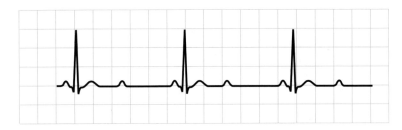

Figure 8.43 **Second degree (2:1)**

Third degree AV block (complete heart block)

Complete block of the atrial impulses occurs at the A-V junction. Another pacemaker distal to the block takes over in order to activate the ventricles. May be caused by:

- Digitalis toxicity
- Acute infection

■ Myocardial infarction
■ Degeneration of the conductive tissue (in the heart).

Key factors in third degree AV block (Figure 8.44):

■ P wave present but there is no relationship between P waves and QRS complex
■ P–R interval is not constant. There are a greater number of P waves than QRS complex, i.e. complete dissociation between P waves and QRS
■ QRS complex is normal
■ Rate   atrial rate is normal but ventricular rate is slow – less than 60
■ R–R relatively constant P–P intervals and R–R intervals.

Treatment – an artificial pacemaker will be inserted to take over the function of the SA node.

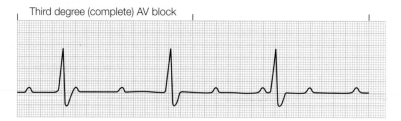

Figure 8.44 **Complete heart block**

Figure 8.45 compares all the heart blocks.

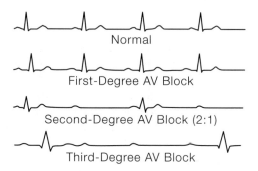

Figure 8.45 **Comparison of the heart blocks**

Asystole

Key factors of asystole (Figure 8.46):

■ P wave absent
■ QRS absent

- Rate none
- No palpable pulse or breathing.

This is a fatal arrhythmia and an emergency (Chapter 10).

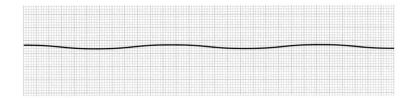

Figure 8.46 Asystole

Neurological assessment

Level of consciousness is a good indicator of neurological changes and clinical deterioration. A neurological assessment should provide the means for diagnosis of neurological deficit and the measurement of progress as it is considered essential in the assessment of the acutely ill patient (NICE, 2007; Resuscitation Council UK, 2015).

A comprehensive neurological assessment should include:

- Level of consciousness
- Cranial nerves
- Motor function
- Sensory function
- Pupillary (pupil) reaction
- Vital signs.

Nurses and medical staff working in neuroscience specialist areas will use this full assessment. Nurses' assessment in other care areas normally includes the level of consciousness, pupillary signs, vital signs and motor function. All changes should be reported immediately to the mentor/nurse in charge. For the purpose of this particular chapter, assessment using the Glasgow Coma Scale (GCS) will be discussed.

The 'D' (disability) in the ABCDE approach involves neurological assessment (Box 8.5). This is normally achieved using the AVPU tool (see below) but for a fuller examination, the Glasgow Coma Scale (GCS) should be used, or in the case of patients with head trauma. Box 8.6 compares the AVPU and the GCS.

Most Trusts dictate that healthcare assistants (HCAs) should not perform neurological assessment as the interpretation of neurological dysfunction is a sophisticated procedure. Though 'simple' to use, the GCS is a complex tool and should be used by experienced practitioners (although this assessment is often delegated to student nurses who are junior and inexperienced in using the tool, increasing the risk of misinterpretation).

Accuracy of assessment is crucial. To identify discrepancies with assessment it is suggested that at shift handover assessment of the patient's GCS is conducted together by nurses on both shifts.

Box 8.5 Reasons for neurological assessment

- Determines subtle and rapid change in the patient's condition
- Helps monitor neurological status following neurological procedures
- Observation of deterioration and in establishing the extent of traumatic head injury
- Helps detect life-threatening situations
- Alerts nurse to seek urgent assistance when required.

(Dawes *et al.*, 2007)

Box 8.6 Association between the AVPU and the GCS

A   GCS 15
V   GCS 12–14
P   GCS 7–9
U   GCS 3.

(Kelly *et al.*, 2004)

AVPU

AVPU is incorporated within the national early warning system (NEWS) assessment tool. This component provides a rapid summary assessment of the patient's level of consciousness (i.e. AVPU scores) or if frequent monitoring is required, the GCS should be used.

A – Alert and oriented. Do not ask questions that provide a 'yes' or 'no' answer. Ask the patient simple open-ended questions in relation to time, place and person
V – Responds to Verbal stimulus
P – Responds to Pain – note if patient moans or withdraws from the stimulus
U – Unresponsive.

The Glasgow Coma Scale (GCS)

The GCS was developed in 1974 by Teasdale and Jennett. It was originally designed to grade the severity and outcome of traumatic head injury but has been extended for all causes of impaired consciousness and coma. This tool should only be used as an assessment of the depth of unconsciousness (this is the scoring). To reduce ambiguity, there is a need to define responses in descriptive terms in addition to numerical scoring. NICE guidelines indicate that the GSC should be used to assess all brain-injured patients and suggests that assessment should be undertaken every 30 min until the GCS reaches

15 or the patient's condition stabilises; clinical experience dictates the latter (NICE, 2007).

The GSC's graphic, visual format ensures uniformity (at local, national and international levels) and should give reliable, quick, concise, visual interpretation of the patient's level of consciousness and hence neurological status over a period of time. Accurate assessment and prompt action when needed can improve the eventual outcome, not just in terms of survival but also minimising the degree of residual neurological deficit. This tool has also been used as a prognostic device during immediate assessment following a head injury. Each section is allocated a numerical score (decreasing indicates neurological deterioration). This numerical scoring allows for a quick conclusion in relation to the severity of the patient's condition, the lower the score, the poorer the prognosis.

The GSC provides a standardised consistent assessment of conscious level by evaluating three behavioural responses: Eye opening (E); Verbal response (V); and Motor response (M) (GCS). The rest of the chart provides information about other observations that could help identify the cause of neurological deterioration. The lowest score achievable is 3 (total unresponsiveness), the maximum is 15 (awake, alert and fully responsive). A score of less than 8 is considered significant with the patient's airway potentially becoming compromised due to reduced level of consciousness, and so requires immediate appropriate airway management (possibly through elective ventilation). Equally, a reduction in motor score by one or an overall deterioration of two is significant and should be reported (NICE, 2007).

Scoring may be misleading in those patients who are hypoxaemic, haemodynamically unstable, having seizures (or are post ictal (post seizure), showing little response), under the influence of sedation, alcohol and drug intoxication. Therefore, it is important to re-evaluate once any underlying acute condition has been corrected.

The use of a total score to describe an individual patient level of consciousness provides a quick overall index of severity of dysfunction. The disadvantage is that it conveys less information than the description of the three responses separately and is liable to be invalid if one component of the scale is not testable. This tool should not be used in isolation; it is good practice to accompany the scores with written commentary (described in simple, objective terms to convey a clear, unambiguous picture of their responsiveness) of the assessment. Reasons for this are discussed later in the chapter. Despite this, it is important NOT to adapt the assessment findings to fit the patients – nurses must record what is seen/heard (without interpretation) but should accompany the score with descriptive assessment information.

Level of consciousness

Normal consciousness relates to the ability to organise thoughts, experience sensations and emotions and perform appropriate mental processes. It depends on the reticular activating system (RAS), which is a densely populated group of neurons that receives input from multiple sensory pathways. It extends from the spinal cord to the lower brainstem, upwards through the mesencephalon and thalamus and is then distributed throughout the cerebral cortex (Hall, 2015). It is responsible for arousal from sleep and maintains consciousness. The arousal reaction is dependent on the stimulation of the RAS. The RAS receives input signals from a wide range of sources, including the senses.

The assessment of the level of consciousness directly assesses the functioning of the brainstem and cerebral cortex in that the person can interact with and interprets the environment.

With any alteration to the level of consciousness (Box 8.7), check the patient's blood glucose to rule out hypoglycaemia (as this is a common cause).

Activity 8.1

Reflect on situations where the patients that you have cared for had an alteration in their level of consciousness. List the causes (if known). Now compare to the list in Box 8.7.

Box 8.7 Causes of decreased conscious level

Metabolic causes

- Hepatic coma
- Electrolyte imbalances (e.g. sodium – hyper-/hypo-neutraemia)
- Uraemic coma
- Diabetic coma (hypoglycaemia).

Drugs

- Sedatives/strong analgesics/anticonvulsants/amphetamines
- Alcohol intoxication.

Increase in brain volume

- Brain tumours/cerebral abscess
- Cerebral oedema from head injury.

Increase in cerebral blood volume

- Haematomas – extradural, subdural, intracerebral, subarachnoid haemorrhage.

Decreased cerebral metabolism

- Hypoxaemia, hypercapnia, acidosis, alkalosis, hyponatraemia.

Circulatory

- Secondary brain injury such as hypoxaemia or ischaemia should be treated as soon as possible to prevent irreversible damage.

Best eye response

This assesses the functioning of the brainstem and reticular activating system (RAS). It must be noted that eye opening is not always an indication of intact neurological function. Individuals in persistent vegetative state (PVS) will open their eyes (they also track movements) as a direct reflex action generated by the RAS. If eyes are open and no blinking is apparent, gently close the eyes and observe if they open.

Communication is paramount, even if the patient has alterations to their level of consciousness. Inform the patient what is to be done and apologise for the need to hurt them.

Level of consciousness is assessed by the patient's response to command to physical stimuli, spontaneously or to command. Scoring is bracketed below:

- *Eyes open spontaneously* (E4) – in the absence of stimulation the patient who is conscious will open their eyes spontaneously (on approach) unless sleeping. It is important not to talk to the patient straight away as this automatically reduces the score to E3
- *Eyes open to speech* (E3) – the patient's eyes open to clear, simple verbal command
- *Eyes open in response to pain only* (E2) – if responses to speech have failed, try physical contact (gently shake or touch the shoulder) first before inflicting pain and then gradually increasing the nature of the pressure.

  There are two forms of painful stimuli: (1) *Peripheral* pressure – pen pressed to the lateral outer aspect of the second or third finger (NOT on the actual nail bed as this can cause damage and bleeding under the nailbed). It is important to rotate the point of stimulation around on each assessme]nt; (2) *Central* stimuli – the trapezius squeeze is the preferred approach. The trapezius muscle extends across the back of the shoulders from the middle of the neck and is held between the thumb and forefingers for a maximum of 10 seconds, note any verbal or non-verbal responses noted (grimacing). Gradually increase pressure. Continual squeezing can cause tissue damage
- *Supra-orbital* pressure – should only be used when the healthcare professional has been trained to do this correctly. Just below the inner aspect of the eyebrow is a small notch through which a branch of the facial nerve runs. Pressure is applied through the flat of the thumb on the supra-orbital ridge under the eyebrow, graduating pressure for approximately 30 seconds. This should not be performed if there is any orbital damage or skull fracture
- Sternal rub and mandibular pressure are inappropriate for repeated assessments due to tissue damage and bruising. Alternative routes should be considered
- *No response* (E1) before scoring, ensure adequacy of painful stimuli. Note – if the patient's eyes are closed, swollen, or if facial fractures or dressings – this is recorded as 'C' (closed) on the chart, obviously reducing the score (E1).

Best verbal response

This provides information about the patient's speech, comprehension and functioning areas of the higher, cognitive centre of the brain (attention, memory, judgement, insight, calculation, abstraction, thought processes and content). This category reflects the patient's ability to articulate and express a reply. Also assess whether they are aware of themselves and their environment.

- *Orientated* to time, place and person (V5) – simple, sensitive language must be used. The type of questions should be consistent with a careful selection of questions that should incorporate factors such as age, culture, language. Avoid using day of the week, date or monarch questions. Patients should be asked to confirm their name, current location, month, season. Assess the patient's response not only in terms of answers but also language, speech and voice qualities (e.g. modulation, articulation and rate). Speech should be spontaneous and well-paced, content should be logical
- *Confused* (V4) – healthcare professionals caring for the patient must determine the characteristics of confused responses as variations in expectation may influence the scoring and making it become inaccurate. Delusional answers may indicate a need for more detailed assessment (mental capacity). Nurses should assess logic and judgement, i.e. does the patient answer questions appropriately?; is there any evidence of reasoning and decision-making abilities?
- Essentially, a confused response is when the patient can formulate sentences but what is said does not make sense in the context of the question. If a person answers one question incorrectly, the score should be V4
- *Inappropriate words* (V3) – are where understandable conversation is absent or limited. The patient does not use sentences to speak, only words. Some patients may have motor dysphasia, where they are unable to utter the words they wish to say. Expressive dysphasia may occur with a stroke; this is where the patient has difficulty in putting words together to make meaning but may have comprehension
- *Incomprehensible sounds* (V2) – there are no understandable words said – only sounds (e.g. moaning, groaning and crying). If the patient has sustained damage to speech centre in the brain and is unable to talk but remains aware and alert, the score must still be recorded as a score of V2
- *None* (V1) – no verbal response to speech or painful stimulus. Note – patients with a tracheostomy or endotracheal tube should be recorded as 'T' with a score of V1. A criticism of the tool is that patients cannot be adequately assessed if they have any kind of communication difficulties related to language (no comprehension of the English language) or pre-existing pathology that might affect speech, e.g. learning difficulties, stroke. Patients with aphasia (unable to speak) have an 'A' recorded on the chart and a score of V1 documented (despite them being alert and orientated).

Best motor response

This tests the area of the brain that identifies sensory input and translates this into a motor response. The intention is to determine the patient's ability to obey a command to localise, and to withdraw or assume abnormal body positions, in response to a pain stimulus. This is the most reliable predictor of outcome/prognosis.

- *Obeys commands* (M6) – the patient obeys simple commands, e.g. squeeze your hand or put your tongue out (Figure 8.47)

- *Localises to central pain* (M5) – localising to pain (peripheral or central) denoted intact sensory system, motor system and cortical processing. It is assessed via response to a central painful stimulus as there is no response to verbal command. It involves higher centres of the brain recognising that something is hurting the patient and trying to remove that pain source. This assessment does not need to be done if the patient already demonstrates this act to an unwanted stimulus, e.g. pulling off the oxygen mask/nasogastric tube
- *Withdrawal from pain* (M4) – the patient bends the arm at the elbow towards the source of the pain, failing to locate the source of pain. Both arms are assessed independently
- *Abnormal flexion to pain* (M3) – flexes/bends the arms towards the trunk. This is also characterised by internal rotation and adduction of the shoulder and flexion of the elbow and is a slower reaction. Abnormal flexion of the elbow and resistance may indicate severe damage to the cerebral cortex
- *Extension to pain* (M2) – extension of the arms, straightens the elbow and internal shoulder and wrist internal rotation may be apparent. An abnormal response is associated with a poorer prognosis. This occurs when motor pathway is blocked/damaged in the brainstem
- *No response* (M1) – no response to painful stimuli. The longer this persists, the poorer the prognosis for the patient.

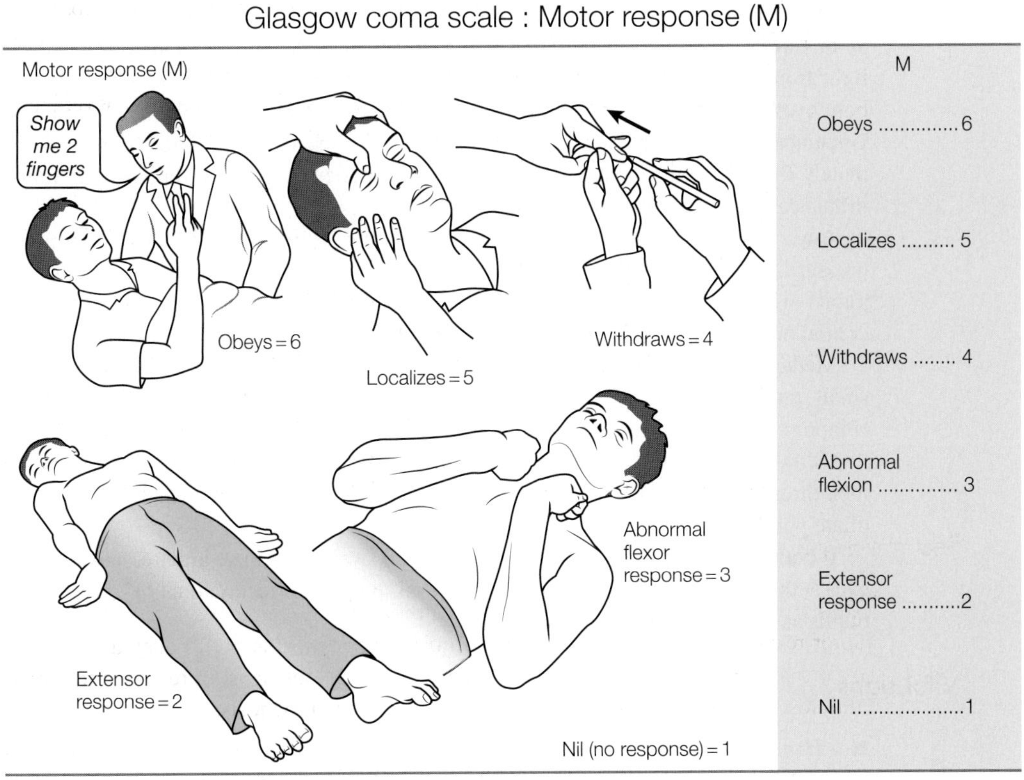

Glasgow coma scale : Motor response (M)

Motor response (M)

Show me 2 fingers

Obeys = 6

Localizes = 5

Withdraws = 4

Abnormal flexor response = 3

Extensor response = 2

Nil (no response) = 1

M	
Obeys	6
Localizes	5
Withdraws	4
Abnormal flexion	3
Extensor response	2
Nil	1

Figure 8.47 GCS motor responses

Limb movements

This assessment can detect weaknesses on one side of the body/limbs (arms/legs) and can give an indication of the extent of the damage to the motor cortex that controls the motor movement. Ask the patient to extend both arms, palms up in front of them with their eyes closed. The weaker arm will rotate palm downwards (pronation).

- Normal power – hold patient's limbs (one at a time) and instruct them to push against your hand or pull you towards them (apply some resistance)
- Mild weakness – *patient is able to counter the resistance but is easily overcome*
- Severe weakness – *patient is able to move limb but not against the resistance*
- Flexion, extension, no response.

Some tools reflect interpretation therefore differ slightly in wording. Frequency of observations is reliant upon clinical judgement and is dictated by the patient's condition.

Pupil reaction

This measurement assesses the second (optic) and third (oculomotor) cranial nerves. This procedure is best conducted in a darkened area (where possible) with a bright shining pen torch. The patient must not be looking directly at light (artificial or direct) as this automatically constricts the pupils. Have the light on and gradually move the light from the outside (head) towards the pupil, noting the pupil's reaction to light in both eyes, noting if it is brisk, sluggish or no reaction. Note the final size of the pupil. Document each eye findings separately. Normal pupil size is considered to be approximately 2–5mm. Nurses need to be aware if the patient has any problems that would influence results, e.g. cataract, eye injuries, false eye.

Any changes in pupil reaction, shape or size are a late sign of raised intracranial pressure (ICP) particularly following head trauma. Sluggish or suddenly dilated unequal pupils are an indication that oedema or haematoma is worsening and the oculomotor cranial nerve is being compressed (herniated) through the foramen magnum.

Medications can influence the size of the pupils and should be documented. Very small pupils (1–2 mm) may suggest the use of opiates, fentanyl or barbiturates. 'Pinpoint' and 'unreactive' indicate damage to the Pons.

'Blown pupils' (large and unreactive to light) follow herniation of part of the temporal lobe through the foramen magnum. However, the use of eye drops such as atropine can dilate pupils.

If both eyes are closed because of gross orbital swelling or there are dressings on both eyes – the letter 'C' (closed) is recorded. Brisk pupils are recorded as '+'. Unreactive pupils as '−' and sluggish pupils as 'S'.

Vital signs

- *Heart rate* – the control of the vital signs (heart rate, blood pressure, respiratory status) is in the brain stem of the medulla oblongata. Changes in intracranial pressure will affect the vital signs. Bradycardia demonstrates signs of raised intracranial pressure (Cushing's response) a vasomotor reflex

■ *Blood pressure* – because of the compensatory mechanisms within the brain, any drop in blood pressure does not cause a drop in cerebral perfusion pressure as the auto-regulation mechanism causes cerebral vasodilatation. If compensatory mechanisms fail (blood pressure falls further), or due to head trauma hypotension may lead to brain ischemia. Hypertension is part of the Cushing's response

■ *Respiration* – initially with raised intracranial pressure, a reduced respiratory rate will occur. As ICP increases, breathing becomes rapid (loss of brainstem functioning). This is the third part of the Cushing's response

■ *Temperature* – control centre in the hypothalamus (brainstem). Pyrexia occurs when thermoregulation fails.

Summary

For many patients, monitoring of vital signs (e.g. blood pressure, pulse, and respiration) is sufficient. However, there will be instances when more advanced modes of assessment are required. This type of information is obtained by the use of technical equipment. Nurses need to be conversant and skilful in using this equipment appropriately and accurately.

References

BAPN (British Association of Paediatric Nephrology) (2008) Haemodialysis clinical practice guidelines for children and adolescents, BAPN. Available at: www.renal.org/guidelines/clinical-practice-guidelines-committee#sthash.T7LWGLv3.dpbs (accessed 1 February 2016).

BTS (British Thoracic Society) Standards of Care Committee (2002) Non-invasive ventilation in acute respiratory failure, *Thorax*, 57: 192–211.

Dawes, E., Lloyd, H. and Durham, L (2007) Monitoring and recording patients' neurological observations. *Nursing Standard*, 22(10): 40–45.

Hall, J.E. (2015) *Guyton and Hall Textbook of Medical Physiology*, 13th edn. St Louis, MO: Elsevier.

Kelly, C.A., Upex, A. and Bateman, D.N. (2004) Comparison of consciousness level assessment in the poisoned patient using the Alert/Verbal/Painful/unresponsive scale and Glasgow Coma Scale. *Annals of Emergency Medicine*, 44(2): 107–113.

NICE (National Institute for Clinical Excellence) (2002) *Guidance on the Use of Ultrasound Locating Devices for Placing Central Venous Catheter*, NICE CG 49. London: NICE.

NICE (National Institute for Clinical Excellence) (2007) *Head Injury: Triage, Assessment, Investigation and Early Management of Head Injury in Infants, Children and Adults*. Available at: www.nice.org.uk (accessed 20 February 2016).

NMC (Nursing and Midwifery Council) (2015) *The Code: Professional Standards of Practice and Behaviour for Nurses and Midwives*. London: NMC.

Resuscitation Council UK (2010) *Peri-arrest Arrhythmias*. London: Resuscitation Council.

Resuscitation Council UK (2015) *Prevention of Cardiac Arrest and Decisions about CPR*. London: Resuscitation Council.

Chapter 9

Oxygenation

Tina Moore

It is a simple and indisputable fact – oxygen is necessary to sustain life. Clinical studies show that a human being can live for days without water, and weeks without food – but without oxygen, biological death begins to occur within three minutes. Oxygen is the miraculous element that permits life to exist and flourish on earth.

(The miracle of oxygen, 2003)

Key concepts

Gas transportation

Pulse oximetry

Oxygen saturation

Oxygen administration

Hypoxaemia

Peak expired flow rate

Nebuliser therapy

Learning outcomes

By the end of this chapter you will be able to:

- Identify the causes of hypoxaemia (below normal oxygen content in arterial blood)
- Describe the signs of hypoxaemia
- Understand reasons for monitoring oxygen saturation, peak flow rate and interpret readings accurately
- List the different types of devices used to administer oxygen and discuss the advantages and disadvantages of each device
- Identify the need for and administer appropriate oxygen and nebuliser therapy
- Demonstrate knowledge of problems associated with administration of oxygen and nebulisers.

Introduction

Oxygen is vital for life. Changes to the patient's respiratory status is one of the early warning signs of physiological deterioration. Subsequently, appropriate assessment and early, effective intervention are paramount. This particular chapter discusses commonly used devices to assess the adequacy of gaseous exchange and improve gas exchange or oxygenation of the tissues. All areas discussed within this chapter apply to the adult, child and those with mental health issues; where appropriate, differences are discussed. At the time of this publication, The British Thoracic Society guidance on the administration of oxygen therapy is currently being updated. It is anticipated that the positions of 'Oxygen Champions' will soon be in place within acute care areas.

It is useful to read Chapter 7 before continuing with this chapter.

Gaseous exchange

Understanding the normal processes involved in gaseous exchange is crucial in order to conduct a meaningful and accurate assessment, thus enabling the correct intervention. The efficiency of this process is dependent upon a close match between the amount of gas reaching the alveoli (ventilation) and the blood flow in the pulmonary capillaries (perfusion). The relationship between ventilation and perfusion in the lungs is measured by calculating the difference between the alveolar and arterial partial pressure oxygen.

At rest, alveolar ventilation is:

Ventilation (V) = 4L/min and perfusion (Q) = 5L/min, resulting in a V:Q ratio of 4:5 (or 0.8)

In a 'perfect lung', gaseous exchange will be evenly distributed (perfectly matched), i.e. all alveoli would receive an equal share of alveolar ventilation and the pulmonary capillaries would receive an equal share of the cardiac output. It must be remembered that these are normal, average healthy adult values, but individual patients will not always match them, even in health.

Transfer of oxygen to the cells

The transfer of oxygen (O_2) from the atmosphere to the cells is a four-stage process (Figure 9.1).

Stage 1 Movement of oxygen into the alveoli

The movement of oxygen into the alveoli involves the mechanism of ventilation. Ventilation is the mechanical movement of gas or air into and out of the lung (inspiration and expiration). Ventilation is usually an involuntary process and involves homeostatic changes that can adjust the breathing rate and volume automatically via the nervous system to maintain adequate gaseous exchange. It is worth noting that ventilation is not the same as respiration. Respiration is the exchange of gases (oxygen and carbon dioxide) during cellular metabolism.

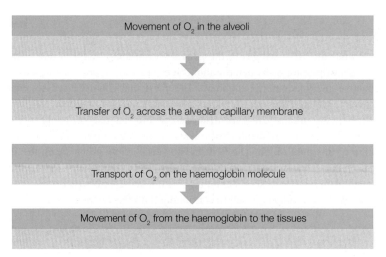

Figure 9.1 **Transfer of oxygen to the cells**

The medulla oblongata (in the brain stem) controls ventilation by the transmission of impulses to the respiratory muscles, causing their contraction and relaxation. Chemoreceptors which are located in the circulatory system (carotid and aortic bodies) and medulla oblongata, sense the effectiveness of ventilation by monitoring the pH status of the cerebrospinal fluid, the oxygen content (PaO_2) and carbon dioxide ($PaCO_2$) content of the arterial blood gas (ABG) (see Chapter 8). These respond to hypercapnia (high carbon dioxide levels); acidaemia (low pH levels) and hypoxaemia (low oxygen levels) by sending impulses to the medulla to alter the rate of ventilation. In chronic obstructive pulmonary disease (COPD), these receptors become insensitive to small changes in $PaCO_2$ and as a result the regulation of ventilation is poor, which means that this group of patients will have a higher than normal $PaCO_2$ level.

The process of breathing to aid the movement of O_2 into the alveoli

At the start of inspiration (the movement of gas from the atmosphere into the alveoli), pressures within the atmosphere and lungs are equal. Gas moves via a pressure gradient, i.e. from an area of high pressure to an area of low pressure. Influences on the pressure gradient include changes in the size of the thoracic cavity. During inspiration (Figure 9.2), the intercostal muscles and diaphragm contract, making the thoracic cavity larger, and contraction of the external intercostal muscles pulls the anterior end of each rib up and out, elevating the sternum. The intra-thoracic pressure is lowered. The pressure gradient is a high area of pressure (atmosphere) to an area of low pressure (alveoli).

Expiration is normally a passive process. The intercostal muscles relax, reducing the size of the thorax and increasing intrapleural pressure. The pressure in the thoracic cavity is now higher than atmospheric pressure, forcing air out. The pressure between the visceral and parietal pleura is always negative (i.e. less that the atmospheric pressure). Negative intrapleural pressure is required to overcome the problem of collapsed alveoli (atelectasis) caused by the surface tension of the fluid lining, the alveoli and the stretch of elastic fibres, that are constantly attempting to recoil.

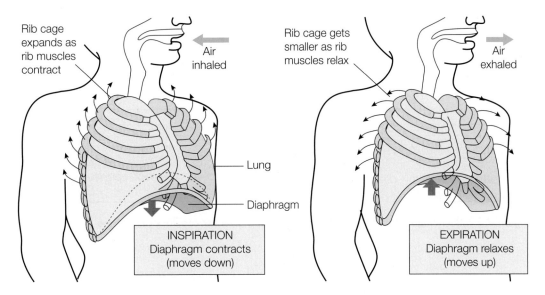

Figure 9.2 **The process of breathing**

As alveolar pressure increases, a positive pressure gradient is established – from alveoli to the atmosphere. In forced expiration, contraction of the abdominal and internal intercostal muscles can increase alveolar pressure, resulting in a very large air pressure gradient. The elastic recoil of the thorax and lungs aids the return to the pre-inspiration volume; if a disease condition, e.g. emphysema, reduces the elasticity of pulmonary tissue, expiration becomes forced even at rest.

Stage 2 Transfer of oxygen across the alveolar capillary membrane

Gas exchange occurs across the alveolar capillary membrane which has a vast surface area, a very thin membrane and a constant supply of both air and blood. These are ideal conditions for oxygen diffusion/transfer. Oxygen will move from an area of high pressure to an area of low pressure until equilibrium is achieved.

Surfactant is secreted by the alveolar cells and maintains its integrity by covering the inner surface of the alveolus and lowering the alveolar surface tension at the end of expiration, thus, preventing atelectasis. Inadequate alveolar ventilation (Figure 9.3) can cause a decrease in the normal pH level, increase $PaCO_2$ and decrease PaO_2.

Inadequate alveolar ventilation = $\downarrow$ normal pH level; $\uparrow$ $PaCO_2$; $\downarrow$ PaO_2

Stage 3 Transport of oxygen on the haemoglobin molecule

Oxygen is transported within the circulation in two ways, approximately 3 per cent is dissolved in plasma and measured clinically by arterial blood gas analysis (ABG) as PaO_2. The remaining 97 per cent is transported by binding with haemoglobin and

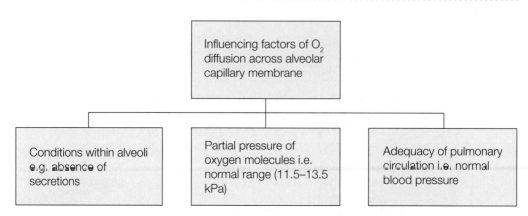

Figure 9.3 **Influencing factors of O_2 diffusion across the alveolar capillary membrane**

is measured clinically by arterial (SaO_2) and peripheral (SpO_2) oxygen saturation. As oxygen diffuses across the alveolar capillary membrane, it dissolves into the plasma where it exerts pressure. As the partial pressure of oxygen increases in the plasma, oxygen moves into the erythrocytes (red blood cell) and binds with haemoglobin until it becomes 'saturated'.

Measurement of haemoglobin concentration is important when assessing individuals with respiratory problems. This is because a decrease in haemoglobin concentration below the normal value of blood reduces PaO_2. Increases in haemoglobin concentration may increase oxygen content, minimising the impact of impaired gas exchange. Respiratory disease impairs gas exchange and an adequate plasma level of PaO_2 is essential for the remaining oxygen to bind with the haemoglobin in order to facilitate tissue perfusion.

$$O_2 \text{ in plasma} = \uparrow O_2 \text{ partial pressure} = \text{movement into red blood cell} = \text{haemoglobin} + O_2$$

Stage 4 Movement of oxygen from the haemoglobin to the tissues/cells

Oxygen enters the tissues by diffusing down the concentration gradient, from high concentration in the alveoli to lower concentrations in the capillaries. This process is influenced by haemoglobin levels (a decrease will reduce oxygen content). This process continues until the haemoglobin binding sites are what is referred to as 'saturated', i.e. full of oxygen (Figure 9.4). Table 9.1 shows the normal haemoglobin values.

$$O_2 \text{ in haemoglobin} \rightarrow \text{tissues diffusion}$$

Pulse oximetry

Pulse oximetry monitoring (oxygen saturation of peripheral capillary blood) is an accepted practice to provide an immediate assessment of the oxygen status of the patient and is now considered the 'fifth' vital sign (BTS, 2008). This device offers a simple,

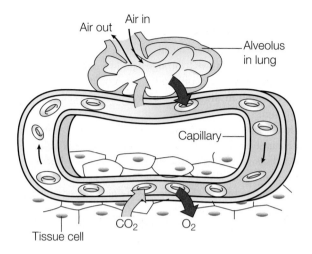

Figure 9.4 Transfer of oxygen to the cells

Table 9.1 Average normal haemoglobin values

Age	Haemoglobin value
Adult male	140–180 gm/L
Adult female	120–160 gm/L
Children	110–130 gm/L
One month old	110–150 gm/L

reliable and quick way to continuously assess and monitor the adequacy of the patient's gas exchange at the bedside. When analysing the effectiveness of oxygen therapy, it is important to note the patient's oxygen saturation levels in the context of the amount of oxygen inspired by the patient. This will provide information on their ability to retain oxygen.

Peripheral oxygen saturation monitoring (SpO_2) does not provide a picture of the overall efficiency of gas exchange in the lungs or tissues, merely the transport of oxygen on the haemoglobin molecules. That is, it does not give information on carbon dioxide levels which is particularly important when determining patient deterioration. In this instance, ABG analysis should be performed together with comprehensive respiratory assessment of the patient.

Continuous SpO_2 monitoring should be used on patients who have problems with their breathing or a change in their respiratory status and for those receiving continuous oxygen therapies.

Rationale for pulse oximetry monitoring

Hypoxaemia (reduced oxygen tension or partial pressure of oxygen in the blood) is defined as an oxygen saturation level of less than 90 per cent (BTS, 2008). However, it is normal to expect transient dips in saturation levels for non-acute patients as low as 90 per cent during sleeping (BTS, 2008).

The diffusion of oxygen is dependent upon a normal airway diameter (airway passages can also become narrowed through sputum, vomit, pulmonary oedema and blood), adequate respiratory rate/depth and a functioning nervous supply. Influencing factors include a reduction in the amount of available oxygen, e.g. someone suffering from smoke inhalation.

There is no doubt that tissues require oxygen for survival. Generally, the aim is to achieve a target saturation of 94–98 per cent for those aged below 70 and children. Patients aged 70 and above may have saturation levels below 94 per cent and not require oxygen therapy. For patients with COPD, and for those at risk of Type 2 respiratory failure, an initial saturation of 88–92 per cent is suggested, pending availability of ABG results (BTS, 2008).

Satisfactory delivery of oxygen to the tissues depends on a number of factors:

- Adequate alveolar ventilation
- Diffusion from the alveoli into the pulmonary vascular system
- Delivery of oxygenated blood via the circulation to cells within tissues.

Respiratory failure is a syndrome in which the respiratory system fails in one or both of its gas exchange functions (oxygenation and CO_2 elimination). In practice, it may be classified as either hypoxaemia or hypercapnia. Type 1 respiratory failure (hypoxaemia) occurs where there is hypoxaemia (PaO_2 less than 8 kPa) and without CO_2 retention. This can be caused by lung problems involving fluid filling or collapse of alveoli, e.g., pulmonary oedema, pneumonia. Hypoxaemia results in tissue dysfunction and if severe enough, organ failure. Equally, hypoxaemia will also result in hypoxia (reduced oxygenation of cells in the tissues) and can result from acute myocardial infarction, severe trauma, anaemia (Box 9.1).

Type 2 respiratory failure (hypercapnic) is where a patient is unable to excrete a sufficient amount of CO_2 with accompanying hypoxaemia ($PaCO_2$ greater than 6 kPa and PaO_2 less than 8 kPa). Causes can include chest wall deformities, overdose, neuromuscular disease, anything that causes shallow breathing and retention of CO_2.

Tolerance for hypoxaemia depends on the body's compensatory mechanisms available and the sensitivity of the patient to hypoxia. If the patient has no additional problems, e.g. cardiac problems or anaemia, then important symptoms may not manifest until the PaO_2 falls below 6.8–7 0 kPa (normal = 11.5–13.5 kPa). If this happens, symptoms such as malaise, light-headedness, vertigo, impaired judgement are likely to occur.

Mild to moderate hypoxaemia is (10.5–5 kPa) can be seen in patients during the peri- and postoperative period. Hypoxaemia often goes unrecognised and its potential to impede recovery (including wound healing and an increased resistance to infection) is often underestimated. Other symptoms include: confusion, tachypnoea, dyspnoea, tachycardia.

Severe hypoxaemia ($PaO_2 < 4.5$ kPa) may cause bradycardia, lethargy, renal blood flow decreases, hypotension, diaphoresis (sweating) and central cyanosis – a bluish, purple discoloration of the lips, mucous membrane of the mouth and tongue. Other signs include coma, convulsions and possibly respiratory arrest.

Box 9.1 Alterations to gas exchange can cause hypoxaemia

- *Low inspired oxygen*: drop in atmospheric pressure associated in high altitudes
- *Alveolar hypoventilation*: causing hypercapnia (CO_2) (e.g. occurs in patients with COPD; patients receiving too much sedation) and shallow breathing following abdominal/thoracic surgery
- *Diffusion abnormalities*: diffusion of oxygen through the alveolar capillary membrane is impaired if the membrane is thickened or there is a decrease in the surface area available for diffusion, e.g. pulmonary oedema
- *Abnormal ventilation (V): perfusion (Q) ratio:* this is the most common cause of hypoxaemia. Hypoxaemia can be caused by either inadequate ventilation of well-perfused areas of the alveoli (reduced oxygen intake), e.g. chest infection, asthma, pneumothorax, acute coronary syndrome or an abnormal V:Q ratio caused by good ventilation with poor perfusion, as seen in the case of pulmonary embolism
- *Atelectasis*: the alveoli become deflated in the event of a collapsed lung (whole or partial) as in the case of critical illness
- *Low haemoglobin concentration*: hypoxaemia results in low arterial saturations and cellular function alterations, e.g. anaemia, sickle cell anaemia.

Clinical significance

Central cyanosis is the blue discoloration of the lips, mucous membrane of the mouth and tongue caused by lack of oxygen in the blood, usually detectable when the arterial saturations are less than 85 per cent, therefore, cyanosis is a late clinical sign. This occurs when approximately 50 g/L of unoxygenated haemoglobin in the capillaries generates the dark blue colour. For this reason, patients who are anaemic may be hypoxemic without showing any cyanosis.

Activity 9.1

Have you cared for an adult or child who has been diagnosed as having hypoxaemia? Reflecting upon the experience, think of answers to the following questions:

- What did their colour look like?
- Describe how they were breathing (think of the rate, rhythm, depth, degree of effort).

Now try and relate your answers to the four stages of oxygen transfer discussed in this chapter.

Treatment for hypoxaemia

Administration of oxygen alone will not help to prevent or alleviate hypoxaemia. Every step should be undertaken to increase gas exchange as follows:

- Position should be upright where possible
- Maintenance of adequate fluid balance/maintenance of adequate blood pressure (to ensure sufficient delivery of oxygenated blood to the tissues)
- Slow, deep breaths (increases tidal volume and hence gas exchange) as hyperventilation decreases the amount of oxygen inspired
- Physiotherapy may be useful
- Supplementary oxygen may be prescribed
- Compliance is essential and is required continuously. If the patient is confused, it may be a symptom of hypoxia
- Non-invasive ventilation – if there no response to the above.

(Moore and Woodrow, 2009)

Watch out

- Look out for other clinical signs – severe hypoxaemia is not excluded by the absence of cyanosis. It will not be present in patients with anaemia, where the haemoglobin level is low or if there is poor perfusion of the capillaries.

While pulse oximetry provides a quick, non-invasive method of monitoring a patient's oxygen status, it is not suitable for monitoring patients with carbon monoxide poisoning as the sensor is not designed to differentiate between oxyhaemoglobin and carboxy-haemoglobin. Pulse oximetry recordings will provide false elevated oxygen saturation (SpO_2) readings.

Likewise, in the case of patients with anaemia, monitoring should be treated with caution because it is the percentage of oxygen saturation that is recorded, irrespective of haemoglobin levels (Box 9.2). Therefore, a saturation of 97 per cent means that 97 per cent of the *total* amount of haemoglobin available in the blood contains oxygen molecules, again falsely elevating the readings.

A pulse oximeter (Figures 9.5 and 9.6) measures the absorption of specific wavelength(s) (some machines have more than one wavelength) of light in oxygenated haemoglobin. A probe or sensor is placed on a site with an adequate pulsating vascular bed. This is usually a finger, but earlobes can be used too. Manufacturer's guidelines should be consulted as to where to place the probe, especially with small children, as malpositioning may interfere with calibration. One side of the probe has energy sources in the form of light-emitting diodes (LED) that transmit red and infrared light wavelengths. These are directed perpendicularly, through pulsating arterial blood, to a semiconductor photo detector on the other side. The amplitude of light transmitted is measured by the monitor. This device is able to differentiate between arterial and venous blood.

Box 9.2 Uses for oxygen saturation monitoring

- For patients with conditions affecting/potentially affecting respiratory status
- During diagnostic testing for patients with acute problems
- Monitoring for potential hypoxaemia caused by invasive procedures (e.g. insertion of a tracheostomy)
- As a baseline – within the first five minutes of initiating oxygen therapy (BTS, 2008)
- Evaluating the effectiveness of oxygen therapy
- Weaning respiratory support (e.g. oxygen therapy, Continuous Positive Airway Pressure (CPAP)) in the absence of ABGs.

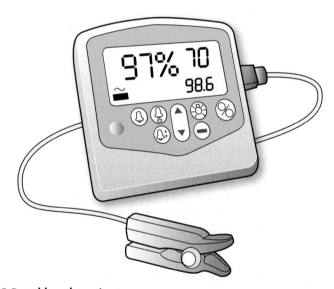

Figure 9.5 Portable pulse oximeter

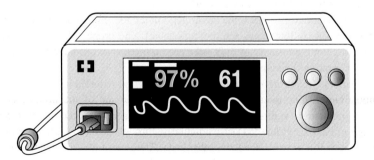

Figure 9.6 Pulse oximeter

Amplitude is dependent upon:

- The volume of arterial pulse (readings will be unreliable in those with peripheral shutdown) (Figure 9.7)
- The wavelength of light used (direct sunlight on the sensor will affect the results)
- The oxygen saturation of haemoglobin (unreliable in anaemia).

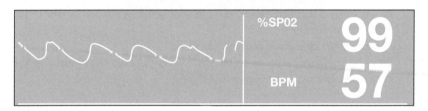

Figure 9.7 Pulse amplitude

Procedure for pulse oximetry monitoring

1   The procedure should be explained to the patient and, where possible, consent gained.
2   Wash and dry hands before and after the procedure.
3   Ensure that the device is working properly (test it out on yourself). Ensure that the probe is the correct size for the patient's extremity. Sensors are sized according to the patient's weight; different manufacturers specify somewhat different ranges. It is important to use the correct size to avoid skin complications and ensure accurate readings.
4   Studies now suggest that the use of dark coloured nail polish (e.g. black, green, blue) does not affect the accuracy of the readings. However, all nail polish should be removed (obtain consent where possible) as this will enable the monitoring of the patient's nail colour (for peripheral cyanosis) and capillary refill time.
5   The skin where the probe is to be placed should be cleaned (following manufacturers' guidelines, some suggest soap and water or alcohol-impregnated swabs) before attaching the probe. Make sure that the skin is also thoroughly dry.
6   Check that the alarm limits set are suited to the patient. For patients requiring continuous pulse oximetry recordings, avoid using the same arm as the blood pressure recordings.
7   Choose an extremity – normally the finger, but the toe, earlobe or bridge of the nose may be used (follow manufacturer's guidance). The probe (Figure 9.8) should be well fitted with constant but light pressure on the tissues so that the energy source cannot bypass the tissues.
8   All patients requiring pulse oximetry monitoring (continuous or intermittent), should have a full comprehensive respiratory assessment taken.
9   Once the machine is turned on, there should be a display – usually with a waveform or bar graph (see Figure 9.7).
10 Alarms should be set – for low saturation and high and low pulse rate – normally these are automatically set to default values when the device is switched on, i.e. oxygen saturation less than 95 per cent (unless COPD, then 92 per cent) (BTS, 2008).

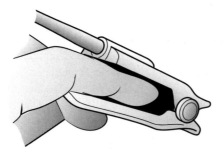

Figure 9.8 Finger probe

11 Readings become unreliable on patients who are moving about a lot, therefore pulse oximetry readings alone should not be relied upon (see Table 9.2). Other clinical assessment data (particularly respiratory) should be noted and acted upon.
12 Document the time and site when the probe is placed (NMC, 2015). Change position of the probe at least every four hours as there is a possibility that pressure sores and damage to the tissue by the heat expelled may occur.

Top tip

If the reading is abnormal and the patient does not show any obvious signs of respiratory distress, never assume that the device is faulty! Try another site first. If the reading is the same, it may mean that the patient has circulatory failure.

Oxygen therapy

The administration of oxygen is used in all practice settings. It is the first line of treatment, particularly in many acute and emergency situations, e.g. patients who are in shock; acute respiratory failure; cardiac arrest; myocardial infarction and low oxygen saturations.

Anecdotal evidence suggests that oxygen is often given without careful appraisal of its potential benefits and indeed side effects, regularly being delegated to junior staff and students. Inappropriate dosage and failure to monitor the effects of oxygen therapy can have serious consequences. Note that oxygen therapy (unless in an emergency situation) should always be prescribed and administered accordingly. Having a target goal for intervention, e.g. oxygen saturation levels are seen as good practice.

Watch out

Despite receiving oxygen therapy, the patient's condition may worsen, e.g. increased dyspnoea, drowsiness. This is because tolerance for hypoxaemia depends on the compensatory mechanisms available and the sensitivity of the patient to hypoxia.

Table 9.2 Problems associated with using pulse oximetry

Potential problems with accuracy of reading	Appropriate intervention
Dark skin decreases the accuracy of pulse oximeters at low oxygen saturation levels (Bickler *et al.*, 2005)	
Poor perfusion/vasoconstriction, caused by weak pulses, hypotension and hypothermia will cause low, intermittent or unavailable readings	Warm extremities with a blanket or a warmer pack (leave for a short time to avoid heat injury)
Sudden movements and restlessness may cause the sensor to become partially dislodged, or cause motion artefact. This will affect the ability of the light to travel from the LED to the photo detector. Rhythmic movement (e.g. seizures, shivering) may also cause problems	Explain the importance of keeping still; if the child is unable to, consider moving the probe to the ear lobe (consult manufacturer's guidelines) as this may be the most suitable place, as movement least affects the probe
Pressure sore/thermal damage	Check position of the probe and condition of the skin every 2 hours. Change probe position every 4 hours (MDA, 2001). Also check the security of the probe
Evidence on the effects of bright light (including direct sunlight, fluorescent lights, surgical lamps) shining directly on the sensor probe interfering with the readings remains inconclusive	Remove the source of light
Optical shunting occurs when the probe is positioned badly and the light goes directly from the light emitting diode (LED) to the photo detector missing the vascular bed	Check position and reposition if indicated
Abnormal haemoglobin can occur with carbon monoxide poisoning due to smoke inhalation. The sensor cannot differentiate between oxyhaemoglobin and carboxyhaemoglobin and will therefore provide a falsely elevated SpO_2 reading	Pulse oximetry should not be used. ABG analysis should be used instead
Anaemia. It is the percentage of oxygen saturation that is recorded, so the haemoglobin levels are immaterial. Therefore a saturation of 97% means that 97% of the *total* amount of haemoglobin in the blood contains oxygen molecules, giving the impression of being 'fully saturated'	Take ABGs
Arrhythmias	Test the equipment on yourself or another healthy person. Correlate the pulse reading with the patient's heart rate (if there is a variance, it could indicate that not all pulsations are being picked up). Send blood for ABG analysis. A replacement monitor may be indicated. An ECG may need to be taken
Intermittent blood flow	Check pulse rate and capillary refill time
Alterations to recordings occur when using an automated blood pressure device (blood pressure cuff) is used on the same limb.	The pulse oximeter sensor needs to be placed on a finger of the opposite side, as blood flow to the finger will be cut off whenever the cuff inflates. Readings will be inaccurate.

Source: Adapted from Moore and Woodrow (2009).

Rationale for administrating oxygen therapy

Oxygen is a colourless, odourless gas that makes up 21 per cent (referred to as air) of the atmosphere. Its administration can be a life-saving intervention but it needs to be undertaken properly and correctly. The need for supplementary oxygen (greater than 21 per cent) should be determined through evaluation of the pulse oximetry monitoring, clinical assessment and possible ABG analysis. It is used to correct hypoxaemia, with respiratory failure being the main reason for such an intervention. Administration also requires care and attention, with the practitioner following procedures for administering drugs. Nurses are encouraged to consult the BTS (2008) guidelines as there is an extensive list of clinical situations there, complete with guidance on the safe administration of oxygen. Oxygen therapy corrects hypoxaemia, reduces the work of breathing and reduces the myocardial workload.

Activity 9.2

- Think about some patients in your care who have required supplementary oxygen therapy. Can you remember what the underlying problem was that required this type of treatment?
- List the type of device(s) you have seen used to administer supplementary oxygen in clinical practice
- From your experiences, what do you think were the advantages/disadvantages in using the devices?

Oxygen-delivering devices are usually classified into two general categories: low-flow systems and high-flow systems. Whether a system is low or high flow does not determine its capability of delivering low verses high concentrations of oxygen and the dosage should be adjusted in accordance with ABG results if available/appropriate.

Low-flow systems (variable performance systems)

Low flow systems depend upon the patient's minute ventilation, peak inspiratory flow rate and oxygen flow rate, therefore they do not always provide all the gas necessary to meet the patient's total minute ventilation requirements. Delivery of oxygen is at a low flow rate and provides variable oxygen concentration to the patient.

This system requires the patient to entrain (draw in air) while gas rich with oxygen is also inspired from a reservoir (mask or bag), making it difficult to estimate exactly how much inspired oxygen a patient is receiving.

If the patient is breathing rapidly (increased minute volume), the concentration of oxygen delivered is decreased. If the patient takes deep, slow breaths, a much higher concentration of oxygen is inspired. Therefore, the concentration of oxygen delivered is dependent on the patient's breathing pattern and minute volume (respiratory rate multiplied by tidal volume = minute volume).

Low-flow systems include: simple face masks (Figure 9.9); nasal cannulae; partial re-breathing mask and non-rebreathing mask.

Simple facemask is calibrated to deliver a flow of up to 60 per cent oxygen. Within the sides of the simple face mask there are relatively large 'ventilation' holes that allow room air in (during inspiration) and release exhaled gases (during expiration). This makes the inspiratory flow greater and more diluted than the oxygen flow rate, resulting in variability in the amount of inspired oxygen. For this device, oxygen flow must be at least 5 L/min to prevent collection and rebreathing of exhaled gas (high in carbon dioxide content).

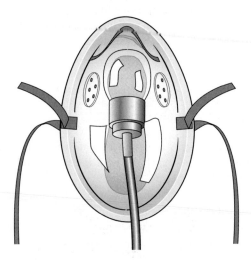

Figure 9.9 Simple face mask

If the face mask does not fit properly, there will be an increase in entrained room air which reduces the inspired oxygen concentration further. The mask should be applied securely over the patient's mouth, nose and chin. The metal piece over the bridge of the nose should be pressed firmly to keep the mask more secure and to create a seal to prevent gas loss. Straps should be adjusted to fit correctly on the patient's face.

Young children may be frightened and agitated when oxygen is administered and feel a sense of claustrophobia. A parent could hold the mask in proximity to or over the child's face instead. This should be documented.

Limitations of access for expectoration of sputum, vomiting, eating and drinking can be problematic.

Top tip

During meal times, patients should have the oxygen via a nasal cannula.

Partial rebreathing mask and bag

For those patients whose are acutely ill or deteriorating, alternative devices should be considered, e.g. a partial-rebreathing bag and mask in order to achieve a greater percentage of oxygen delivery (Figure 9.10). By adding a reservoir bag to the face mask, an extra supply of oxygen is administered, i.e. higher than 60 per cent. The reservoir bag fills with oxygen, thus providing an oxygen reservoir for the patient to inspire. The bag should deflate by only one-third on inspiration (to prevent the accumulation of CO_2 in the reservoir bag). If this does not occur, the oxygen flow rate should be adjusted accordingly and the deflation of the reservoir bag closely monitored.

Watch out

Remember, a high oxygen flow rate will cause drying and irritation of the eyes. Artificial eye drops may need to be prescribed.

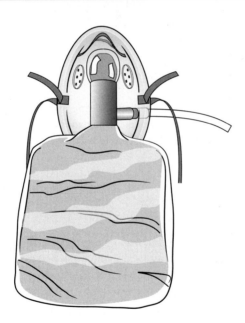

Figure 9.10 **Partial rebreathing mask and bag**

Non-rebreathing bag and mask

This device is designed to supply high concentrations of oxygen from a reservoir mask and is used for all patients with shock, major trauma, sepsis or other critical illnesses (BTS, 2008). The flow rate should be 10–15 litres. During inspiration the side port valves of the mask close and the valve between the bag and mask connection opens, allowing inspiration of approximately100 per cent oxygen (Figure 9.11). The opposite occurs during expiration. These valves are designed to prevent exhaled gas from entering the reservoir bag, eliminating the rebreathing of expired gas.

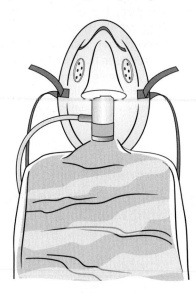

Figure 9.11 **Non-rebreathing bag and mask**

Again the reservoir bag should not collapse during inspiration (suggesting flow rates are insufficient to meet the patient's ventilatory demands). If this occurs, the patient may struggle against the one-way valve and therefore the work of breathing is increased, leading to tiredness and exhaustion.

Top tip

All masks should be well fitting but may give patients a sense of claustrophobia. You may need to let the patient get used to the mask first by placing and holding it gently on their face for a few minutes before tightening the straps. If the strap is too tight, you will not be able to move two fingers inside the strap.

Nasal cannulae

Nasal cannulae (Figure 9.12) are simple, unobtrusive devices, preferably used in medium dosage administration (BTS, 2008). They are particularly useful for patients who are unable to tolerate a mask or who are eating and drinking, coughing, expectorating copious amounts of sputum or vomiting. It is a lightweight and flexible plastic tubing with two prongs entering the nose. For application, direct the prongs inwards, following the curvature of the nasal passages, the tubing can be hooked behind the patient's ears.

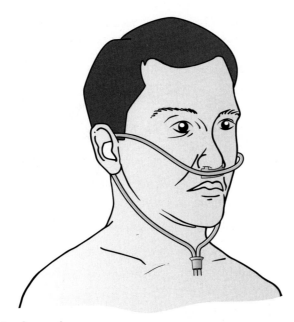

Figure 9.12 Nasal cannulae

Top tip

A nasal cannula is not effective for patients who are 'mouth-breathers', e.g. patients who have complete or partial nasal obstruction.

The nasal cannula is capable of delivering a flow of oxygen ranging from 24–44 per cent, depending on the amount of flow in litres. However, it is advised that manufacturer's guidelines are always followed. Disadvantages include discomfort, caused by crusting and drying of the nasal cavity due to dry oxygen.

Note that the maximum flow rate is 6 litres but up to 4 litres is considered the norm. If the flow rate is too high, it can cause trauma, epistaxis (bleeding from the nose) and drying out of the mucosal membranes.

The nasal cavity and around the sides of the nose should be inspected regularly for pressure sores. Gauze padding can be placed around the ears between the patient's skin and tubing to help minimise the risk of pressure sores. Humidification can also help with drying and irritation. Nasal care should be given with cotton buds.

High-flow systems (fixed performance masks)

Venturi mask

A Venturi mask allows a fixed flow of oxygen (Figure 9.13). This is achieved through kinetic energy (speed of movement), facilitated through a jet adapter (often colour-coded)

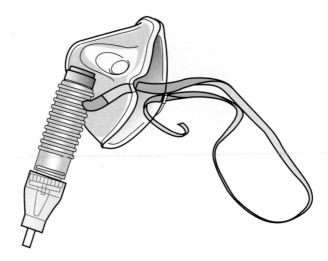

Figure 9.13 **Venturi mask**

(Figure 9.14) that is positioned between the mask and the tubing to the oxygen source. Oxygen rates are set above the normal respiratory flow rate and are available in the following colour-coded concentrations: 24%, 28%, 35%, 40% and 60%.

The Venturi mask is used for patients who require an accurate concentration of oxygen. Delivery of oxygen concentration is more accurate using this system as it is not altered by variations in ventilation, thus making blood gas analysis more meaningful. Through this system, a consistent flow of oxygen should be sufficient to meet all of the patient's minute ventilation requirements.

In conditions such as COPD, the delivery of excessive oxygen could depress the respiratory drive. Therefore, caution needs to be taken when administrating oxygen to such patients. Normally, CO_2 levels influence the respiratory centre to increase the rate and depth of breathing, resulting in the increase in the excretion of carbon dioxide. Patients with COPD retain carbon dioxide (raised $PaCO_2$ levels), thus depend upon hypoxia to stimulate their respiratory drive (known as the 'hypoxic drive'). In these instances, the use of fixed performance masks are particularly useful (BTS, 2008). They are also viewed as effective for patients with variable, deep, irregular, shallow breathing

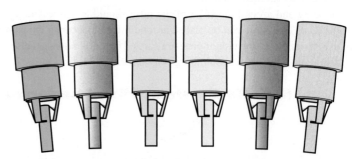

Figure 9.14 **Jet adapters for a Venturi mask**

patterns. However, if a patient with COPD is severely hypoxaemic, they should still receive appropriately higher dosages of oxygen.

Don't forget!

Hypoxaemia! It is highly dangerous and is responsible for many cardiorespiratory arrests and thus a sudden and profound risk to life. Failure to correct hypoxaemia for fear of causing hypoventilation and carbon dioxide retention is unacceptable clinical practice. This is why the patient should be closely monitored for signs of hyperoxia (too much oxygen).

Tracheostomy mask

Within general care areas there may be the opportunity to care for a patient requiring oxygen therapy via a tracheostomy (see Chapter 14 on tracheostomy care). The tracheostomy T-piece or mask is attached by corrugated 'elephant' tubing to the oxygen outlet/humidifier (Figures 9.15 and 9.16). Patients are encouraged to cough to remove mucus from the airway. If they are unable to do so, then suctioning should be administered. Remember, the patient's normal air filtering/arming system has been bypassed, so there is more likely to be an increase in mucous formation. Humidified oxygen should always be given where possible. There may be an initial flow rate set at 10L/min usually, unless there are contraindications, e.g. COPD until the patient's condition stabilises or the oxygen levels improve.

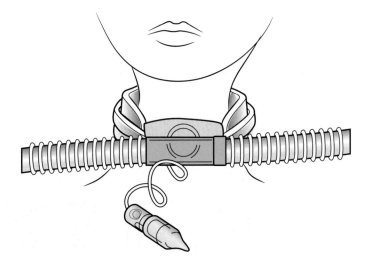

Figure 9.15 **Tracheostomy T-piece with elephant tubing**

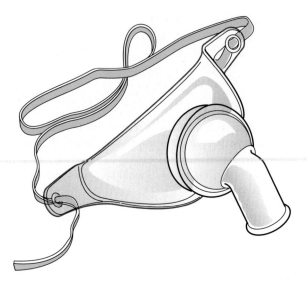

Figure 9.16 Tracheostomy mask

Watch out

Water can accumulate in the corrugated tube, particularly at the 'loop' and requires regular monitoring and emptying. Failure to do so may cause the water to drain accidentally into the patient's airway.

If the flow rate is not regulated properly, this can become a low-flow system.

Humidification

Oxygen is a dry gas and can cause drying out of the upper airways. It is considered to be unnecessary to use humidification for short-term oxygen therapy or low-flow rates, i.e. 4 litres/minute or less (BTS, 2008). If the patient is to have oxygen for longer than 24 hours and complains of the drying out of their nasal passage and mouth, then humidification should be administered, using a humidifier (Figure 9.17).

Don't forget!

Water can accumulate inside the mask, particularly when humidification is used. This should be checked and removed/wiped periodically for patient comfort and prevention of the inhalation of water. Skin areas should be assessed frequently for skin abrasions and pressure sores.

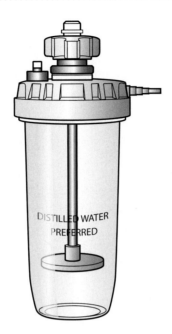

DISTILLED WATER PREFERRED

Figure 9.17 **Humidifier**

Continuous positive airway pressure (CPAP)

CPAP is a non-invasive respiratory support. Its aim is to improve oxygenation/exchange of gases in the alveoli when conventional devices are ineffective. In order to provide safe and appropriate care, nurses should undergo extra training. Students have to work under the close supervision of a qualified nurse and must never be in a position when they are left to care for these patients alone. Variations may be seen in the community for patients with obstructive sleep apnoea.

Procedure for administering CPAP

1 Explain the procedure to the patient, where possible, gain consent.
2 Wash hands before and after procedure.
3 Select the correct type of face mask (ordered by doctor) and correct size – there are full face masks, masks covering the nose and mouth (Figures 9.18 and 9.19) and nasal prongs.
4 In hospitals, the masks shown in Figures 9.18 and 9.19 are the ones mainly used. Ensure that the top of the mask rests on the bridge of the nose and the bottom should rest on the chin, this should ensure there is no air leak into the eyes or out of the mask.
5 It is the responsibility of the qualified nurses or physiotherapists to assemble the CPAP circuit. The oxygen or air flow rate should be adjusted to obtain the positive end expiratory pressure (PEEP) level specified by the doctor. Usually a flow rate of 25L/min will generate a PEEP of 5cmH$_2$O.
6 If possible, the patient should sit as upright as they can tolerate or is clinically safe;

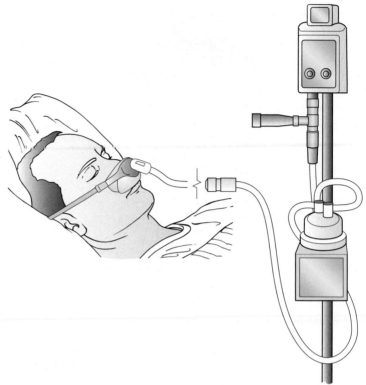

Figure 9.18 **CPAP mask and circuit**

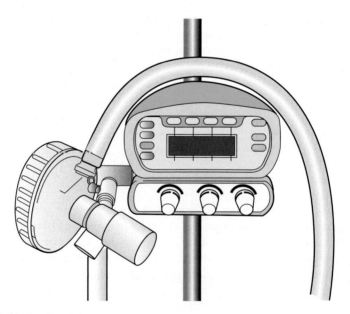

Figure 9.19 **CPAP circuit**

this position helps with lung expansion and should aid in the improvement of ventilation and gas exchange.

7   Hold the mask to the patient's face for a few breaths to familiarise them with the device and reduce anxiety.

8   If the patient is cooperative, attach the head straps and adjust to a comfortable fit.

9   Titrate the oxygen as prescribed.

10   Once the patient is stable, reduce cardiovascular/respiratory observations from every 15 to 30 minutes, then increase/decrease observations according to the patient's condition (see Chapter 7).

11   Continuous pulse oximetry and ECG monitoring should be in place (see Chapter 8). Generally, an ABG is taken one hour following intervention and then monitored very closely thereafter.

12   Once the patient is stable, then weaning from the device should be discussed.

13   If the patient's condition does not improve or there are signs of deterioration, possible transfer to ICU should be considered.

Figure 9.20 shows a CPAP in operation and Figure 9.21 shows an NIV nasal prong mask.

Box 9.3 Potential complications of CPAP

■   *Anxiety and confusion*: as the mask has to fit tightly for maximum effect, this can be a very frightening experience for the patient (especially for a child or those with mental health problems). The degree of co-operation required from the patient should never be underestimated. Patients who suffer with claustrophobia may find it particularly difficult. Constant communication, reassurance and encouragement, reinforcing the benefits of the therapy by the nurse are required

■   *Potential airway obstruction* from retained secretions: due to the tight fit of the mask, the patient will not be able to remove it easily in order to expectorate any secretions. Patients will need very close monitoring and the mask should be removed to allow the patient to cough and expectorate when required

■   *Abdominal distension* with the risk of aspiration: insertion of a naso-gastric tube for the purpose of aspiration and free drainage may help prevent this

■   *Dehydration and malnutrition*: the patient is at high risk due to their difficulty in breathing and the design of the mask makes them unlikely to be able to maintain an adequate oral intake (fluid and food). IV fluids and nasogastric feeding are likely

■   *Hypotension:* in patients with severe hypovolaemia, CPAP can reduce venous return, therefore reducing cardiac output and blood pressure

■   *Pressure sores*: ensure that the mask is the correct size and fits according to the manufacturer's guidance. Remove the mask every two hours to relieve pressure and assess the skin, inspect the ears, chin and bridge of the nose for the fit of the mask. Consider the use of protective dressings

■   *Drying of conjunctiva*: insertion of artificial eye drops four hourly may help

■   *Drying of oral and nasal mucosa*: perform regular mouth care and consider nasal drops.

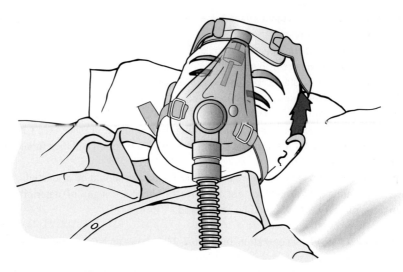

Figure 9.20 CPAP face mask

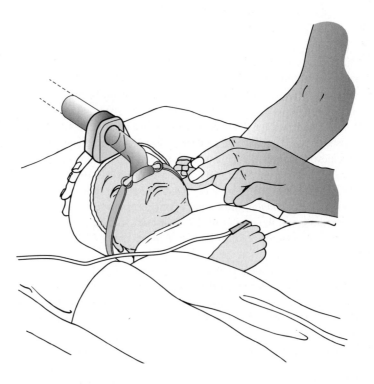

Figure 9.21 Nasal prong mask

Monitoring the patient receiving supplementary oxygen

Despite receiving supplementary oxygen, patients can and do deteriorate, sometimes rapidly, requiring more invasive intervention. For this reason, it is essential that patients are closely monitored for signs of deterioration as well as improvement.

Treatment guidelines should be based on achieving target PaO_2 and SpO_2 rather on administering predetermined concentrations or flow rates of inspired oxygen as determined by the BTS (2008). Trust guidelines should reflect these recommendations, which provide useful guidance for a variety of acute and critical problems.

As discussed, oxygen is classified as a drug, outside of the resuscitation situation, it should always be prescribed, stating the flow rate, delivery system, duration and monitoring of treatment (Box 9.4). The use of oxygen must be documented clearly for each patient and nurses/healthcare professionals should sign on the prescription chart each time it is administered. When oxygen is being administered, the patient should be positioned upright (if possible), to maximise lung expansion.

A full respiratory assessment, as discussed in Chapter 7, together with a respiratory auscultation (Chapter 8) should be undertaken and the patient closely monitored. The delivery systems used should also be recorded in the patient's monitoring charts.

Monitoring therefore should include:

- Clinical signs – a comprehensive respiratory and cardiovascular assessment
- Continuous pulse oximetry monitoring should be started within the first five minutes of initiating oxygen therapy
- Arterial blood gas
- The dangers of hypercapnia should never be ignored and nurses need to monitor the patients for this, e.g. flushing and warm peripheries (vasodilatation), bounding pulse, drowsiness, confusion and coma.

A guide to the safe administration of oxygen

Here is a list of questions that should help you provide safe and effective care when involved in the administration of oxygen. Answer the following questions; the answers have already been discussed in this chapter.

- How can inadequate tissue oxygenation be recognised?
- When is acute oxygen therapy appropriate and at what dose?
- How is oxygen best delivered? Is humidification necessary?
- What are the dangers of oxygen therapy?
- What assessment and monitoring are necessary?
- Is the outcome of the disease improved?
- When should oxygen therapy be stopped?

Peak flow meter

Some respiratory disorders will cause an alteration to airway resistance and lung compliance. A peak flow meter is a small hand-held device that measures how fast a

Box 9.4 Risks of oxygen therapy

These include:

- *Combustibility* – oxygen supports the combustion of other fuels. Extreme care should be taken, particularly during advanced cardio-pulmonary resuscitation. A no smoking policy exists, particularly in areas where oxygen is used
- *Absorbed atelectasis* – high concentrations of oxygen that is administered for relatively long periods of time may cause the alveoli to collapse. This is due to the absorption of gas into the bloodstream. Nitrogen, a relatively insoluble gas, normally maintains a residual volume within the alveolus and therefore keeps the alveoli open and functioning properly. Nitrogen provides a certain amount of surface tension that prevents the collapse of the alveoli. When people are hospitalised or have undergone surgery and general anaesthesia, large amounts of oxygen are usually administered. This decreases the nitrogen concentration in the air and leads to absorption atelectasis. When the alveolar oxygen is then absorbed into the pulmonary capillary, the alveolus collapses, partially to total collapse. Surfactant production is reduced; making the alveoli lose its integrity and more prone to collapse
- *Hyperoxia* (oxygen toxicity) – pathological changes within the lung occur depending upon the amount of exposure and oxygen tension of inspired air. Therefore, a flow of oxygen of more than 50 per cent is considered toxic (Pierce, 2007). Symptoms include early to mild tracheobronchitis; depression of the mucocilliary function (leading to impaired mucous clearance); prolongation of non-productive cough; substernal pain and nasal stiffness. Atelectasis can develop due to oxygen replacing nitrogen and diminishing lung compliance
- *Carbon dioxide narcosis* – carbon dioxide is normally the primary stimulant driving the respiratory system. However, in patients with chronic hypercapnia (as in COPD), hypoxaemia becomes the major respiratory stimulus. Generally, the patients receiving oxygen therapy should be observed for signs of respiratory depression (shallow, slower breathing)
- *Discomfort* – oxygen is a dry gas that can dehydrate exposed membranes, resulting in a dry mouth. Oral fluids and mouth care can help. Humidification will also reduce these effects. The patient should be well hydrated so monitoring a fluid balance is essential. Humidification can also mobilise secretions and enhance patient comfort. Regular nasal and eye care also aids comfort
- *Infection control* – face masks/tubing should be changed. Readers need to refer to their local policies for guidance.

person can blow air out of the lungs when there is forceful exhalation, after maximum inhalation (Figure 9.22). This measurement is called the 'peak expiratory flow' (PEF). The peak flow meter helps to assess the airflow through the airways and thus helps to determine the degree of obstruction. Often dosages of the drugs are adjusted according to the peak flow readings.

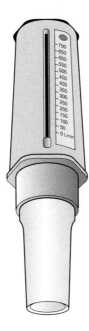

Figure 9.22 **Peak flow meter**

Rationale for recording peak expiratory flow

Peak flow is recorded for the following reasons:

- Management of symptoms of asthma
- To aid the diagnosis of asthma
- Monitoring the progression of the disease and to evaluate treatment.

There are two major types of peak flow meters: the low-range peak flow meter for small children between 4 and 9 years of age, and for adults with severely impaired lung function; and the standard-range peak flow meter for older children, teenagers, and adults. This can be seen in any setting.

Adults have larger airways than children. If given a low-range peak flow meter, they will continually have maximum peak flow rates even when suffering from severe shortness of breath. This may jeopardise proper management, they therefore need the much larger standard range.

Normal peak flow rates vary according to age, height, and sex (Figures 9.23 and 9.24). However, a patient's normal score should be within 20 per cent of a person of the

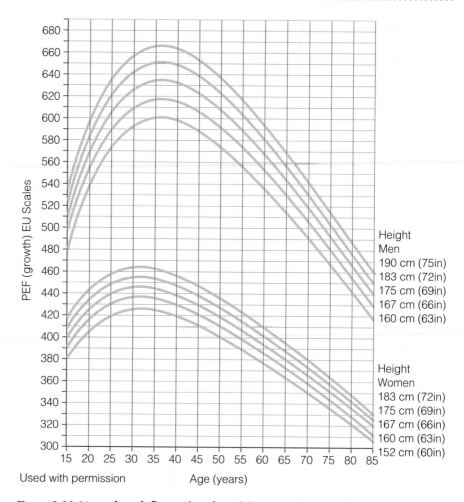

Figure 9.23 Normal peak flow values for adults

same age, sex, and height who does not have asthma. There are published standardised normal values which were calculated by comparing asthmatics with a set of age- and sex-matched controls.

Procedure for recording peak flow

1 Explain the procedure and the rationale for the skill. Gain consent from the patient. Demonstrate the skill, giving very clear instructions.
2 The patient ought to have their own device, if not one way flow disposable mouth pieces are used with it. They should be sitting in an upright position to maximise lung expansion and forced expiratory pressure.
3 Wash and dry hands before and after the procedure.
4 The red cursor along the side of the device should be set at zero. It is important that your hand should not be touching the cursor as it will not move on expiration.

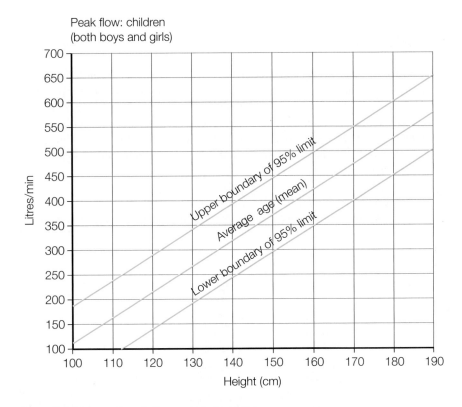

Figure 9.24 **Normal peak flow values for children**

5   Place the disposable mouth piece securely at the top of the device.
6   The peak flow meter should then be held horizontally in front of the mouth. Instruct the patient to take a deep breath on inspiration, close the lips firmly around the mouthpiece, making sure there is no air leak around the lips.
7   The patient should then breathe out as hard and as fast as possible using full effort.
8   Where the cursor stops should be noted.
9   Return the cursor to zero and instruct the patient to repeat this sequence twice more, thus obtaining three readings. Resting in between if needed.
10 The highest score of all three measurements should be recorded.
11 Remove and discard the disposable mouth piece.
12 Document and report the results (NMC, 2015).

Nebuliser therapy

Nebuliser devices provide the administration of drugs via inhalation. This is usually through a face mask but can also be delivered through a mouthpiece (Figure 9.25). You will see this device used mainly for problems with the lower respiratory tract.

Case study 9.1

Mr Sharp, 70 years old, was transferred to your ward after being admitted through Accident and Emergency Department (A & E) with shortness of breath, exacerbation of chronic obstructive pulmonary disease (COPD). Mr Sharp has suffered from COPD for 35 years, the underlying cause is emphysema. He continues to smoke 60 cigarettes a day and there is no sign of him giving this up. He currently has a productive cough. Part of his treatment is to have oxygen administered via a nasal cannula.

■ What would be your priorities in caring for Mr Sharp?
■ What information would you give him regarding his oxygen administration?

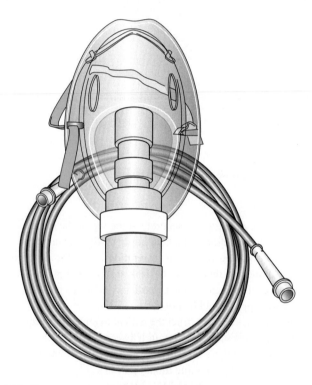

Figure 9.25 Nebuliser – storage chamber and mask

Oxygen therapy during nebulised treatments

Normally nebulised treatment is given via air, but can be delivered through oxygen if the patient has moderate to severe hypoxaemia. Constant observations of the patient are required for signs of hyperoxia. The cylinder should have a minimum flow rate of

6 L/min. Once the nebuliser therapy is complete, the patient should be changed back to their usual device.

When nebulised bronchodilators are given to patients with hypercapnic acidosis (see Chapter 8), they should be given with compressed air. If necessary, supplementary oxygen should also be give (concurrently) by nasal cannulae at 2–4 L/min in an attempt to maintain an oxygen saturation of 88–92 per cent. Once nebuliser therapy is complete, then controlled oxygen therapy (via a Venturi mask) should be given (BTS, 2008).

Rationale for performing nebuliser therapy

Bronchodilators are commonly administered through this device, to reduce, relieve and prevent bronchoconstriction and increase the gas flow to the alveoli. Other drugs administered are mucolytics to facilitate mucus drainage from the bronchi and lungs, or corticosteroids to decrease bronchial inflammation. Antibiotics may also be prescribed via this route. Sometimes the desired effect has an opposite effect on patients, i.e. bronchial constriction may occur. If the patient states that the nebuliser therapy is not working or you hear additional/worsening wheezing sounds, turn off the nebuliser immediately and report it to the nurse in charge.

It is advisable that the patient has not eaten anything prior as nebulisation may induce a feeling of nausea.

Procedure for administering nebuliser treatments

1   Explain the procedure and the rationale for administration. Gain consent from the patient. Some patients may experience side-effects of the medication, e.g. tremor, tachycardia, dizziness, dry mouth, irritation to the eyes. These should be explained.
2   Wash hands before and after the procedure.
3   Where appropriate, teach and encourage deep breathing exercises to maximise the effects of the drug. The patient should be encouraged to cough after the administration of the drug. Nebuliser therapy may loosen secretions and therefore a sputum pot and tissues should be available.
4   The patient should be sitting in an upright position to aid deep breathing exercises during administration.
5   Before administration of the drug, take a peak flow reading (if patient is able and it is appropriate).
6   Open the storage chamber of the nebuliser mask (unscrew the bottom) and insert the solution, reattach the storage chamber (the mask is also attached). Ensure the attachments are secure.
7   Normally air (via a cylinder) is used to drive the gas/medication into the lower airways. Please note that a fine spray/mist and a hissing sound will occur if done correctly and the flow is high enough. Oxygen can be used as the driving gas but caution is required for patients with COPD.
8   If the patient is severely hypoxaemic, supplementary oxygen may be prescribed during nebuliser therapy. This should be delivered via a nasal cannula. Monitor the patient's respiratory status closely (Chapter 7).
9   Check that the device is working first before attaching the mask to the patient's

face. For the child/patient who feels claustrophobic and those patients who are very anxious, let them feel the moisture/steam first by putting the mask very gently next to their face. Do not apply the straps of the mask yet. Once they have got used to it, then gently strap on the mask. Diversion therapy or play may also be required.

10 The patient may also require oxygen saturation monitoring throughout this procedure.

11 A gas flow rate of 6–8 litres is required. This should be delivered until the storage chamber is almost empty (there may be a little residue left in the chamber). Generally, you should expect the time for administration to be 7–10 minutes.

12 Post-nebuliser peak flow assessment (normally after 30 minutes) should also be performed in order to evaluate the effectiveness of the drug administered.

13 Any residue should be discarded and the nebuliser mask and storage chamber should be washed, dried and placed by the patient's bedside for future usage.

14 Observe the patient's eyes, as the mist/moisture may cause some irritation.

15 Document findings/administration (NMC, 2015).

Summary

A large number of acute/critically ill patients will require supplementary oxygen therapy. Nurses need to be conversant with the correct administration techniques. Administration also involves evaluating the effectiveness of oxygen therapy through continuous monitoring of oxygen saturation. Pulse oximetry monitoring offers a quick and non-invasive means of assessing the adequacy of oxygenation to the tissues.

References

Bickler, P.E., Feiner, J.R. and Severinghaus, J.W. (2005) Effects of skin pigmentation on pulse oximeter accuracy at low saturation. *Anesthesiology*, 102(4): 715–719.

BTS (British Thoracic Society) (2008) BTS guideline for emergency oxygen use in adult patients. *Thorax*, 63(Supplement VI): vii–68.

Medical Devices Agency (2001) *Tissue Necrosis Caused by Pulse Oximeter Probes*, SN2001. London: MDA.

Moore, T. and Woodrow, P. (2009) *High Dependency Nursing Care: Observation, Intervention and Support for Level 2 Patients*. London: Routledge.

NMC (Nursing and Midwifery Council) (2015) *The Code: Professional Standards of Practice and Behaviour for Nurses and Midwives*. London: NMC.

Pierce, L. (2007) *Management of the Mechanically Ventilated Patient*, 2nd edn. St. Louis, MO: Elsevier.

The miracle of oxygen (2003) Available at: www.oxygenmiracle.com/main.htm (accessed 12 February 2016).

Chapter 10

Emergency management and resuscitation

José Hernandez-Padilla and Fiona Suthers

Survival rates after in-hospital cardiac arrest remain unacceptably low worldwide. Early recognition of deteriorating patients, subsequent activation of the emergency protocol in place, fast initiation of CPR and prompt use of a defibrillator have been linked to positive outcomes after these fatal events. As nurses are usually the front-line professionals dealing with peri-arrest and cardiac arrest events in hospital settings, they are expected to be competent in performing all these actions. Unfortunately, research often suggest that nurses and nursing students lack ability to effectively do so.
(Hernandez-Padilla et al., 2015; Perkins et al., 2015)

Key concepts

Early recognition of sick patients
First aid
Basic life support
Airway management
Early defibrillation
Advanced life support
Post-resuscitation care
Bleeding
Shock

Automated external defibrillator
Burns
Fractures
Seizures
Choking
Anaphylaxis
Cardiopulmonary resuscitation
(adult/child)
Recovery position

Learning outcomes

By the end of this chapter you will be able to:

- Perform a full assessment on patients who are deteriorating
- Recognise a cardiac arrest, activate the emergency procedure in place and initiate cardiopulmonary resuscitation

- Demonstrate knowledge and understanding on how to effectively manage a patient's airway using basic techniques and adjuncts
- Provide emergency first aid to a variety of situations (including shock, burns, seizures and choking)
- Recognise and discuss the treatment for an anaphylactic reaction
- Identify the need for and discuss post-resuscitation care and advance life support.

Introduction

When a clinical emergency situation arises, nurses are expected to perform at their best in order to preserve the person's life and promote recovery. However, clinical emergencies comprise a wide range of events in which a specific set of skills is required depending on the situation. This chapter will discuss protocols and strategies to effectively manage those patients suffering from the most common life-threatening clinical conditions.

Early recognition of the sick patient (pre-arrest)

Early recognition and timely intervention of an acutely ill patient and the subsequent activation of the emergency procedure in place may prevent cardiac arrest. Clinical assessment skills are paramount to enable healthcare professionals to effectively act upon early signs of deterioration. The use of a track and trigger score-system, in combination with the adoption of the ABCDE approach as a systematic way for assessing deteriorating patients, can improve outcomes for those who are critically ill (NICE, 2014).

Rationale for assessing a sick patient

By following a structured approach to assess sick patients, a whole picture of their clinical condition can be drawn, and measures to prevent cardiac arrest can be taken (ibid.). Reasons for using a systematic approach when assessing a sick patient include:

- Saving a substantial amount of time during the assessment process
- Facilitating the early recognition of a critically ill patient and the early activation of the emergency system in place
- Gaining enough clinical information about the patient, as this enables early implementation of the appropriate treatment in order of priority
- Preventing, overall the occurrence of cardiac arrest events.

Track and trigger score-system

Different track and trigger score-systems have been developed and each setting may use their own version, but familiarity with these tools is essential. However, most track and trigger score-systems are represented in an observation chart that includes measurement of respiratory rate, pulse oximetry (SpO_2), temperature, blood pressure, pulse, level of consciousness and blood glucose level.

In a track and trigger score-system chart, depending on the deviation from what is considered to be 'normal', registered vital signs will receive points. Once the chart is completed, a total score needs to be calculated by adding all the individual points. Your clinical responses must be appropriate and based on standardised information that is often found on the back of the track and trigger score-system chart used (Royal College of Physicians, 2012).

ABCDE approach

A sick/acutely ill patient is someone whose vital signs deteriorate to the extent where it is recommended either to increase the frequency of monitoring or to escalate the clinical care. This is considered to be an emergency situation and help must be summoned and the assessment suggested below must be performed (Adam *et al.*, 2010; Royal College of Physicians, 2012).

- Track and trigger score-system charts must be used immediately when a patient is feeling unwell or you suspect clinical deterioration (vital signs) (Box 10.1)
- Nurses are expected to rapidly and accurately take and record the observations included in a track and trigger score-system chart
- Further actions will depend on the total score obtained; therefore, it is crucial that nurses are familiar with the track and trigger score-system used within their Trusts
- Concerns about patients' clinical deterioration must be escalated immediately and continuous ABCDE assessment performed until more senior staff are available (Table 10.1).

The early recognition of clinical deterioration is a key element in the prevention of cardiac arrests. Using a track and trigger score-system will help to easily and quickly identify objective signs of deterioration. In addition, using the ABCDE approach to assessing acutely ill patients will help in finding clinical problems and promptly treating them, even before medical help arrives.

Watch out

What is normal for one person might not be normal for someone else. The patient's baseline (initial observations) should be known before considering raising clinical concerns.

Don't forget!

Track and trigger score-system + ABCDE approach assessment = potential prevention of cardiac arrest.

Table 10.1 The ABCDE approach

A Airway	▢	Assess whether the airway is open, clear or obstructed.
	▢	A patient's airway is open if he can speak.
	▢	A noisy airway indicates some level of obstruction (e.g. stridor, gurgling).
	▢	If your patient cannot speak and the airway is silent, suspect complete blockage (choking).
	▢	If there are concerns about the patient's airway:
		▢ Try to reposition them (e.g. recovery position if unresponsive and breathing or sitting up right if conscious) and consider using airway adjuncts (i.e. airway management).
		▢ Dial 2222 (in-hospital emergency number).
B Breathing	▢	Measure respiratory rate.
	▢	Assess respiratory depth and rhythm.
	▢	Look for the use of accessory muscles.
	▢	Assess chest movements. Are they bilateral?
	▢	Measure oxygen saturation levels using a pulse oximeter (Chapter 9).
	▢	If concerned about the patient's breathing:
		▢ Sit the patient up (if conscious) or put him into recovery position (if unconscious and breathing).
		▢ Appropriate intervention. Give 15 litres of high-flow oxygen using a non-rebreathing mask.
		▢ Dial 2222.
C Circulation	▢	Assess colour and temperature of the skin.
	▢	Measure pulse.
	▢	Take blood pressure.
	▢	Check the capillary refill time.
	▢	Measure the urine output.
	▢	Perform an ECG if possible.
	▢	If you are concerned about your patient's circulation:
		▢ Appropriate interventions (e.g. lay patient flat and elevate the limbs if the blood pressure is too low).
		▢ Dial 2222.
D Disability	▢	Assess level of consciousness using the *AVPU* method.
		▢ A – Alert
		▢ V – Only responsive to Voice
		▢ P – Only responsive to Pain
		▢ U – Unresponsive
	▢	Assess pupils' size, equality and reactiveness.
	▢	Check capillary blood glucose level (CBG).
	▢	Measure tympanic temperature.
	▢	Assess pain using the *PQRST* approach.
		▢ P – Provocation/palliation.
		▢ Q – Quality/quantity.
		▢ R – Region/radiation.
		▢ S – Severity scale.
		▢ T – Timing.
	▢	If concerned about the patient's neurological condition:
		▢ Appropriate interventions (e.g. give glucose if capillary glucose reading is below 4 mmol/dl).
		▢ Dial 2222.
E Exposure	▢	Physical examination from head to toe.
	▢	Ask for permission and maintain patient's dignity, if a child, involve parents.
	▢	Get information about the patient's history:
		▢ Allergies.
		▢ Conditions.
		▢ Medication prescribed/taken.
		▢ Possible side-effects of this medication.
	▢	If concerned about the patient's physical symptoms:
		▢ Appropriate interventions (e.g. apply pressure and elevate the limb to stop bleeding).
		▢ Dial 2222.

First aid

Rationale for using first aid to respond to an emergency

Accidents can happen when least expected and their consequences could potentially be fatal for the patient. Healthcare professionals may witness or be the first responder to an accident, and must ensure that they are capable of providing effective emergency first aid. This occurs in the interim of time before more qualified staff and appropriate equipment are available. The sudden, unexpected and potentially life-threatening nature of an accident will require immediate and effective provision of help.

Reasons for providing emergency first aid include:

- To preserve the life of both the patient and the healthcare professional
- To prevent the situation from worsening
- To promote the recovery of the patient.

Provision of emergency first aid aims to preserve life, to prevent the situation from worsening and, if possible, promotes recovery. Acting fast, calling for help immediately and using conservative treatment are the key elements to achieve these goals when providing emergency first aid to shock, bleeding, burns, fractures and seizures. These problems are likely to be seen in an accident and emergency department or urgent care centres.

Bleeding

When there is a breakage in the continuity of a blood vessel, blood loss occurs. The amount of blood loss will depend on the type of vessels affected (Table 10.2) and the extension of the injury (Barraclough, 2014). The main aim is to minimise blood loss.

Table 10.2 Types of bleeding

Type of bleeding	Identification cues		Treatment	
Arterial	Blood spurts in a synchronised rhythm with the heart rate.	S	Sit or lay down	This will prevent the patient from falling in case they lose consciousness.
	Blood is bright red.	E	Examine	Examine the injury and remember its characteristics for when you need to report the incident.
Venous	Blood oozes out the wound.			
	Blood is dark red.			
		E	Elevate	Elevate the wound above the level of the heart. Gravity will reduce the blood loss.
Capillary	Blood trickles from the wound.	P	Pressure	Direct – continuous for 10 minutes.
	It is easier to stop than the previous two.			Indirect – compress the brachial or femoral artery. Dressings – apply sterile dressing firmly without compromising the blood flow to the rest of the limb.

Shock

Shock could be defined as a life-threatening condition caused by a lack of oxygen supply to the body tissues, which is usually a consequence of a fall in the patient's blood pressure. The aim is to improve the amount of blood supply to the main organs (heart, lungs and brain).

The most common types of shock are:

- *Hypovolaemic shock*: caused by bleeding (internal or external), gastrointestinal problems related to diarrhoea and vomiting or extensive burns, haemorrhage.
- *Cardiogenic shock:* caused by myocardial infarction, cardiac failure or tension pneumothorax.
- *Anaphylactic shock*: caused by untreated life-threatening allergic reaction.

Common signs and symptoms of hypovolaemic and cardiogenic shock are shown in Table 10.3.

Table 10.3 Common signs and symptoms of hypovolaemic and cardiogenic shock

	Physiological reaction	*Signs and symptoms*
Stage I	Adrenaline is released and compensatory mechanisms are activated	■ Increased heart rate ■ Slightly decreased or normal blood pressure ■ Pale and/or clammy skin
Stage II	Compensatory mechanisms begin to fail	■ Fast and weak pulse ■ Low blood pressure ■ Fast and shallow breathing ■ Cyanotic, clammy and sweaty skin ■ Light-headedness, dizziness and weakness ■ Decreased consciousness and/or confusion ■ Nausea and/or vomiting
Stage III	Neurological problems start to occur due to lack of oxygen supply to the brain	■ Deep, slow and laboured breathing (air hunger) ■ Absence of peripheral pulses ■ Unconsciousness

Source: Barraclough (2014).

Don't forget!

- Shock symptoms + bleeding/fluid loss = hypovolaemic shock
- Shock symptoms + chest pain and impending doom = cardiogenic shock.

Immediate responses to signs of shock are:

- Treat the possible cause of shock (e.g. anaphylaxis, bleeding)
- Lay the patient flat and elevate the lower limbs, keeping them raised
- Notify nurse in charge/doctor immediately
- Make sure you keep the patient warm without overheating them
- Continue to monitor the patient using ABCDE approach
- Get ready to initiate CPR in case the patient deteriorates further.

Watch out

Internal bleeding can be a hidden life-threatening condition. If your patient has suffered any trauma or presents signs of shock, also look for bruises, swelling, pain and any other symptoms that may indicate internal bleeding (e.g. coughing or vomiting blood).

Burns

A burn is defined as the damage caused to the body tissues after entering into contact with extreme heat. The severity of a burn may differ depending on the age of the patient, the size of the burn, its cause, its location and its depth (Barraclough, 2014) (Table 10.4).

Fractures

A fracture is a type of injury in which discontinuity of a bone is caused by direct, indirect or twisting forces. A fracture could be manifested by the following symptoms:

- Pain in the area, which worsens when mobilised
- Bruising in the area, which is a consequence of injured tissues
- Swelling over a bone due to the body's inflammatory response to damage
- Deformity on the limb or area affected
- Crepitus (a grating feeling when mobilising the fracture), due to friction between rough ends of the latter
- Loss of power in the affected limb.

Procedure for providing first aid for fractures

The basic treatment of a fracture MUST always be very conservative.

1   Perform the Primary Survey (see Table 10.7).
2   Instruct the patient to immobilise the fracture or use your hands if needed.
3   If the patient is safe, DO NOT mobilise them unless they go into shock.
4   Don't allow them to have anything to eat or drink.

Table 10.4 Types of burns

Cause	Examples	Treatment
Dry heat	Direct contact with a flame, hot metal or even friction	▪ Perform the Primary Survey (see Table 10.7) ▪ Use luke warm running water, for at least 10 minutes, to cool the burn ▪ Remove jewellery (watches, rings, bracelet) and clothing while cooling, only if they are not stuck to the skin ▪ Protect the wound. Use clingfilm or a non-adherent dressing pad and secure it with a bandage ▪ Patient will be assessed by a nurse or doctor
Wet heat	Contact with boiling water or any other very hot liquids	▪ Treat it exactly the same as a dry heat burn
Chemical	Sulphuric acid or any other chemicals that can corrode and burn the skin	▪ Perform the Primary Survey ▪ Try to brush the chemical off the skin if possible ▪ Rinse the burn with running cold water for at least 20 minutes ▪ Try to safely remove contaminated clothes if they are not stuck to the skin ▪ Patient will be assessed by a doctor
Radiation	Sunburn or tanning pools	▪ Perform the Primary Survey ▪ Remove the patient from the source of the burn ▪ Cool the burn with cold water for 10 minutes. Instruct the patient to have a cold shower or bath when possible ▪ If level of consciousness is unaffected, advise the patient to take small sips of water. ▪ Monitor patient for widespread blistering ▪ Patient will be assessed by a doctor
Electrical	Electrical shock	▪ Perform the Primary Survey ▪ Ensure safety and switch off power supply ▪ Try to cool down the entry and exit wound, as well as the pathway between them. Use water for at least 10 minutes. ▪ Follow recommendations given to treat a dry heat burn ▪ Patient will be assessed immediately by a doctor

Seizures

Sometimes wrongly referred to as fit or convulsion, a seizure could be defined as a sudden disturbance in the electrical activity within the brain. Depending on which part of the brain is affected, symptoms may vary from 'auras' to 'tonic-clonic' convulsions.

Possible signs and symptoms of a seizure include:

- Lack of response to external stimuli
- Repetitive and unusual movements
- Localised stiffness or twitching
- Déjà vu and/or aura experience
- Violent generalised jerking and/or muscle rigidity
- Rolling eyes and/or aggressive behaviour
- Skin on the face becomes blue and lips cyanotic
- Gasping and laboured breathing (air hunger).

Procedure for immediate response to a someone having a seizure

1 Make the surrounding area to the person safe or, if conscious, direct them to a safe environment and sit them on the floor.
2 Keep talking to the patient (hearing is the last sense to leave).
3 Protect their head by placing something soft and padded under it (e.g. pillow, rolled blanket).
4 Note the start time and the duration of the seizure and inform the nurse/doctor in charge if:
   a It is the first time the person experiences a seizure
   b The seizure has lasted longer than 5 minutes
   c The person does not recover the level of consciousness after 5 minutes.
5 Document the incident (NMC, 2015).

Choking

When someone's airway is completely obstructed by a foreign body, the person will:

- Be unable to speak or cough
- Try to grasp their throat
- Become pale and cyanotic at late stages
- Be very distressed
- Become unconscious if unresolved.

(Perkins et al., 2015; Resuscitation Council (UK), 2011)

Procedure for dealing with someone who is choking

1 Encourage the patient to cough.
2 If they cannot cough or they stop coughing, shout for help and get ready to give up to five back blows.
3 Tell the patient to bend forward and hold onto a steady table, chair or wall (Figure 10.1 (a)).
4 If the patient is unable to hold onto any of the above, put your arm across their chest (Figure 10.1 (b)).
5 With the palm of your hand, hit the patient firmly in between the shoulder blades.
6 Check if the object causing the obstruction has come out after the back blow.

7   Repeat the procedure up to five times if nothing comes out.
8   If after giving five back blows, the airway is still completely obstructed and the patient cannot cough, perform up to five abdominal thrusts.
9   Stand behind the patient and make a fist with your dominant hand. Put your arms around the patient's upper abdomen and locate the middle point between the xiphisternum and the umbilicus. Place the fist of your dominant hand on this anatomical point and grasp it with the other hand (Figure 10.1 (c)).
10 Push firmly inwards and upwards (Figure 10.1 (d)).

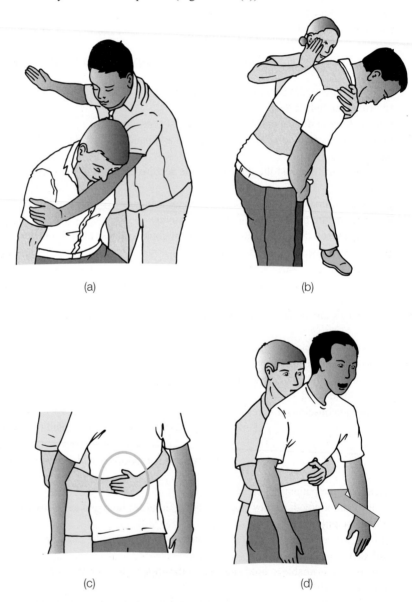

(a)   (b)

(c)   (d)

Figure 10.1 **Dealing with someone who is choking**

11 Check if the object causing the obstruction has come out after the abdominal thrust.
12 Repeat the procedure up to five times if nothing comes out. If after one cycle of five back blows and five abdominal thrusts, the airway continues to be obstructed, send someone to call 2222 and continue alternating up to five back blows with up to five abdominal thrusts.
13 If the patient becomes unconscious, initiate CPR.
   a NEVER perform abdominal thrusts on children under the age of 1 year. Substitute them for up to five chest thrusts instead
   b NEVER perform abdominal thrusts on a heavily pregnant woman. Substitute them for up to five back blows instead
   c If abdominal thrusts are implemented, the patient should be assessed for internal damage/bleeding.
14 Document procedure and findings (NMC, 2015).

Anaphylaxis

According to the European Resuscitation Council's (2015) guidelines, anaphylaxis occurs when a hypersensitivity reaction becomes life-threatening due to the severity of a systemic overwhelming inflammatory response in the human body (Truhlář *et al.*, 2015).

Anaphylactic reactions are always triggered by allergens. The most common are: *food* (nuts, shellfish, fish, eggs, additives); *drugs* (penicillin and other antibiotics, NSAIDs, aspirin); and *venom from stinging insects* (honeybees, wasps, hornets). Typically and if untreated, they will cause cardiac arrest after 30–35 minutes. Shock due to insect stings will be expected after 10–15 minutes and death after hypersensitivity reaction to intravenously administered drugs will most often occur within 5 minutes (Resuscitation Council (UK), 2011).

Rationale for recognising and treating anaphylaxis

The sudden onset of anaphylaxis, its rapid progression and its severe symptomatology, will always require prompt recognition, urgent treatment and close monitoring. Anaphylaxis is a life-threatening and rapid-onset condition caused by a severe allergic reaction. Its symptoms can vary widely, but problems related to airway, breathing and/or circulation are often accompanied by skin problems. Treatment of anaphylaxis includes rapid IM injection of adrenaline 1:1000 solution, which can be repeated if the patient does not improve (Resuscitation Council (UK), 2011; Truhlář *et al.*, 2015).

Reasons for using the ABCDE approach to recognise anaphylaxis include:

- Gains time in the process of diagnosing and treating the anaphylactic reaction
- Avoids making mistakes when identifying typical symptoms of an anaphylactic reaction
- Allows one to proceed with the correct treatment as soon as possible
- Prevents, overall, the occurrence of fatal consequences.

Procedure for immediate response to someone having a severe anaphylactic reaction

1   Put the patient in a comfortable position.
2   If there are *problems with the patient's airway and/or breathing*, then sit them upright.
3   In the *absence of airway/breathing problems but if there are problems with circulation* (e.g. low blood pressure), lie them flat and elevate their lower limbs, this helps with reducing the workload of the heart.
4   *Problems with the airway and/or breathing, in conjunction with low blood pressure.* Try to compensate by laying the patient back as far as they can tolerate and raise the legs.
5   Continuously reassure the patient by giving information on what you are doing.
6   Obtain information about the patient's past medical history including allergies, conditions and medication either given or taken. Gather information about food intake in the few hours prior to the episode and consider exposition to a possible allergen.
7   Use the ABCDE to assess the patient.
8   On assessing, the following signs and symptoms may be shown by a patient suffering from anaphylaxis (Table 10.5).
9   Document procedure and findings (NMC, 2015).

Table 10.5 ABCDE for anaphylaxis

Initial	Definition	Symptoms
A	Airway	Swelling, hoarseness, stridor
B	Breathing	Cyanosis, fast and shallow breathing, wheeze, fatigue, $SpO_2 < 92\%$
C	Circulation	Hypotension, fast and weak pulse, pale and clammy skin, light-headedness
D	Disability	Confusion, drowsiness, anxiety, convulsions, loss of consciousness, coma
E	Exposure	Patchy/generalised red rash, urticaria, angioedema

Don't forget!

When trying to establish anaphylaxis, *REMEMBER!!* If your patient shows life-threatening problems with their airway and/or breathing and/or circulation, in conjunction with any skin and/or mucosal changes, you must immediately start treating the situation as an anaphylactic reaction.

Treatment of anaphylaxis

Early treatment of an anaphylactic reaction is crucial for improving the patient's outcomes (Resuscitation Council (UK), 2011; Truhlář *et al.*, 2015). A nurse who has undergone additional training and been assessed as competent can administer the drugs as an emergency and without prescription. Drugs can also be administered as part of prescribed treatment from the doctor.

- Immediately consider removing the trigger if possible (e.g. stop intravenous infusions)
- Give high-flow oxygen, up to 15 litres if SpO_2<95%, using a non-rebreathing mask
- *Adrenaline* is the first line drug in the treatment of anaphylaxis and should be administered promptly. Check if the patient has any known allergy to adrenaline.

NB: nurses have to be suitably trained and assessed as competent in order to administer adrenaline in an emergency.

- If the patient has any known allergies, they may carry an auto-injector of adrenaline. Instruct or assist them to use it. Give the auto-injector yourself if your patient is unable to do it by themselves.

Procedure for administering an auto-injector of adrenaline

1   Read the instructions on the actual device.
2   Remove the cap, which is a safety release.
3   Hold the device firmly by making a fist around it.
4   DO NOT place your thumb at either end of the device.
5   Choose a big muscle (e.g. antero-lateral part of the thigh) and stab the auto-injector in a 90° angle.
6   Do not worry about removing clothing; the needle will go through it.
7   Hold the auto-injector there for 10 seconds and release the pressure after that.
8   Give a gentle and brief massage to the zone. This may help with absorption of the drug.
9   Document procedure and findings (NMC, 2015).

Procedure for dealing with an anaphylactic reaction

1   If an auto-injector is not available, give an intramuscular (IM) injection of adrenaline 1:1000 solution. Beware that the dosage will vary depending on your patient's age. See the summary table (Table 10.6). If the patient's condition does not improve, the dose of adrenaline can be repeated after 5 minutes.
2   If their condition worsens, the adrenaline can be given before 5 minutes, and given when the patient's condition was noted to deteriorate.
3   In the instance that the patient becomes unconscious but is still breathing, put them into the recovery position.
4   If the patient stops breathing, commence CPR.

Table 10.6 Adrenaline dosages by age

Doses of IM adrenaline 1:1000 for anaphylaxis treatment	
Adult	500 micrograms IM (0.5 mL)
Children > 12 years	500 micrograms IM (0.5 mL)
Children 6–12 years	300 micrograms IM (0.3 mL)
Children < 6 years	150 micrograms IM (0.15 mL)

Problems related to the airway and/or breathing and/or circulation, in conjunction with skin problems must be treated as an anaphylactic reaction.

■   Treatment of anaphylaxis requires immediate IM injection of adrenaline 1:1000 solution

■   Emergency services need to be alerted immediately upon recognition of anaphylaxis and patients should be mobilised as little as possible

■   Adrenaline doses can be repeated after 5 minutes if the patient does not improve after the first injection. If this is the case, get ready to initiate CPR.

Don't forget!

Clinical manifestations of anaphylaxis may vary considerably, which make its diagnosis rather difficult. If in doubt, treat your patient with an adrenaline injection (unless allergy to this drug has been stated).

Box 10.1 Symptoms that should be noted

■   *Severe asthma*: Similar airway and/or breathing problems to those which are typical in anaphylaxis. Patients may show symptoms of neurological problems related to a lack of oxygen supply to the brain. However, although a fast heart rate might be present, blood pressure does not usually drop as dramatically as it would do in anaphylaxis

■   *Septic shock*: Do not get confused between petechial/purpuric rash and urticaria/red rash. In conjunction with low blood pressure, the former could be an indicator of septic shock, whereas the latter may indicate anaphylaxis

■   *Faint*: May be caused by a vasovagal episode, i.e. after immunisation. If this is the case, your patient will not show rashes, laboured breathing or swelling.

■   *Panic attack*: Fast and laboured breathing must not be confused with an anaphylaxic reaction. Patients who have previously experienced an anaphylactic reaction may panic when they think it is happening again. Although your patient may present flushing skin. On assessment, they will not be presenting with low blood pressure, red rashes or angioedema

■   *Non-allergic urticaria*: A red rash or urticaria, in isolation, does not mean anaphylaxis. Proceed with your ABCDE assessment to establish the correct diagnosis.

Basic life support

Cardiovascular diseases are the biggest killer in Western countries, with both ischemic myocardial and cerebral episodes leading the charts of most common causes of death (WHO, 2014). A sudden and severe ischaemic episode of this nature could lead to cardiac arrest if not rapidly treated. Should anyone go into cardiac arrest, they will collapse immediately as a consequence of their heart's inability to effectively eject blood out and therefore to provide enough oxygen and nutrients to the rest of the body organs. Cellular death commences from the moment this occurs and provision of good quality basic life support positively influences the patient's chances of survival.

Rationale for performing basic life support

Basic life support precedes advanced emergency assistance and it might need to be implemented in a variety of situations, e.g. unconscious and breathing or cardiac arrest events.

Reasons for applying basic life support include:

- Maintaining airway patency if unconscious
- Reducing the risk of aspiration amongst unconscious patients in case of vomit or regurgitation
- Delaying and/or preventing brain damage in the interim before defibrillation and advance life support are available.

Procedure for basic life support

According to the European Resuscitation Council's (2015) guidelines, after finding a collapsed patient, apply early recognition of whether they are breathing. If absent, call 2222 and initiate CPR, including the use of an Automated Electrical Device (AED) as soon as this becomes available (Perkins *et al.*, 2015). Perform the Primary Survey (Table 10.7).

When performing the Primary Survey on a child or infant, beware of the following modifications:

1 *Response:* Check response by gently stimulating them (e.g. flicking their palms of hands/feet).
2 *Airway:* When dealing with an infant's airway you must keep the head in a neutral position. In children, you must tilt the head back and lift the chin cautiously. DO NOT hyperextend the neck.
3 *Breathing:* Infants and children breathe faster; therefore in a 10-second period, you should see between three breaths (children) and five breaths (infants) if the patient is breathing effectively.

Table 10.7 Primary Survey

D	Danger	*Check for danger* by: ▪ Looking around and making sure it is safe for you to approach the patient.
R	Response	*Assess level of responsiveness* by: ▪ Shouting at the patient: 'Open your eyes, please!' ▪ Gently squeezing the patient's shoulders.
S	Shout	*Shout for help* or press the emergency bell ▪ DO NOT leave the patient to make an emergency call.
A	Airway	*Open the patient's airway* using head tilt–chin lift manoeuvre (and note modifications).

B	Breathing	*Assess breathing* taking the following into consideration:
		▪ Maintain head tilt–chin lift during the assessment.
		▪ Put your head closer to the patient's head and:
		  1 Look for chest movements.
		  2 Listen for normal respiratory sounds.
		  3 Feel for warm air on your cheek.
		▪ Assess for up to 10 seconds.
		▪ Disregard agonal breathing at this point.
		▪ Your patient must effectively breathe, at least, twice for you to say he/she is adequately breathing.

C	Circulation/CPR	*If you are on your own:* ▪ And the patient is effectively breathing, put them into recovery position, make an emergency call 2222 and identify/treat any life-threatening circulatory problems. ▪ If the patient is not breathing, the emergency call must be made/summon help first before starting CPR. ▪ Start CPR as soon as possible *If you have a helper with you/if help has arrived:* ▪ If the patient is effectively breathing; send the helper to urgently contact the nurse in charge/doctor. Put the patient into recovery position and try to identify/treat any circulatory problems. ▪ If the patient is not breathing, you must commence CPR while you send the helper to make the emergency call.

If the patient is not breathing or you are unsure whether they are, YOU MUST initiate cardiopulmonary resuscitation (CPR). Early recognition of a cardiac arrest and rapid initiation of CPR can improve chances of survival. If after performing a Primary Survey, the patient is not breathing normally, the hospital resuscitation team must be alerted and CPR must be initiated immediately (Figure 10.2). Follow the sequence of 30 chest compressions to 2 rescue breaths on adults and 15 chest compressions to 2 rescue breaths on children. If the patient shows signs of life, stop CPR and reassess breathing. If the patient is breathing effectively, put them into the recovery position.

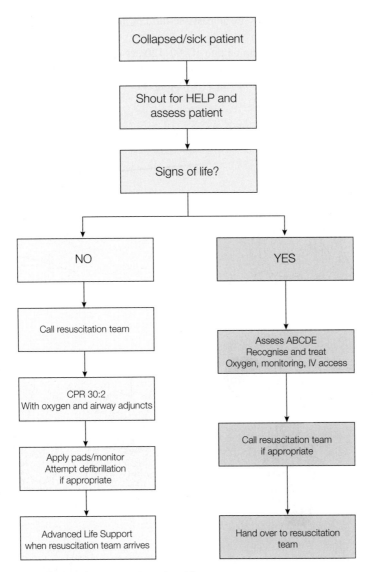

Figure 10.2 **In-hospital resuscitation algorithm**
Source: Adapted from Gwinnutt *et al.* (2015).

Procedure for chest compressions (Adult)

1   Place the heel of your dominant hand on the lower third of the patient's sternum (Figure 10.3 (a)).
2   Put your other hand on top, interlock both hands' fingers and lift them up (Figure 10.3 (b)).
3   Lean over the patient's body until you get your shoulders, elbows and wrists aligned. Lock elbows and press down without bending them (Figure 10.3 (c)).

4   Depress the patient's chest by at least one-third of the total chest depth (Figure 10.3 (d)).
5   Aim to achieve a compression rate of 100–120 per minute (Figure 10.3 (e)).
6   Do 30 chest compressions and give 2 rescue breaths (Figures 10.3 (f) and 10.3 (g)).
7   Document procedure and findings (NMC, 2015).

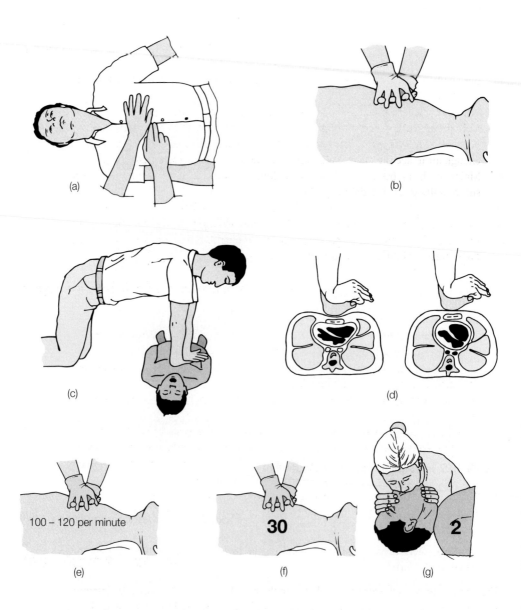

Figure 10.3 **How to perform CPR**

Don't forget!

As applying a single precordial thump is unlikely to revert a shockable rhythm, its use should only be considered if a witnessed cardiac arrest due to ventricular fibrillation (VF) or pulseless ventricular tachycardia (pVT) occurs and if it could be done without delaying defibrillation.

Procedure for giving rescue breaths

1   Put one hand on the patient's forehead to pinch the nose (index and thumb) (Figure 10.4 (a)).
2   With the other hand, maintain chin lift ensure the mouth is open (Figure 10.4 (b)).
3   Hold your breath, place your lips around the patient's mouth making sure there is a good seal and blow in. When giving the rescue breath, blow in steadily and provide enough air to see the chest rising (approximately 1 second (Figure 10.4 (c)).
4   Maintain 'head tilt–chin lift' while looking at chest to check whether air has successfully gone into the lungs (Figure 10.4 (d)).
5   Repeat the process and give another breath (Figure 10.4 (e)).
6   In total, the process of stopping chest compressions, giving the two breaths and resuming chest compressions, should not take longer than 5 seconds. Continue with the sequence of 30:2 (Figures 10.4 (f) and 10.4 (g)).

Procedure for paediatric basic life support

1   Initiate CPR with five rescue breaths.
   a   In infants, follow recommendations given above to open the airway and provide mouth-to-mouth/mouth-to-nose breaths
   b   In children, follow recommendations given above to open the airway and provide mouth-to-mouth breaths.
2   Assess breathing for up to 10 seconds. If the patient is not breathing effectively, initiate CPR.
3   Provide 15 chest compressions with same depth and rate as described for adults.
   a   In infants, locate the lower half of the sternum and use the tips of the fingers
   b   In children, locate the lower half of the sternum and use one or two hands (depending on your ability and the size of the child).
4   Give two rescue breaths considering the aforementioned modifications.
5   Continue with the sequence of 15 chest compressions to two rescue breaths.
6   Document procedure and findings (NMC, 2015).

Airway management

The human airway is the air passage between the mouth/nose and the lungs. Maintaining airway patency is indispensable for life. An obstructed airway would imply a reduction in the amount of air inhaled and therefore in the oxygen supplied to the brain. This would result in a life-threatening situation that must be addressed immediately.

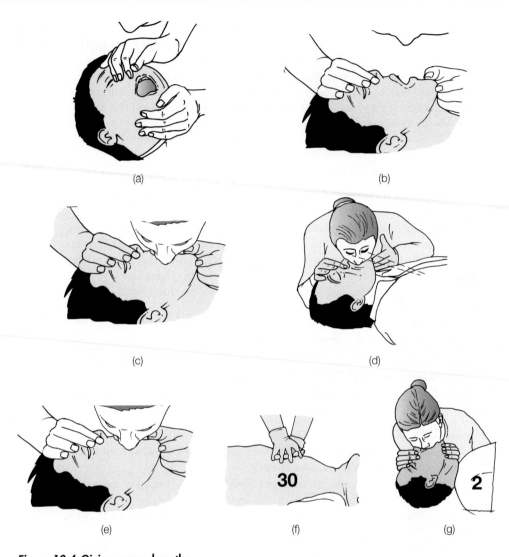

Figure 10.4 Giving rescue breaths

Don't forget!

CPR must continue until one of the following occurs:

- ■ *The patient shows signs of life* – stop CPR and reassess breathing for up to 10 seconds
  - ■ If the patient is breathing effectively, place them into recovery position
  - ■ If the patient is NOT breathing effectively, resume CPR.
- ■ *Exhaustion* – stop quickly to rest but recommence CPR when possible
- ■ *The emergency team arrives* – and they are ready to take over.

Rationale for performing airway management

Potential causes for airway obstruction include (Resuscitation Council (UK), 2011):

- Foreign bodies
- Displacement of the tongue, soft palate or epiglottis as result of loss of consciousness
- Blood or vomit resulting in aspiration by those with decreased level of consciousness
- Oedema or inflammatory processes affecting the airway (e.g. anaphylactic shock).

The aim of airway management is:

- To ensure airway patency and breathing continuity in patients with decreased level of consciousness
- To enable the provision of artificial ventilation support for those unable to effectively breathe by themselves
- To be able to clear someone's airway when this is completely obstructed by a foreign body.

Procedure for managing the airway

Applying basic manual manoeuvres such as 'head tilt-chin lift' or 'jaw thrust' to open your patient's airway will allow you to move their tongue forward, reducing its ability to obstruct the natural air passage (Resuscitation Council (UK), 2011).

The *head tilt and chin lift* (Figures 10.5 (a) and (b)) can be applied in unconscious patients without suspected spinal injury:

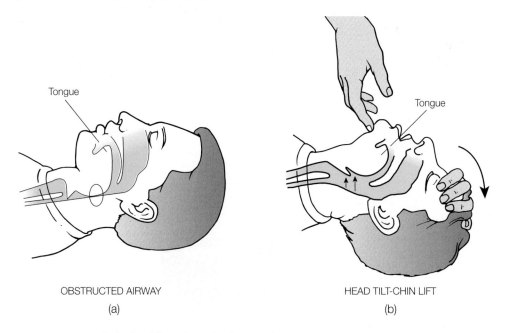

Tongue

Tongue

OBSTRUCTED AIRWAY

(a)

HEAD TILT-CHIN LIFT

(b)

Figure 10.5 **Head tilt-chin lift to clear an obstructed airway**

1 Place one hand on the patient's forehead and tilt it back.
2 Simultaneously, place two fingers under the bony part of the chin and lift it up, keeping the mouth open.
3 You must hyperextend the neck.

The *jaw thrust* (Figures 10.6 (a)–(c)) can be applied to unconscious patients with suspected spinal injury:

(a)

(b)

(c)

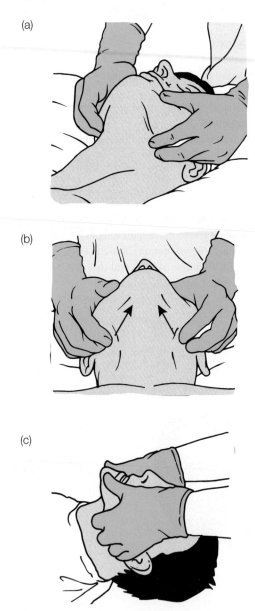

Figure 10.6 Jaw thrust manoeuvre

Jaw thrust (continued)

1   Place your hands on the patient's cheekbones with your thumbs facing downwards resting on the chin (Figure 10.6 (a)).
2   Find the angle of the jaw and place your index and middle finger behind it (Figure 10.6 (b)).
3   Lift the lower part of the jaw by applying pressure upwards and forward with your fingers.
4   Open the mouth by gently pushing the chin downwards (Figure 10.6 (c)).

Using basic airway adjuncts (Resuscitation Council (UK), 2011)

There are different kinds of airway adjuncts that can be used (Table 10.8): oropharyngeal (Figure 10.7) and nasopharyngeal (Figure 10.8).

Procedure for oropharyngeal airway insertion

1   Measure the airway adjunct and choose the appropriate size.
2   Open the patient's mouth and insert the airway 'upside down' (Figure 10.9a).
3   Push the airway down until you feel resistance (soft palate).
4   Turn the airway adjunct 180° and keep pushing down.
5   The oropharyngeal airway adjunct must rest on your patient's teeth (Figure 10.7).
6   Document procedure and findings (NMC, 2015).

Table 10.8 Airway adjuncts

Airway device	Indications	Contraindications	Measurement
Oropharyngeal	Unconscious patients without gag reflex	Activation of gag reflex upon insertion	From the angle of the jaw to the height of front teeth
Nasopharyngeal	Any semi-conscious or unconscious patients	Major head trauma with suspected skull fracture	From the tragus or the angle of the jaw to the nearest nostril

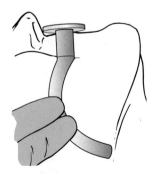

Figure 10.7 Oropharyngeal airway adjunct

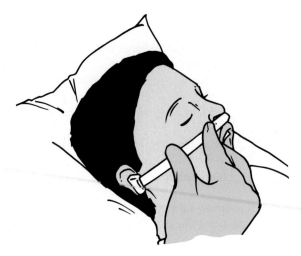

Figure 10.8 Nasopharyngeal airway adjunct

Procedure for nasopharyngeal airway insertion

1   Measure the airway adjunct and choose the appropriate size.
2   Choose the right nostril and confirm patency.
3   Lubricate the exterior part of the airway adjunction.
4   Hold the airway with the thumb, the index and the middle finger of your dominant hand.
5   Apply pressure on the patient's nose tip with the thumb of your other hand. This will enlarge the nostrils.
6   Insert the airway vertically downwards (it may need slight twisting), curving it towards your patient's feet (Figure 10.9b).
7   Document procedure and findings (NMC, 2015).

NB: If an obstruction is found while attempting this on the right nostril, try with the left nostril.

Basic techniques to support ventilation

There are some basic techniques to support patient ventilation (Resuscitation Council (UK), 2011), such as a pocket mask (Figures 10.9 (a)–(g)).

Procedure for inserting a pocket mask

1   Get the mask out of the case and pop it open with your thumbs (Figure 10.9 (c)).
2   With the patient lying in supine position, place the mask on their face around the nose and the mouth (Figure 10.9 (d)).
3   Put both hands around the mask. Make a tight seal around the mask by pressing down with both hands. DO NOT pinch the mask (Figure 10.9 (e)).
4   Perform head tilt-chin lift while applying the seal (Figure 10.9 (f)).
5   Give rescue breaths by blowing through the valve of the mask (Figure 10.9 (g)).

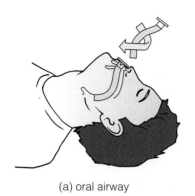

(a) oral airway

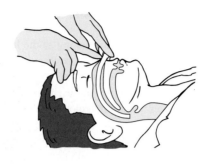

(b) nasopharyngeal airway

Figure 10.9 **Airway support**

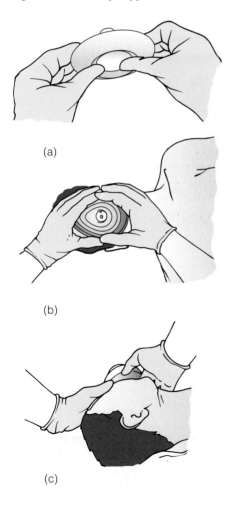

(a)

(b)

(c)

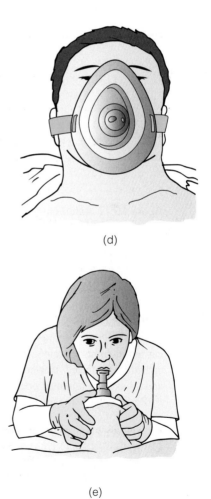

(d)

(e)

Figure 10.10 **Manoeuvres to insert a pocket mask**

Early defibrillation

For effective functioning of the heart, both the electrical and mechanical activity of the myocardium have to work synchronously. Severe problems related to one or the other may cause the patient to go into cardiac arrest. When this occurs, oxygen supply to the brain is stopped and early defibrillation may be the key element to successful resuscitation without neurological damage (Perkins *et al.*, 2015).

In the event of cardiac arrest, an automated external defibrillator (AED) (Figure 10.10) has the potential to revert certain cardiac arrhythmias causing this fatal condition. Early use of defibrillation has been linked to increased chances of successful resuscitation, therefore, AEDs should be used as quickly as possible. Although using an AED does not require previous training, it is very important to consider and ensure safety at all times when operating it.

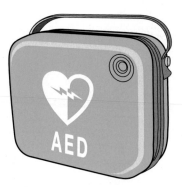

Figure 10.11 **Automated external defibrillator (AED)**

Rationale for performing early defibrillation

When someone goes into cardiac arrest, there are four possible arrhythmias that might be preventing the person's heart from effectively ejecting blood out (Table 10.9).

The AED also has the ability to detect those arrhythmias that have the potential to be reverted by delivering an electrical current through the myocardium. Furthermore, it can autonomously decide whether to charge an electrical shock or not, depending on the arrhythmia detected. However, for safety reasons, an AED cannot deliver the shock itself and it has to be a human operator who does it.

Reasons for using an AED early include:

- It has the potential to revert the arrhythmia that caused the cardiac arrest
- Being safe and easy to use in all settings
- It allows the delivery of an electrical shock even when people are not medically trained.

Table 10.9 **Shockable and non-shockable rhythms**

Shockable rhythms	Non-shockable rhythms
VF (Ventricular Fibrillation)	Asystole
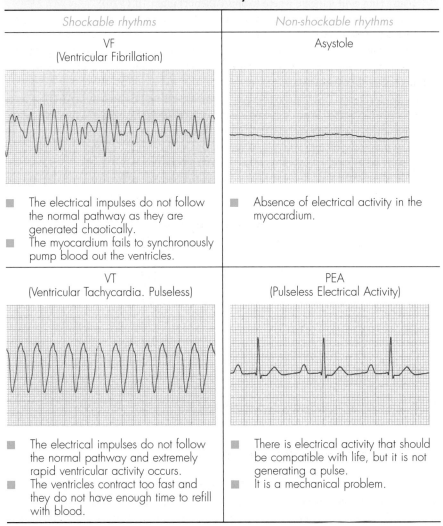	
■ The electrical impulses do not follow the normal pathway as they are generated chaotically. ■ The myocardium fails to synchronously pump blood out the ventricles.	■ Absence of electrical activity in the myocardium.
VT (Ventricular Tachycardia. Pulseless)	PEA (Pulseless Electrical Activity)
■ The electrical impulses do not follow the normal pathway and extremely rapid ventricular activity occurs. ■ The ventricles contract too fast and they do not have enough time to refill with blood.	■ There is electrical activity that should be compatible with life, but it is not generating a pulse. ■ It is a mechanical problem.

Procedure for defibrillation

In a resuscitation attempt, should you have access to an AED, you must start using it immediately. Follow the recommendations below to safely and effectively use an AED (Perkins *et al.*, 2015):

1 As soon as the AED is available, it takes priority. Start using it.
2 Open the case and get the AED out.
3 Switch the AED on. It will give you instructions (Figure 10.11 (a)).
4 Follow the AED prompts in the same order as given (Box 10.2).

5   Apply defibrillation pads to the patient's chest. Look at the pictures on the actual pads. They will indicate where to apply them (Figure 10.11 (b)).

6   If another rescuer is doing CPR, find a way to apply the pads without stopping the chest compressions.

7   When the AED starts analysing the patient's heart rhythm, make sure nobody touches the patient. Give verbal instructions (e.g. 'Don't touch the patient. It is analysing the heart rhythm').

8   If the AED says, 'No shock advised'; resume CPR immediately.

9   If the AED says, 'Shock advised'; make sure everybody stands back. Give verbal instructions (e.g. 'Shock advised. Stand clear. It is charging.').

10   Put your finger on top of the shock button and look around the patient, while waiting for the AED to say, 'Shock now' or 'Deliver shock now'.

11   When the AED gives the prompt to deliver the shock, ensure that verbal command is also given (e.g. 'Stand clear! I am about to deliver shock') and keep visual contact with those surrounding the patient.

12   Once you are sure nobody is touching anything the patient is in contact with, give final instructions (e.g. 'Delivering shock now') and press the button. (Figures 10.11 (c) and 10.11 (d)).

13   Resume CPR immediately following standard guidelines.

14   Continue CPR until the AED instructs you to stop or the patient shows signs of life.

15   If the patient does not show signs of life, the AED will restart the process every 2 minutes. Follow the steps above.

Box 10.2 Using an AED

■ Pads can only be applied to patient's bare skin. The chest will have to be fully exposed

■ The patient's chest must be dry

■ Shave any excessive hair from the chest (only the areas where the pads will be applied)

■ If the patient is wearing a bra, it will need to be removed (it is recommended to cut through the centre, exposing the entire chest)

■ Remove or move out of the way any jewellery (e.g. long necklace) in the area of the chest where the pads will be applied

■ If there are any body piercings in the area of the body between both defibrillation pads, try to tape them (without delaying the delivery of the shock). DO NOT apply these pads on top

■ If the patient has an implanted artificial pacemaker or internal defibrillator, DO NOT apply the pads on top

■ If, for any reason, defibrillator pads have to be applied in an alternative position; remember that there must be, at least, one pad distance between both pads

■ The person using the AED must visually check and verbally ensure that the delivery of the shock is done safely and rapidly.

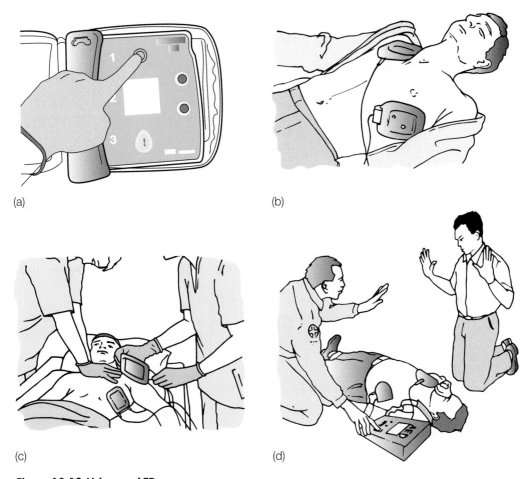

(a)

(b)

(c)

(d)

Figure 10.12 Using an AED

Considerations when using an AED

Before applying the defibrillation pads to your patient's chest, you must consider the following important safety considerations (Perkins *et al.*, 2015):

▪ If the patient is lying in a puddle of fluids, ensure that no-one is standing in the fluids when delivering the shock

▪ If using supplemental oxygen, make sure it is taken away from the patient at least one metre before shocking. Instruct other bystanders to put it behind their back when stepping back.

If using an AED with children, the procedure will be adapted to the child (Box 10.3). Place one pad on the sternum (centre of the chest) and the other one at the back (in between the shoulder blades) (Figure 10.13).

> ## Box 10.3 Using AED with children
>
> 1 AEDs should not be used in children under 1 year
> 2 AEDs can be used normally with children older than 8 years
> 3 AEDs with paediatric pads should be used in children between 1 and 8 years. If paediatric pads are unavailable, use normal adult-size pads, but consider changing their position as shown in Figure 10.12
> 4 Place one pad on the sternum (centre of the chest) and the other one at the back (in between the shoulder blades).

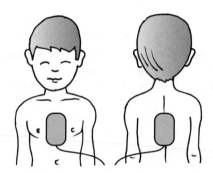

Figure 10.13 Using an AED on a child

Advanced life support (ALS)

Advanced life support (ALS) is an extension of basic life support based on the implementation of several more complex life-saving protocols and algorithms. The provision of advanced life support is dependent on the availability of advanced medical equipment and senior members of staff with sound clinical knowledge and skills. Apart from focusing on aspects already discussed in this chapter (CPR, defibrillation, airway management), ALS includes the use of IV drugs and the diagnosis and treatment of the possible causes of cardiac arrest.

Rationale for providing advanced life support

Basic life support is hardly ever enough to restore the return of spontaneous circulation (ROSC) in those who fatally went into cardiac arrest. Often, the implementation of ALS protocols is crucial to successful resuscitation.

Reasons for providing ALS include:

- Finding out what was the cause of the cardiac arrest and treating it, in order to revert the fatal condition
- Increasing, overall, the chances of successful resuscitation.

Recognition of cardiac arrest and alertness of the emergency team (see Primary Survey in Table 10.7), initiation of CPR, early use of a defibrillator or AED, airway management and post-resuscitation care are discussed in this chapter. However, although nurses who are not advanced life support providers will not get directly involved with it, the use of protocolled drugs and the diagnosis and treatment of the reversible causes of a cardiac arrest during a resuscitation attempt need to be briefly reviewed.

According to the Resuscitation Council (UK) guidelines (Gwinnett *et al.*, 2015), ALS can be summarised in the algorithm in Figure 10.13 (Soar *et al.*, 2015a).

Use of drugs in advanced life support

Continue with CPR while giving drugs.

- Adrenaline:
  - In shockable rhythms, give adrenaline after the third shock
  - In non-shockable rhythms, give adrenaline immediately
  - Give a dose of 1 mg of 1:10000 solution
  - Give adrenaline in IV bolus + IV flush (20–30 ml of 0.9% sodium chloride or 5% dextrose)
  - Elevate the limb and give a massage to facilitate the drug reaching the heart
  - Repeat the dose every 3–5 minutes.
- Amiodarone:
  - Only use in shockable rhythms after the third shock
  - Give an initial dose of 300 mg
  - Give amiodarone in IV bolus + IV flush (20–30 ml of 0.9% sodium chloride or 5% dextrose)
  - Elevate the limb and give a massage to facilitate the drug reaching the heart
  - An IV infusion of 900 mg over 24 hours can be given if the patient does not respond to previous treatment.

Soar et al. (2015b)

Reversible causes of cardiac arrest

The four 'Hs'

- *Hypoxia:* arterial blood gases (ABG) can provide valuable information; however, provision of 100 per cent oxygen supply is standard procedure in all resuscitation attempts. Bilateral chest movements must be achieved when ventilations are given
- *Hypovolaemia:* history and/or physical examination may indicate severe haemorrhage. When hypovolaemia is suspected to be the cause of cardiac arrest, fluids must be given immediately to restore the intravascular volume
- *Hypo/Hyperkalaemia and other metabolic disorders:* such as hypocalcaemia or acidaemia can be diagnosed using results of a full blood test and/or ABG, or even a 12-lead ECG. The treatment will differ depending on the actual disorder (e.g. calcium chloride is given for hypocalcaemia and hyperkalaemia)
- *Hypothermia:* diagnosed by using a low-reading thermometer, if hypothermia is

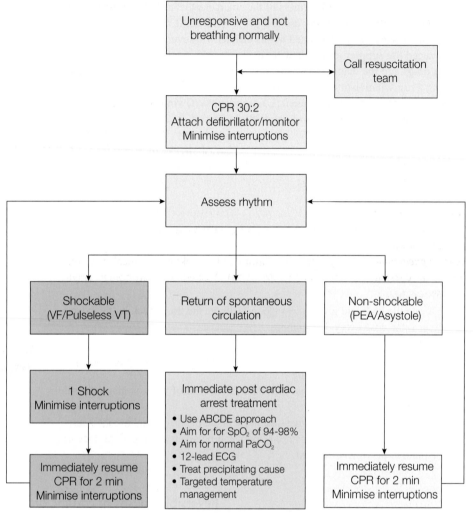

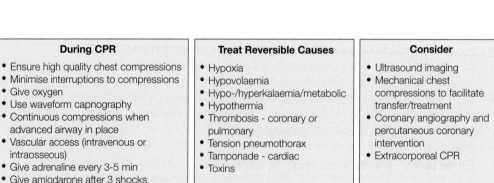

Figure 10.14 Advanced life support algorithm

stated as a possible cause, the patient needs to be warmed up slowly (0.5° C per hour) and from the inner to the outer (e.g. using warm IV fluids). CPR must be continued until the patient's temperature reaches 35°C.

The four 'Ts':

- *Thrombosis:* diagnosed through full blood test, 12-lead ECG and history. If thrombosis is suspected to be the cause of the cardiac arrest, thrombolytic drugs must be given and the resuscitation attempt must be prolonged 90 minutes after their administration
- *Cardiac Tamponade:* can only be diagnosed for using transthoracic echocardiography. The only solution to cardiac tamponade is emergency pericardiocentesis and early cardiac surgery
- *Toxins:* very difficult to diagnose without previous history to the event. Treatment is often supportive and antidotes can be given if the toxic substance causing the arrest is known
- *Tension pneumothorax:* diagnosed using ultrasound or looking at clinical symptoms (unilateral chest movements, trachea deviation). Treated with emergency needle decompression.

Soar *et al.* (2015b).

Watch out

IV drugs during a cardiac arrest can only be prescribed and given by ALS providers with experience in doing so.

Procedure for putting the patient in the recovery position

The recovery position ensures airway patency and reduces the risk of aspiration among those who are unconscious, but breathing effectively.

1   Remove glasses and watch/jewellery from the far arm (Figure 10.15 (a)).
2   Move the near arm out, so you can kneel closer to the patient (Figure 10.15 (b)).
3   Bring the patient's far arm across their chest and hold the back of their hand against the cheek (Figure 10.15 (c)).
4   Keep on holding the hand against the patient's cheek (Figure 10.15 (d)).
5   Keep your other hand on the external side of patient's knee and pull on it firmly and quickly against you, rolling them onto their side (Figure 10.15 (e)).
6   Use your other hand to grasp and pull up the knee until the foot is flat on the ground (Figure 10.15 (f)).
7   Tilt the patient's head back and rotate the head towards the ground (Figure 10.15 (g)).
8   Place the upper leg in such a way that the hip and the knee are bent at 90° angles (Figure 10.15 (h)).

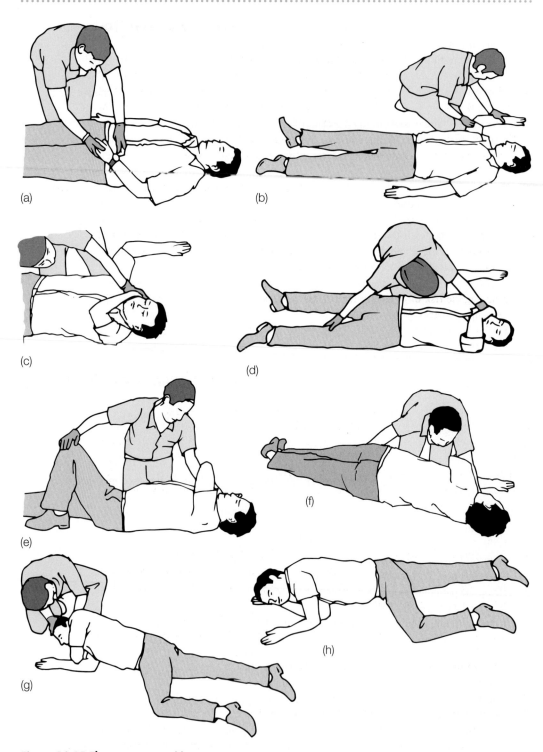

Figure 10.15 The recovery position

Post-resuscitation care

There is a possibility that, if the cardiac arrest is caused by a shockable rhythm and this is treated with early defibrillation, the patient will recover immediately as cerebral perfusion is restored. Unfortunately, the ROSC after a cardiac arrest does not mean that the patient is out of risk and, in fact, post-resuscitation care is always needed. Senior members of staff who are specialised in the field often provide this care.

However, if the ROSC occurs before the emergency team arrives, qualified nurses must provide post-resuscitation care in the interim of time before staff arrive.

Rationale for providing post-resuscitation care

When people go into cardiac arrest, the aim is to resuscitate them as soon as possible. If we succeed in the achievement of ROSC, the subsequent goals are going to be related to establishing and maintaining stable haemodynamic, cardiac and cerebral functions.

Reasons for providing post-resuscitation care include:

- reducing the risk of reoccurrence of cardiac arrest;
- preventing further deterioration;
- finding the cause of the cardiac arrest and treating it;
- promoting full recovery of the patient.

Procedure for post-resuscitation care

If your patient shows signs of ROSC after using an AED, where possible, follow these recommendations (Resuscitation Council (UK), 2011). Achievement of ROSC does not imply that the patient following a cardiac arrest is out of risk. Provision of post-resuscitation care aims to find out the cause of the arrest and implement the appropriate treatment to prevent reoccurrence of cardiac arrest. Nurses have to perform a full assessment using the ABCDE approach and treat, to the best of their knowledge, any problems encountered.

1 Stop the resuscitation attempt and assess breathing.
2 If the patient is breathing, turn them to one side to protect the airway, (recovery position). Nurses will have to protect the patient's airway and fully assess them using the ABCDE approach, treating any encountered problems to the best of their knowledge as they go along.
3 Reassure the patient all the time, even if they remain unresponsive.
4 Inform the emergency team of the changes and provide an update of the current situation.
5 Give 15 litres of high-flow oxygen using a non-rebreathing mask.
6 A 12-lead ECG to be performed as soon as possible.
7 Assess the patient using the ABCDE and record all the observations.
8 Communicate findings/problems to the nurse in charge or doctor.
9 Continue assessing, reassessing and recording all relevant clinical observations following the ABCDE approach until the emergency team arrives and takes over from you.

10   DO NOT sit the patient up. This may cause the blood pressure to drop drastically provoking cardiac arrest.

11   DO NOT turn the AED off or take the defibrillation pads off the patient's chest at any time unless instructed by the doctor.

12   Document findings (NMC, 2015).

Summary

Early recognition and timely intervention are paramount to prevent progression to cardiac arrest. This can be supported by the use of the ABCDE as a systematic approach to assessing the patient. In the event of a cardiac arrest, timely intervention and effective technique should help with a more successful outcome.

References

Adam, S.K., Odell, W. and Welch, J. (2010) *Rapid Assessment of the Acutely Ill Patient*. Oxford: Wiley-Blackwell.

Barraclough, J. (2014) *Emergency First Aid Made Easy: A Comprehensive First Aid Manual and Reference Guide*, 8th edn. Bradford: Qualsafe.

Gwinnett, C., Davies, R. and Soar, J. (2015) In-hospital resuscitation. Available at: www.resus. org.uk/resuscitation-guidelines/in-hospital-resuscitation (accessed 18 February 2016).

Hernandez-Padilla, J.M. *et al.* (2015) Effects of two retraining strategies on nursing students' acquisition and retention of BLS/AED skills: a clustered randomised trial. *Resuscitation*, 93: 27–34.

NICE (National Institute for Health and Care Excellence) (2011) Anaphylaxis: assessment to confirm an anaphylactic episode and the decision to refer after emergency treatment for a suspected anaphylactic episode. Available at: www.nice.org.uk/guidance/cg134/resources (accessed 2 January 2014).

NICE (National Institute for Health and Care Excellence) (2014) Acute patients in hospital overview. Available at: www.pathways.nice.org.uk (accessed 25 October 2014).

NMC (Nursing and Midwifery Council) (2015) *The Code: Professional Standards of Practice and Behaviour for Nurses and Midwives*. London: NMC.

Perkins, G.D., *et al.* (2015) Section 2. Adult basic life support and automated external defibrillation. *Resuscitation*, 95: 81–99.

Resuscitation Council (UK) (2011) *Advanced Life Support*, 6th edn. London: Resuscitation Council (UK).

Royal College of Physicians (2012) National Early Warning Score (NEWS): Standardising the assessment of acute illness severity in the NHS. Report of a Working Party. London: RCP.

Soar, J. *et al.* (2015a) Adult advanced life support algorithm. Available at: www.resus.org.uk/ resuscitation-guidelines (accessed 18 February 2016).

Soar, J. *et al.* (2015b) European Resuscitation Council Guidelines for Resuscitation 2015. Section 3. Adult advanced life support. *Resuscitation*, 95: 100–47.

Truhlář, A. *et al.* (2015) European Resuscitation Council Guidelines for Resuscitation 2015: Section 4. Cardiac arrest in special circumstances. *Resuscitation*, 95: 148–201.

WHO (World Health Organisation) (2014) The top 10 causes of death. Fact sheet no. 314. Available at: www.who.int/mediacentre/factsheets/fs310/en/index3.html (accessed 12 December 2014).

Part III

Organisational
aspects of care

Chapter 11

Moving and handling

Sinna Ramonaledi

Imagine that you are at the patient's bedside (in the community or a hospital). The bed does not have an adjustable height and there is a small bedside locker. You have to bend to attend to the patient's personal care needs. You stoop to pick up items off of the floor (such as slippers) and toiletries from the lower shelves of the locker. In the sluice room you stretch and tiptoe to get items from high shelves. When transferring the patient from the bed to the chair, you stoop, bend, twist and stretch, in addition to adopting awkward and static standing postures. These repetitive poor and complacent techniques for handling of patients and loads cause cumulative stress on the back.

Key concepts

Legal framework

Promoting healthy back or spine

Anatomy of the spine and spinal cord

Ergonomics – natural body movements

Biomechanical principles

Risk assessment

Essential skills for manual handling

Equipment

Learning outcomes

By the end of this chapter you will able to:

- Identify relevant laws and regulations and discuss their impact on moving and handling practices
- Gain an understanding of the employer's and employees' legal responsibilities in work places

■ Describe the anatomical structure and functions of the spine with specific reference to body posture and movement
■ Understand and apply biomechanical principles for efficient handling to minimise risks for musculoskeletal disorders (MSD)
■ Demonstrate the knowledge and application of risk assessment during practice
■ Understand and use essential or core moving and handling manoeuvres.

Introduction

The above scenario is an illustration that manual handling activities can indeed cause injury, back pain and other musculoskeletal disorders, in the short and long term, if not purposefully thought through, to ensure safe performance and practices.

In healthcare settings moving and handling activities are an indispensable part of caring, as most conditions of ill health impair patients' mobility or confidence to mobilise. Assisting patients to move safely or be positioned comfortably is fundamental in managing symptoms, like pain, breathing and airway difficulties. However, spontaneous actions can cause nurses to engage in poor handling practices, which involve bearing the patient's full body weight, inappropriate holds and unintentional exposure. Manual handling procedures not only have inherent potential risks for injuries to nurses, but can also compromise the patient's autonomy, dignity, comfort and safety. Care delivered without due consideration for the patient's quality of life and independence, or the safety of the health professional, is not sustainable (HSE, 2001). These practices can only be improved by purposeful, holistic patient assessment and meticulous plans, which focus on implementing safe techniques. This particular chapter provides principles of back care and practices, but do read and note local policies and guidelines.

Rationale for moving and handling

Handling procedures which use forceful body power during patient care are evidenced as major causes of injuries and musculoskeletal disorders (MSD) among nurses. This is regarded as controversial practice. Despite available professional guidelines for good practice, safe handling is often found not to be role-modelled consistently in some clinical settings. If these areas are used as placements for pre-registration nurses, what naturally follows is that they emulate such practices and become vulnerable to developing back injuries.

Despite statistics showing lower incidences of MSD among healthcare professionals (HSE, 2011), there is still a need for them to engage in best practices. Such practices will prevent back injuries and promote patients' comfort and dignity while empowering them to gain independence.

NHS providers are proactive in supporting staff's safety with policies that include 'no lifting' statements, based on individual professional judgement during patient care. This is further supported by the provision of equipment which facilitates ergonomic approaches to promote efficient handling, safety and comfort for both patients and nurses. These approaches can, however, be more effective, if accompanied by the nurse's understanding of the law and its impact on practice, and the structure and functions of the human spine. This knowledge should be integrated with the application of biomechanical principles during practice. The importance of holistic risk assessment of the patient's handling needs should be emphasised as an integral part of good knowledge and practice.

Don't forget!

Comprehensive knowledge and insight could enhance the nurse's patient handling skills and reinforce the importance of reflecting on problem-solving. It could also help nurses to challenge complacent attitudes towards handling practices and contribute to further reduction in back injuries.

Promoting a healthy back or spine

Eating a balanced diet, keeping active, sleeping sufficiently and using effective strategies to cope with life and work stressors, should enable nurses to maintain healthy lifestyles. This is essential for coping with the demands of clinical practice (e.g. standing for long periods or assisting in mobilising and positioning). This may prove challenging with patients who have illnesses such as low mood, depression, where they do not eat properly, adopt the wrong posture and have difficulty with sleep. Keeping healthy also involves taking care of our backs and spines. These are strong, yet delicate parts of the skeletal and nervous systems. Injured nerves do not always recover fully. Injuries to the back can and do have a debilitating impact on the person's quality of life. Symptoms such as chronic pain, inability to sit or walk and incontinence can have depressing effects on the mind as well as the debilitating effects on the body.

During moving and handling activities, the part of the body that facilitates movement is the spine. To use the spine efficiently, good posture which principally engages muscles of the arms (biceps and triceps), legs (quadriceps) and the buttocks (gluteus maximus) provides the power to assist in moving and handling safely and with ease. It is therefore essential that nurses understand the structure and functions of the spine or vertebral column, and how in association with other body parts, it has inherent capacities for safe body posture and movement.

Take time to look at the NHS web link video which shows good sitting postures: www.nhs.uk/Livewell/workplacehealth/Pages/howtositcorrectly.aspx

The spine (vertebral column)

The spine is part of the skeletal system forming an intricate and tough frame which gives the human body its shape. It is situated at the back (posterior) of the skeleton and can be likened to the central pillar of a house. It is strong and holds the head upright as well as supporting and carrying the weight of the body while acting as an the anchor to other parts of the skeleton. It is made up of a series of 33 irregular ring-like bones called vertebrae. The vertebrae are inter-connected and stacked on top of each other and thus also called the vertebral or spinal column. It extends from the base of the skull to the pelvis (Figure 11.1).

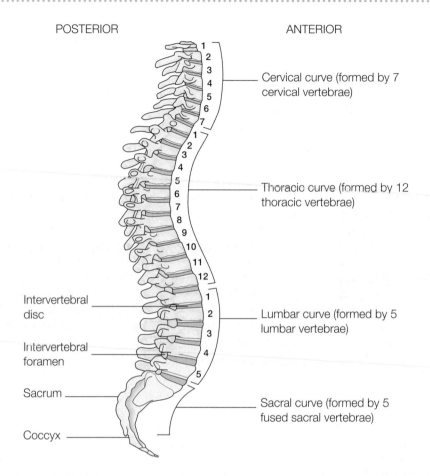

POSTERIOR   ANTERIOR

Cervical curve (formed by 7
cervical vertebrae)

Thoracic curve (formed by 12
thoracic vertebrae)

Intervertebral
disc

Intervertebral
foramen

Lumbar curve (formed by 5
lumbar vertebrae)

Sacrum

Sacral curve (formed by 5
fused sacral vertebrae)

Coccyx

Right lateral view for showing four normal curves

Figure 11.1 **Normal spine**

The spinal column is an S-curved structure which facilitates stability and flexibility of the trunk. When viewed from the front (anterior), or the side, it shows four curves, two concave (lordoses) and the other two convex (kyphosis). The two concave curves are at the cervical and lumbar regions and the two convex are at the thoracic and sacral regions. The concave curves are more flexible and thus vulnerable to injuries during moving and handling activities, if their natural ranges of movements are unconsciously and wrongly exaggerated by awkward postures.

The vertebrae

The vertebrae are inter-connected by facet joints, these bones are small in size at the cervical (neck) region and gradually enlarge, being the largest at the lumbar area where they tolerate most of the body's weight and endure a lot of the stress, or pressure, during

Watch out

Allowing children to playfully hang on the nurse's neck or the small of the back (lumbar area) can increase the risk of injuries. In all health settings one needs to be aware that the patient could become unpredictable, even after well-explained moves, they may still look for support and hold on to the nurse's neck or small of their back, resulting in injuries.

manual handling activities. Despite their differences in size and shape the vertebrae have similar characteristics (Figure 11.2).

Intervertebral discs are situated between adjacent vertebrae separating them and acting as a cushion to prevent friction, absorb shock and pressure from jarring movements and manual handling activities. They consist of an outer flexible and strong fibro-cartilage cover called the annulus fibrosus. The annulus fibrosus surrounds and protects the spongy, pulpy compressible and highly elastic interior called the nucleus pulpous. The discs consist of 90 per cent water but with ageing, the water content reduces. They become hard and less compressible, making adults susceptible to back pain and injuries. They also form a quarter of the length of the spine and the pressure they absorb during the day slightly reduces its height by the end of the day.

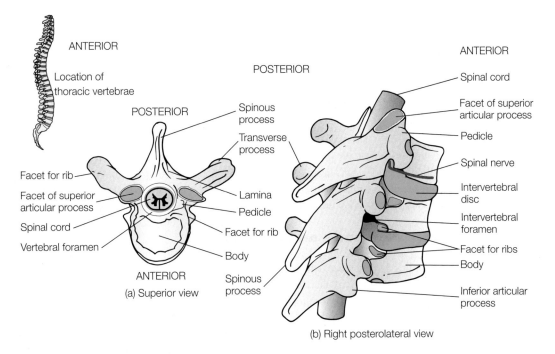

Figure 11.2 **Normal vertebrae**

The discs form strong joints on both sides of the vertebral bodies, allowing cushioned and flexible movements of the spine. However, repetitive stress or exceptional twisting, bending and stooping, can weaken the annulus fibrous, resulting in protruding or bulging of the disc's spongy interior called a prolapsed, slipped or herniated disc. This could put pressure on adjacent spinal nerves, causing intense pain, stiffness and numbness or sciatica to the part supplied by the nerve which is usually the leg (Figure 11.3).

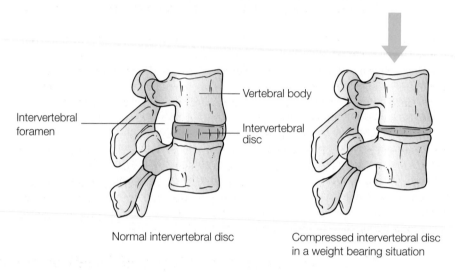

Vertebral body

Intervertebral foramen

Intervertebral disc

Normal intervertebral disc

Compressed intervertebral disc in a weight bearing situation

Intervertebral disc

Figure 11.3 **Comparing a normal and abnormal intervertebral disc**

Soft tissues of muscles, tendons and ligaments enhance the stability and strength of the spine. The muscles are firmly linked to the spine by tendons and support its upright posture. The ligaments are strong fibrous bands connecting vertebrae together and strengthening their joints. These structures together assist the spine during manual handling activities but, despite their strength, are susceptible to injury. Good posture during handling should support these soft tissues, by engaging the stronger muscles of the abdomen, buttocks, legs and arms.

Ergonomics and body movements

Ergonomics is a science which specialises in the study of the relationship between workers and designs of their working environments. It is based on a person-centred approach of working environments in which tasks or work activities, equipment and systems of work are designed to fit the individual, rather than traditional approaches, where the individual is expected to physically adapt to the given working environments (Hignett *et al.*, 2015). Ergonomics ensures that tasks, equipment, information and the environment suit each worker.

It emphasises the harmonious matching of natural human body postures and movements to tasks people do and the equipment used to accomplish work or life activities safely. In healthcare settings, employers are required to provide equipment to help nurses to maintain good posture when undertaking nursing activities with and for patients. Commonly used equipment such as beds and hoists are height-adjustable, making it easier for nurses to work at ergonomic levels, with optimum capacity to help the patients safely.

Biomechanical principles for efficient moving and handling practice

Biomechanics is related to ergonomics and they complement each other in promoting healthy back and natural postures. It is the 'application of physical laws of mechanics' to understand the human body movements. Newton's Laws of Motion are applied to appreciate the effects of forces on the human body. This science aims to understand human performance and movements by exploring the relationship between external forces and anatomical structures of bones, joints, muscles and ligaments (Polak, 2011).

The impact of force from lifting heavy loads or adopting poor postures is attributed to the cause of pain, intervertebral disc degeneration and collapse. Understanding the application of the biomechanical principles can be useful, especially in reducing these risks, by adopting natural postures during all activities. The principles are applicable and adaptable to any contexts in all fields of nursing practice. They are based on the use of the body's centre of gravity, creating a stable leg base for balance, keeping the head up and bending the knees slightly, to maintain the natural spinal curves.

Risk assessment in moving and handling practice

Risk assessment involves a careful examination of what might cause harm, injury or illness to any individual. In moving and handling practice, risk assessment will help the nurse to make informed clinical decisions and provide reasons for the interventions to be undertaken.

The Moving and Handling Operation Regulation 1992 (MHOR) (amended 2004) highlights the duty of the employer to engage in risk assessment in the workplace to prevent and reduce potential injuries from manual handling activities 'as far as reasonably practical'.

In addition, HSE (2004) has suggested a hierarchical process, which could be used to control and reduce injuries in workplaces by doing the following:

- *Avoid.* Hazardous manual handling activities should be avoided (MHOR, 1992)
- *Assess.* When avoiding such activities is challenging, 'a suitable and sufficient assessment' of potential hazards should be done to reduce the risks for harm or injury
- *Reduce.* A safe system of work and strategies to reduce the risks of injury should be put in place, such as educating the staff and providing appropriate equipment, such as hoists
- *Review.* The risk assessment must be reviewed regularly to ensure the strategies to prevent injury remain effective and relevant.

Risk assessment includes recorded plans and interventions to reduce the risks before and during handling. Meanwhile every nurse is expected to be competent in undertaking a personal risk assessment before and during implementing any planned handling decisions and interventions.

A patient handling risk assessment (PHRA) is a legal document like a care plan, which shows the patient's handling needs, goals, plans and safe interventions. Personal risk assessment tools are available, e.g. TILEE (Task to be done; Individual capabilities/skills of the nurse/nurses to do the task; Load/patient to be handled; Environment handling interventions are taking place; Equipment required).

Essential or core skills for moving and handling of people

Like other nursing skills, effective and safe moving and handling skills have elements of manual dexterity (psychomotor), application of evidence-based relevant knowledge (cognition) and having appropriate attitudes (affect), to ensure patient's dignity. In order for effective problem-solving and decision-making to occur, a sound knowledge base is imperative. Competent performance of handling skills requires an awareness that written documents are guides that should be adapted to the patients' mobility and capabilities, their ill-health, holistic needs and human rights. During moving and handling procedures, nurses' attitudes should also demonstrate a duty of care and accountability to prevent injury to self and others during practice. These attitudes can also be supported by listening, empathetic and respectful communication skills.

Handling skills need to be adapted appropriately to the context at hand to meet the patients' needs safely and with dignity. Brooks and Orchards (2011) suggest a framework for safer person handling (Box 11.1) to be considered for every moving and handling procedure.

Box 11.1 Adapted framework of safer person practice (Brooks and Orchards, 2011)

Preparations by the nurse

- *Identify* a clinical rationale (reason) for the moving and handling procedure
- *Refer* to patient's handling risk assessment documents, assess their cognitive, emotional and physical capabilities and how they are usually assisted. What equipment and number of nurses are required?
- *Make* decisions and judgements of appropriate handling interventions needed
- *Undertake* a careful personal risk assessment to identify potential risks for injury for all involved
- *Seek* advice from other professional if needed
- *Consider* legal and moral issues to safeguard human rights and cultural preferences for the patient during the procedure

- *Support* decisions with knowledge of professional guidelines and employers' policies
- *Use* appropriate communication skills and caring attitudes to implement handling plans in partnership with the patients and colleagues
- *Engage* staff with appropriate skills and identify a leader to coordinate the procedure
- *Ensure* that team members are wearing suitable clothing and footwear
- *Consider* how to apply biomechanical principles to the context of the current situation.

Preparation of the environment and equipment

- *De-cluttering or clearing* any obstructing furniture and dangers, ensuring the environment is warm, well lit, clear and spacious
- Floor surfaces should be safe for using the equipment
- Before using any handling equipment check it.

Preparation of the patient

This will be performed during every moving and handling procedure and will not be repeated when discussing specific procedures below.

- The nurse will introduce him/herself to establish a trusting working relationship if the patient does not know him/her
- Provide the patient with information to understand why they have to move and how they are going to move and gain consent to cooperate
- Assess the patient's cognitive, emotional and physical capabilities to complete the task (patient risk assessment document will highlight some of this information)
- If applicable, the use of normal body movements should be encouraged first as these are natural and will facilitate autonomy
- Support the patient verbally by teaching, instructing and supervising to complete the movement independently
- If the patient is unable to complete the move independently despite help and supervision, the nurse will introduce equipment
- Continuously inform the patient of what is happening and reassure them to alleviate any distress
- Praise and encourage the patient positively to help and handle gently, promoting comfort and dignity
- Make patient comfortable
- Document the procedure to ensure other nurses can follow the same method (NMC, 2015).

Activity 11.1

▪ Reflect on the moving and handling practices that you have learnt during your time in clinical practice
▪ Now compare your observations and experiences with the procedures discussed in the rest of this chapter.

Essential handling skills to assist ambulant patients

Ambulant patients (adults and children) have weight-bearing capacities and are able to stand up, supported by the spine to carry their body weight through the legs. These patients also have good upper body strength and control and are also able to sit balanced and upright. This enables them to shuffle the bottom/buttocks to the front of a chair or towards the edge of a mattress and push up to stand with hands on the armrests of the chair/mattress on the bed. They may also have strength and control of leg and thigh movements like kicking and pushing or lifting up or down and have the ability to maintain their feet firmly on the floor.

Despite having weight-bearing capacity, patients may or may not walk, depending on their physical conditions (ill health, pain), psychological and mental state (confused, anxious, fear, loss of confidence, mental health issues, depression). They may need assistance and encouragement to do so.

Procedure for assisting ambulant patients

First, follow the framework for safer handling (Box 11.1).

1   If the patient is sitting upright on a chair, instruct the patient to put their hands on the armrests of the chair, to sit upright and lean forward with head up and facing forward.
2   They should shuffle their bottom or buttocks towards the front until they are in the middle of the chair.
3   Feet position should be feet hip width apart, wide, firm and flat on the floor and under the knees. Ensure the patient is wearing non-slip footwear.
4   Patient puts the strong foot slightly back to help push up when standing up.
5   Patient keeps the head up and looks ahead.
6   To create a momentum or energy to stand, both the nurse and the patient will gently rock back and forwards on the command described below to initiate the movement to stand. If the patient is susceptible to dizzy spells, assess and both agree on the best way to initiate standing, e.g. leaning with the nose over the knees and slowly push slightly forward and up instead of rocking. Abandon standing to walk, check the patient's blood pressure (Chapter 7), the patient's condition may dictate that they are returned to bed.
7   The command will be 'Ready, Steady, Stand'. On 'Stand', the patient pushes their

hands off the armrests and uses the strong foot to propel their body upwards and stands.

8   The nurse should stand closer to the patient on the weaker side (if present) or two nurses stand on either side (see Figures 11.4 (a) and 11.4 (b)).

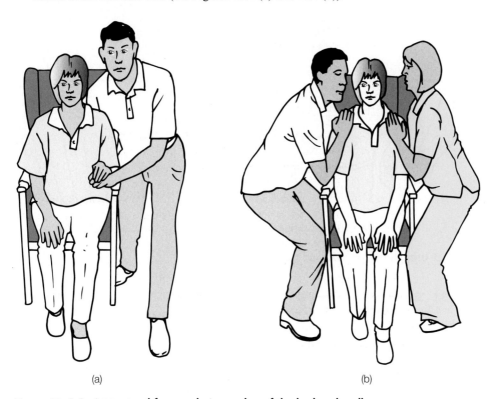

(a)   (b)

Figure 11.4 **Assist to stand from a chair or edge of the bed and walk**

9   When the patient is up and steady, the nurse/nurses offer their palm (with the thumb bent to the middle of the palm or thumb close to the index finger, Figures 11.5 (a) and 11.5 (b)) to palm hold, or the back of a clenched fist for the patient's hand support. These holds avoid the risk of injury to nurses' thumbs if gripped firmly by the patient especially during a fall.
10   Allow the patient to stand calmly for a while, to feel stable and ready to start the walk.
11   Ask the patient if they are ready to walk and clearly instruct to 'walk', then, steadily catch up with their pace to avoid pushing them.

The nurses' position in this procedure.

1   The nurses adopt a lunge position on the side of the patient, and look forward to the direction of standing or face the patient.
2   Stand as close as comfortable to the patient sitting forward in the chair.

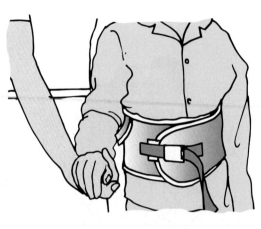
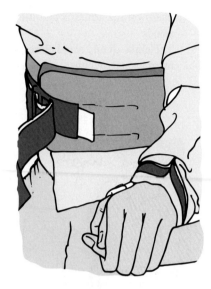

(a) Child handling belt   (b) Adult handling belt

Figure 11.5 **Using handling belts and palm to palm hold**

3   Support with one hand on the front of the patient's shoulder and the other on the lower back or the hip furthest away to prompt standing.
4   Give instructions to stand as above and stabilise by transferring body weight with the back leg brought forward and the front one to step forward. Side-step if facing the patient.
5   Keep close to the patient, but stand slightly behind the nearer hip and place a supportive hand at the further hip or lower part of the back.
6   Offer palm to palm or clenched fist support for both hands, to be ready for walking.
7   Instruct the patient to take the first steps to avoid pushing them.
8   Encourage the patient to adopt safe postures by looking ahead while walking.
9   Reassure the patient praising their efforts and communicate directions and reassure throughout the walk.
10 Keep assessing the patient's condition for coping safely with the walk.
11 If the patient is not coping, abandon the procedure and help the patient to sit on a wheelchair and transport to the destination.
12 On reaching the chair, the nurse and the patient should take side steps to be parallel to the seat of the chair.
13 When the patient feels the chair on the back of their legs, then they can reach for the armrests of the chair using one hand at a time and lower themselves slowly, to sit down.

Procedure for using handling belts

Handling belts (see Figures 11.5 (a) and 11.5 (b)) are used around patients' waists and have either buckles like a car seat belt or Velcro to fasten securely. They have handles to enable (preferably) two nurses to have safe holds to assist the patient to stand and walk. The belts are designed in various sizes. Without the belt, nurses will bend or slant to reach the opposite hip or back of patients when assisting with standing and walking. They can also be suitable aids when patients are uncomfortable with being touched as part of cultural or personal preferences.

First, follow the framework for safer handling (Box 11.1).

1   The belt is placed around the patient's waist after they have shuffled to the front of the chair or the edge of the bed.
2   The nurses position themselves close to the patient, to support them for standing.
3   Each nurse holds the belt handle on the opposite hip and supports the patient on the front of shoulder, ready for standing (arms are not put through the loops to avoid being trapped during a fall).

Top tip

To ensure comfort, handling belts cannot be used on patients with stomas, abdominal wounds, PEG tubes or any type of catheters around the abdomen. The belts are useful on patients who have wider girths, as this presents a challenge for nurses to adopt safe postures.

Moving and handling procedures specific to children

It is easy to underestimate children's body weight and be complacent in planning to carry or assist them during handling. However, it is not necessarily the weight of the child causing problems but the repetitive nature of handling them, which could have a damaging effect on the spine. Risks are also compounded by the children's unpredictable behaviours like jumping in excitement or throwing themselves on the floor when upset and being uncooperative. It is therefore imperative that biomechanical principles are applied even when handling children.

Ambulant children need to be encouraged to move independently with supervision. For instance, as children grow up, it is helpful to provide a step (with appropriate height) for them to use to climb onto chairs, toilet seats and into push chairs under supervision. This will avoid stooping to lift their full body weight from lower to higher heights.

Safe postures are necessary for handling children, e.g. raising cot heights and lowering the sides, then sliding a child on the mattress nearer and assuming a stable base before lifting the child out. While playing with children on the floor, stooping can be reduced by kneeling and sitting on a mat or bean bag. Prolonged kneeling can be uncomfortable and cause knee damage. It could be relieved by a cushion or a small stool between the back of the thighs and calves, to spread the body weight and avoid over-flexion of knees (Alexander and Johnson, 2011).

When carrying small children, it is important to know their weight and assess their behaviours and mobility skills. The child should be carried close to the body, with whole arms and hands. Lifting on a hip should be avoided to prevent back injuries.

Walking with aids

Procedure for using walking frames

Walking frames are used for rehabilitation in adult care after falls, injury and illness. They can give confidence to frail patients and support to those who cannot carry their body weight fully due to painful hips or knees.

Before using a walking frame, the nurse is required to check that it is in good working condition, so as to accomplish the task safely. Checks include:

- If it is the right height for the patient, shown by elbows having a slight flexion and being able to straighten adequately to support the patient's body weight when placed in front.
- The ferrules (covering on the legs) should be intact with non-slip rubber rings to ensure stability and balance.
- Handgrips are undamaged.
- The frame is steady and firm with the patient's name on a label.

First, follow the framework for safer handling (Box 11.1).

1   While preparing and assisting the patient to stand (as discussed in the procedure for assisting ambulant patients), the nurse places the frame at their side but not too close to block moving forward during the transfer of the body weight or too close in front of the patient, as they may rush to hold on it.

2   After the patient has stood up, place the frame in front of them and instruct them to put both hands on the handgrips.

3   The nurse stands on the side and slightly behind, with a reassuring hand on the patient's shoulder if needed.

4   Instruct the patient to take equal steps one at a time, towards the frame, if the frame is at a safe distance. If it is too close, instruct the patient to put the frame a step in front, before stepping forward towards it.

5   The patient can lean slightly onto the frame and take his or her body weight through the arms and walk equal steps, one at a time, to be in line with the back legs of the frame or at the centre of the frame.

6   Encourage the patient throughout the walk, to continue this pattern until they reach a chair at the destination

7   To sit, the patient is instructed to walk parallel and close to the seat of the chair.

8   Start turning the frame slowly, so that it is in front of the patient, after reaching the level of the furthest armrest of the chair (this will help bring the patient close to the chair and avoid walking backwards).

9   When feeling the chair behind their legs, instruct the patient to reach for both the rests of the chair, ONE hand at a time and bend the knees and move backwards to sit.

10 For children (and indeed adults) the frames are specialised to meet the patient's needs, e.g. walking frames with wheels (Figures 11.6 (a) and 11.6 (b)). These walking frames may also have wheels with brakes on the four legs. The child

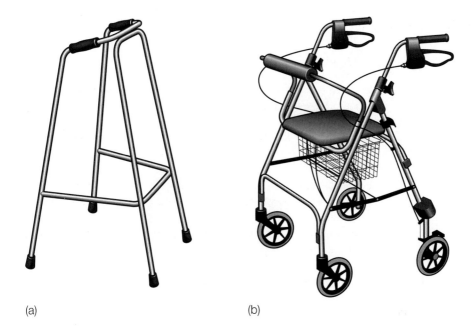

(a)   (b)

Figure 11.6 (a) Walking frame (Zimmer); (b) frame/walker with wheels

pulls the frame behind him or her, thus being able to be close to tables and other children if needed. There may also be a seat on the walker to allow a rest during the walk.

Procedure to transfer patients using a stand aid

Some ambulant patients may be able to stand and carry their body weight confidently but have difficulties walking due to various physical and mental conditions, e.g. breathing difficulties, swollen painful legs, and delusions. For such patients, to continue rehabilitation to gain independence, a stand aid can be used to facilitate transfers from one seated position to another (Figure 11.7). The equipment has a turntable which can be rotated 360 degrees and forms the platform for the patient to stand on. The shin pad provides protection and support for the patient's legs. The equipment is height-adjustable to suit different patients and has a foot pedal brake to secure the turntable when the patient is standing on it. The risk of falling backwards can be avoided by establishing if the patient will be able to stand independently for a short time and with the support of a nurse.

Two nurses *must* undertake the procedure with one helping and encouraging patient and the other operating the equipment.

First, follow the framework for safer handling (Box 11.1).

1   The patient who is sitting on a chair or bed prepares for standing as described earlier.

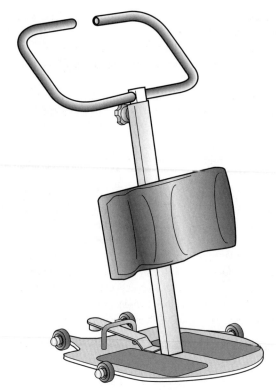

Figure 11.7 **Stand aid**

2   Instruct the patient to shuffle their bottom forward to the front of the chair or near the edge of the bed and to place the feet wide.

3   The nurse operating the stand should swivel it into the space between the patient's feet.

4   Patient puts their feet on the footprints or non-slip squares on the stand, or the feet are slid with slide sheets by the nurse, if too painful or swollen for the patient to lift their feet.

5   The first nurse holds the nearest handling bars firmly and with a good base of support and places the front foot on the pedal brake to stabilise the equipment.

6   Instruct the patient to place one hand on the arm of the chair or mattress to push up and the other on the nearest handling bar of the stand to pull up.

7   The other nurse supports the patient to stand (see Figures 11.4 (a) and 11.4 (b)).

8   When the patient is standing stable on the stand, the nurse operating the equipment takes off the brake and gently swivels the stand 90 degrees while talking and reassuring the patient (diverting attention from looking at the floor, as the swivelling might make the patient dizzy). If the dizziness is problematic, abandon, sit patient in a chair (as discussed earlier) check the patient's blood pressure (Chapter 7). The patient's condition may dictate that they are returned to bed.

9   If it is safe (patient's condition allowing) to continue, the other nurse pushes a wheelchair or the bed, to ensure the patient can feel behind the legs.

10   When the patient can feel the wheelchair/bed behind the legs, then the brakes for either equipment are applied.
11   The nurse operating the stand puts the brakes back on (to steady the equipment).
12   Instruct the patient to put hands on either armrests of the wheel chair or on the mattress and slowly sit down.
13   Feet are lifted off the turntable, or the nurse slides them off. The stand is swivelled away and foot plates of a wheelchair put in place, to rest the patients' feet.
14   Ensure that the patient is comfortable.

Procedure to assist semi-dependent and dependent patients in and around the bed

The patient's condition may impair their ability to move or position themselves independently. Some patients rely on nurses partially or completely, to be safely moved and repositioned, to ensure comfort and good skin integrity.

Currently different brands of electric profiling beds are used in practice settings as part of ergonomic equipment provision (HSE, 2010b). Profiling beds minimise and avoid risks from handling procedures, as they can be manipulated to support the patient to sit up with pillows (Figure 11.8). The knee-break position can prevent patients slipping down the bed (Brooks and Orchard, 2011), while strong and steady bed sides can be used by semi-dependent patients, to roll onto their side, with minimal help.

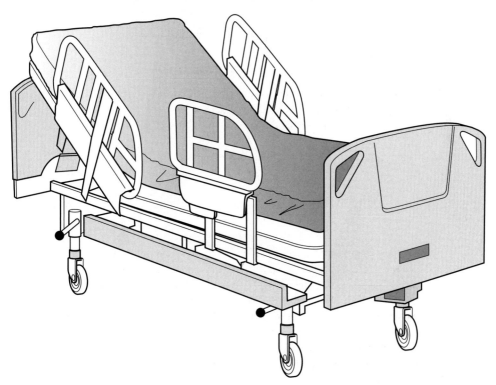

Figure 11.8 Electric profiling bed

The types of equipment that can be used to promote independence while in bed are the rope ladder (Figure 11.9) and transfer boards (Figure 11.10). Sliding sheets can also be used to help move the patient up the bed.

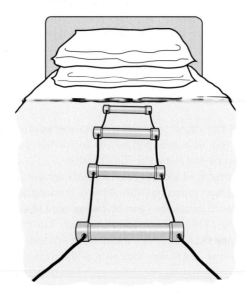

Figure 11.9 **Rope ladder**

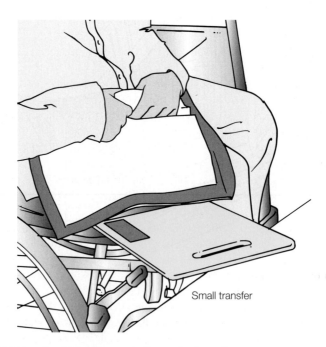

Small transfer

Figure 11.10 **Transferring using a small transfer board**

Before using the equipment, the patient should be taught and encouraged to sit up using natural body movements. Holding with a hand, on each safety side of the bed and digging a preferred heel on the mattress, the patient can pull their chest up to the sitting position. Then putting one hand at a time, behind the hip, balance and adjust their sitting position comfortably.

Rope ladders are simple devices used to enable the patients with upper body strength and stability to pull themselves up to a sitting position while in or on the bed. They are attached to the stable bottom part of the bedstead for safety. This is performed by a physiotherapist. The ladder should be checked to establish if it is secure, by pulling on it before the patient uses it.

Procedure using a small transfer board

This is a steady solid plastic or wood device with a safe working load of 130 kg (20 stones). It is used to bridge gaps between two surfaces, e.g. bed to chair or chair to chair. It is designed to promote patient independence for seated transfers from bed to chair, or vice versa, by providing a low friction glide between the surfaces. The patient needs a balanced, sitting ability with good upper body strength.

First, follow the framework for safer handling (Box 11.1).

1 Ensure the bed brakes are on and position the chair parallel to the bed with the seat level with the patient's bottom.
2 Place the chair slightly lower than the bed for gravity, facilitating a gently decline. Apply the brakes on the chair for safety.
3 Instruct the patient to shuffle the buttocks towards the edge of the bed and level with the chair seat.
4 Instruct patient to lean on the hand which is still on the bed and the nurse places the board under the bottom, to secure one anti-slip pad firmly on the bed and the other on the seat (bridging and minimising the gap between the bed and chair).
5 The patient places their hand, first, in the middle of the board and slides onto the board. The hand can be placed on the opposite armrest of the wheelchair, then to pull and slide further towards the seat.
6 If the patient is wearing clothes which grip on the board, a small sliding sheet can be placed on the transfer board.
7 Ensure that the patient is comfortable on the wheelchair, with feet resting on the foot plates.

Slide or sliding sheets are efficient low-friction devices used in moving patients easily and safely on beds, floors and chairs. They avoid skin damage due to friction and eliminate the manual lifting of patients as they are versatile and can be used to move patients up or down, turn them to their sides in beds, transfer them laterally and slide from tight awkward spaces when fallen (Figure 11.13).

Patients can use slide sheets independently to move in beds, they are manufactured in various widths, lengths and materials or fabrics. Paper-made slide sheets with a light silicone coating for sliding are used and discarded if contaminated or wet. Others are made of fabrics suitable for patient-specific use only, i.e. for the same patient and

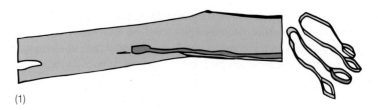

(1)

Figure 11.11 **Extension straps**

discarded if soaked in body fluids as they cannot be laundered. Some fabrics are for long-term use and can be laundered, however, this type could be a risk for cross-infection if used communally.

Examples of slide sheets would be flat slide sheets with/without handles (Figure 11.12), they can be used in pairs or singly if folded and lateral transfer board (Patslide) (Figures 11.13 (a) and 11.13 (b)).

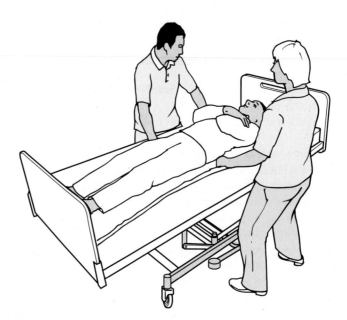

Figure 11.12 **Flat sheets with/without handles**

The types of sliding sheets used are:

- Roller sheets which are tubular with open lateral sides. Some may be padded. Movement is achieved by rolling the top layer close to the patient and allowing it to slide on the bottom layer
- Lateral transfer slide sheets with/without extension loops.

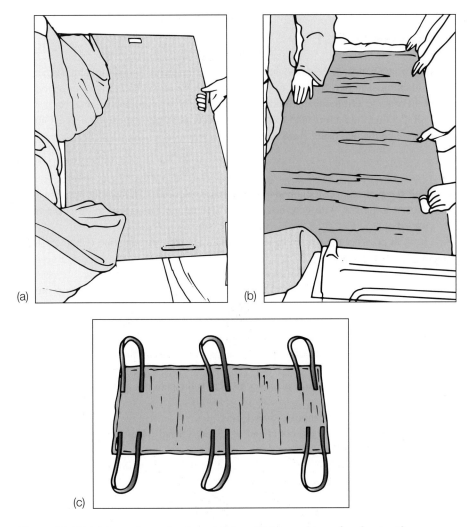

Figure 11.13 (a) Lateral transfer board; (b) and (c) lateral transfer sheet with handholds or loops

Procedure for inserting and removing slide sheets to move a patient up the bed

Two nurses should work together, standing on each side of the bed with safety sides down to be near the patient.

First, follow the framework for safer handling (Box 11.1).

1   Ensure the bed brakes are on and adjust the height of the bed to nurses' waists or pelvic crest for comfort (Brooks and Orchard, 2011).
2   If one nurse is taller, then turn the patient towards the taller nurse (they will have a better reach given their height advantage).

Case study 11.1

Mrs Lydia Scott is 70 years old and lives with her husband. She is frail and has had an abdominal hysterectomy a day ago. She is in moderate pain, has been incontinent of urine and has slipped down the bed. Mrs Scott requires personal care.

Reflect on the factors that need to be considered to provide care and assist her to move up the bed using sling sheets.

3   Pull the patient over their body with comfortable levers (allows the nurse who is shorter in height, with comfortable levers, to nudge the patient towards the taller nurse).

4   Instruct or assist the patient to adopt a modified recovery position (Chapter 10) to be easier to turn.

5   Instruct or assist patient to turn their head in the direction of the turn.

6   The patient's arm on the side of the turn is placed palm up on the pillow to protect the face.

7   Instruct the patient to bend the knee of the far leg. If the patient is unable to do so, a small slide sheet is used to bend the knee.

8   Both nurses adopt a walking stance (one foot in front and the other back) position of a stable base.

9   The nurse towards the turn places arms across the patient's body and put hands on the shoulder and hip.

10   The other nurse superimposes their hands.

11   The patient is told on the command of 'Ready, Steady, Turn' the nurses will turn themselves to an appropriate side.

12   On the command the nurse towards the turn gently pulls the patient towards themselves while the other gently nudges away.

13   The procedure should be done slowly and smoothly, ensuring the patient is not too close to the edge of the bed.

14   The nurses maintain their natural postures by transferring their body weights to the back leg for the one pulling and the front leg for the one nudging.

15   To support the patient and maintain the turn, the nurse should continue to hold the patient on their shoulder and hip appropriately and adopt feet-wide position for a stable base (the lower bed safety side can be pulled up if a patient is anxious or nervous about the procedure. The bed safety side will give them something to hold on to).

Procedure to insert slide sheets

1   Fold clean, appropriate body width and length, tubular or a pair of slide sheets with handles on top, into a longitudinal half and place parallel to the back of the patient.

2   Place the sheets from the head to below the ankles of the patient.

3   The top half fold is folded as quarters towards the patient's back (allowing easy retrieval).
4   Instruct the patient to roll on their back before being turned to the other side.
5   Pull and straighten the sheets.
6   The patient is encouraged and supported to roll onto their back again in the middle of the slide sheets (see Figure 11.12).
7   Move patient up the bed.
8   Make the patient comfortable and remove the slide sheet (Instructions below).

Procedure to remove slide sheets from under the patient

First, follow the framework for safer handling (Box 11.1).

1   After positioning the patient, examine the slide sheets to decide the side with large or small material on which the patient is lying.
2   Remove slide sheets from the side with large or more material (as there is less material left to pull out) and less possibility of changing the patient's position.
3   Use natural hollow areas below the ankles, knees and under the neck (avoid the lumbar area as it is where most of the body weight is situated) to lunge and gently push an arm between the two sheets or layers of a tubular sheet.
4   The nurse on the opposite side should feed the corners of the pair of sheets into the hand of the nurse removing them. Alternatively, the nurse removing the sheet grabs the bottom layer of the tubular sheet.
5   The nurse pulling out the slide sheet should place a free hand on the patient's knee area to support them and avoid the change in position. Then gently scoop and diagonally pull the sheets towards the waist of the patient. Stop when resistance is encountered (to prevent sliding the patient).
6   Repeat the procedure from under the patient's neck, supporting the chest area, scoop and pull the sheet, stopping at the waist.
7   The slide sheets remaining under the patient's waist are gently eased from side to side to avoid sliding the patient.
8   The patient is positioned comfortably and the safety bed sides are pulled up if indicated.

Procedure to transfer a dependent patient from bed to trolley

Lateral transfer board. This equipment is made of steady and slightly flexible plastic and designed to accommodate the full length of the body. The board is used to bridge gaps between two beds or a bed and a stretcher or theatre trolley. It has a sliding side and the other side has a non-slip properties. For safe practice, the board is used with a lateral transfer slide sheet (Figure 11.13 (b)), which has three pairs of loops for ergonomic holds. The sheet can also be a flat sheet with handles and extension straps are attached for long hand holds. Alternatively, a disposable paper transfer slide sheet perforated on the sides for handholds (Figure 11.13 (a)) can be used. The long hand-holds and extension straps avoid bending and stretching during the procedure. Independent patients can undertake lateral transfers with assistance from the nurses, if they can sit and have upper body strength and control. Highly dependent patients should be lying flat on the back.

First, follow the framework for safer handling (Box 11.1).

1   A clinical decision for the use of three to four nurses will be made by the nurse leading the transfer, depending on the patient's condition.

2   If a patient is unconscious, one nurse is needed to control the head and maintain the airway, another to control legs and two on either sides of the bed for a smooth safe transfer.

3   After adjusting the bed height and putting the brakes on, the patient is turned away from the direction of the transfer supported by one or two nurses.

4   Two nurses insert the transfer board and transfer the slide sheet (as described above, procedure for inserting slide sheet). If flat sheets are used, extension straps should be attached.

5   Position the patient again on their back, ensuring that they are fully on the equipment (including the pillow if needed).

6   The height of the trolley is raised to slightly below the bed height and pushed towards the bed to bring them together.

7   Put the trolley brakes on (for safety).

8   Transfer is achieved by all nurses in the direction of the procedure and near the patient adopting a walking stance base of support.

9   Nurses on the transfer direction should hold onto the loops/extension straps of the transfer sheet, while the nurses on the far side place hands on the patient's shoulder and hip.

10   On the 'Ready, steady, slide' command, the nurses with their hands on the patient nudge the patient towards the trolley, while the nurses holding the slide sheet loops, gently pull the patient.

11   The procedure has to be gentle and slow, with nurses transferring their body weight appropriately, to avoid stretching and overarching their backs.

12   To ensure safe control, the leader can command 'STOP', when the patient reaches the middle of the board.

13   The nurses near the trolley will leave the long leverage of straps and grab hold of the slide sheet close to the patient, reposition the walking stance base of support and 'slide' the patient to the middle of the trolley.

14   Pull up the safety rail of the trolley.

15   The nurse next to the bed will slowly swivel the board to the bed.

16   Take the bed brakes off and push the bed away from the trolley then remove the slide sheet using the natural hollow areas. Put the brakes back on.

17   Make the patient comfortable and pull the trolley rail up for the safety.

Hoists

Hoists are a vital part of moving and handling people in order to avoid hazardous manual handling activities. On average, 120 incidents per year are reported to the Medicines and Healthcare products Regulatory Agency (MHRA) (HSE, 2011). They also have inherent risks of back injuries for nurses, when safe postures are ignored during practice.

Patients are also vulnerable to injuries, due to human errors and equipment failures during hoisting.These risks can be eliminated, when nurses have good knowledge and competent skills to use hoists safely and conscientiously apply biomechanical principles. In practice settings, hoists can be electric or battery-operated (Figure 11.14).

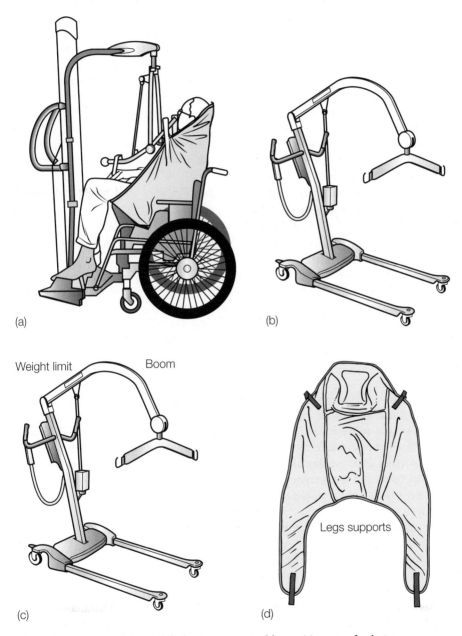

(a)

(b)

Weight limit   Boom

(c)

Legs supports

(d)

Figure 11.14 (a) and (b) Mobile battery-operated hoist; (c) parts of a hoist; (d) a universal sling

The three main types of hoists are:

- *Fixed hoists* – they are mounted on walls or floors and are particularly convenient where there is a lack of space, in bedrooms and bathrooms.
- *Overhead hoists* – these are useful in solving space and flooring problems and promoting user independence. Their use contributes to safe carer postures and fewer back strains due to operational heights.
- *Mobile hoist (passive or active)* – they are in different sizes and safe working loads capacities. The active varieties are rehabilitative and facilitate patients with weight-bearing capacity and balance, to stand or relearn to walk. Passive hoists lift full body weights of dependent and fallen patients and are operated by the nurse. These are the common hoists in practice settings.

Nurses should be familiar with the construction and workings of a hoist and be able to check if they are in good working order before use. Box 11.2 provides a checklist.

Box 11.2 Hoist check list

- Check the weight limit of the hoist, which is on the boom, for the suitability of carrying the patient's weight
- The hoist should have a sticker, indicating the last date of maintenance, which is usually every six months
- The battery should be full and the lowering and lifting functions working
- Note the position of the emergency lowering device
- Ensure the legs can be manipulated to open or close and that the spreader bar is in good condition.

The nurse needs competent skills to check the integrity of the sling parts (Figure 11.14 (d)) and to measure the size for an individual patient patient (PUWER, 1998). Slings come in different sizes and types and are made of different materials or fabrics. The different types include the general purpose universal, hammock style, toilet, full body, amputee and stretcher slings. It is important that the sling is compatible with the hoist brand and the speader bar. The manufacturer's guidance needs to be followed accurately. This includes guidance on how to measure the size for an individual patient.

Procedure for applying the sling on a patient

First, follow the framework for safer handling (Box 11.1).

1   Ask the patient to roll onto their back or assist patient onto their back.
2   Roll the patient onto their side.
3   Fold the sling in half with all the labels and handles on the outside.
4   Position along the back of the patient from the coccyx (lower back). If there is a head support, align the neck seam to the base of the neck.

5   Fold the top half into a quarter and fold in the clips for patient comfort.
6   Roll the patient onto their back, then the other way, for the other nurse to access the sling.
7   Unroll the rest of the sling and adjust to be comfortable.
8   Push the hoist nearer and so it is visible to the patient from the front, lower to the desired height and attach the sling and hoist the patient.
9   Communicate with and reassure the patient all the time while observing for signs of discomfort or anxiety.

Read the Health & Safety Executive (2011) guidance on using hoists at: www.hse.gov.uk/pubns/hsis3.pdf

Moving and handling of patients who are obese

Obesity is a contemporary global challenge for health and social care provision, with its incidence gradually increasing in the world populations. Bariatrics is a branch of medicine which specialises in studying the causes, management and other issues of obesity. This can affect mobility difficulties, resulting from altered centre of gravity, limiting a wide range of movements and dimished ability to flex at the waist due to enlarged girths. Patients may also suffer from pain in the knees and other supporting joints and are vulnerable to poor skin intergrity. Secondary cardio-vascular, respiratory and other conditions could exacerbate the patients' mobility problems with dyspnoea and other symptoms. There are many causes of obesity, but issues with nutrition and lifestyle get more attention, which sometimes divert attention from the patients' complex health and mobility needs, by laying the blame on them for their obesity.

Society can create stigma and prejudice in relation to people who are obese through media reporting and television. This can contribute to a clouding of professional judgement when dealing with obese patients. In handling practice, such attitudes can heighten the risks for injuries to both nurses and patients, due to unrealistic expectations of the patient's mobility abilities. With the increasing rate of obesity, it is important that nurses understand the multiple causes of obesity and its impact on the patients' quality of life. This could foster a problem-solving and non-judgemental approach, to meet the patients' handling needs, based on individual risk assessment and engagement of interprofessional team members and inter-agency collaboration, to bring together the expertise and resources to ensure patient safety. This in turn facilitates empathetic and dignified care of the patient. There is also a need for different practice settings and wards to share accurate and appropriate information. It allows staff adequate time to consult other professionals for support and advice, e.g. back care advisors, tissue viability nurse. Risk assessment and handling procedures will need to be undertaken with the aim of providing fair and dignified care. The ward team need to be able to think about the best approaches to patient care and address staff fears and attitudes, which could impact on the quality of patient care.

The moving and handling legal framework

Health and safety laws are cornerstones in encouraging nurses to reduce and avoid risks of injuries, to patients and themselves during practice. The laws set guidance and duties for both employers and employees, to ensure safe workplaces and practices. Within moving and handling, laws describe safe standards of work, risk assessment processes and the appropriate use of suitable equipment for good handling practice. They provide recommendations to facilitate humane and dignified practices for all people in health and social care settings. The area of health and safety laws and regulations is very broad and only the essential aspects related to everyday practice will be highlighted within the remit of this chapter. Application of all laws in practice is supported by NMC (2015) and employers' policies.

Furthermore, if conflicts are encountered during practice, laws provide the opportunity to reach 'balanced decisions', to highlight that sometimes the human rights of both the patient and the staff need to be considered in a fair manner. As in some handling situations, both can be equally susceptible to injuries. For instance, using 'orthodox' and 'drag' lifts (Figures 11.15 (a) and 11.15 (b)), can cause back injuries to the nurse, damage to the patients' skin due to friction, discomfort or dislocation of the shoulder. However, a patient may prefer these manoeuvres to being hoisted via a mechanical device.

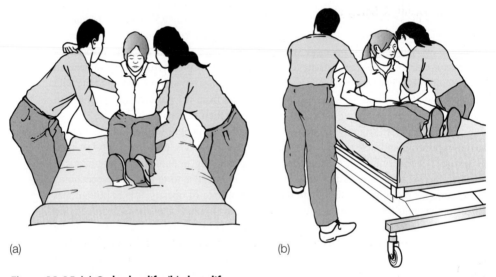

(a)   (b)

Figure 11.15 (a) Orthodox lift; (b) drag lift

It is imperative that nurses develop a sound knowledge of key laws and regulations, pertaining to moving and handling and understand their impact on practice. This knowledge and understanding will assist them to practise within their capabilities and competence, guided by NMC (2015), the law and the employer's policies. The nurses will also appreciate the need to work in collaboration with other professionals, such as physiotherapists or nurse specialists (e.g. tissue viability nurse), to meet the patient's complex handling needs.

Clinical significance

Despite the NMC recognising students as 'responsible', but not accountable for professional actions and omissions, the law states that all care workers are equally accountable when engaging in healthcare practice. More specifically within health and safety in particular, ignorance is not a defence (Dimond, 2011).

Key policy and legislation as applied to moving and handling

Box 11.3 presents the key legislation in this area.

Box 11.3 Key policy and legislation as applied to moving and handling

The Acts, Regulations and Policies relevant to moving and handling practice are:

- The Health & Safety at Work Act (HASWA or HASAWA)1974
- Manual Handling Operations Regulations 1992 (MHOR)
- Reporting of Injuries, Diseases and Dangerous Occurrences Regulation 2013 (RIDDOR)
- Management of Health & Safety at Work Regulations 1999
- Provision & Use of Work Equipment Regulations 1998 (PUWER)
- Lifting Operations and Lifting Equipment Regulations 1998 (LOLER)
- Human Rights Act 1998
- Disability Discrimination Act 1995
- Mental Capacity Act 2005
- NMC Professional Code of Conduct 2015
- Local policies.

Health and Safety at Work Act (HSWA or HASAWA) 1974

This Act has a fascinating history in Britain, inspired by protection of children in factories during the Industrial Revolution and poor regard of miners' health and safety. The aim of the Act is to ensure 'health, safety and welfare of people at work, and to protect people, other than those at work against risks to their health and safety arising out of work activities'. The employer is urged to promote safe workplaces, 'so far as is reasonably practicable'. Meanwhile, employees are expected to collaborate and comply with the employer's policies and safe systems of the work to support safety initiatives (HSWA 1974).

The employer has a legal duty of care not to place the employee under undue and unnecessary risk of injury. If the court of law proves that the employer failed in this duty, there are usually consequences. The legal case in Case study 11.2 illustrates this clearly:

Case study 11.2

Legal case 1 'Ignorance is no defence in handling practice'

In 1997, a student failed in a manual handling claim. While using a 'drag lift' with a healthcare assistant to transfer a patient from a chair to a commode, the patient's knees buckled. The assistant rushed to hold the commode in place and the student nurse bore the patient's full weight and injured her back. The student nurse admitted she knew the drag lift was not a safe procedure to move a patient up the bed, but was never made aware that it should not be used for assisting a patient to stand up.

Reading the above, think through why this situation might have arisen. Some pointers include:

▪ Was a risk assessment of the patient's capabilities and potential risks done? If so, was it read and understood, to help choose a safe procedure to transfer?
▪ Did the student apply biomechanical principles when moving the patient, as posture and base of support are poor during this procedure?
▪ Drag lifts have potential risk for injury to patients and nurses whatever the circumstances. Were you aware of this?

If the patient was the claimant, which safety and human rights issues could have been considered? Also, consider the following:

▪ Fear and psychological trauma of the procedure
▪ Safety and well-being endangered when buckling, with potential risk of a fall
▪ Being asked to stand when not capable of doing so, on the day.

The Lifting Operations and Lifting Equipment Regulation 1998 (LOLER) and Provision and Use of Work Equipment Regulation 1998 (PUWER)

These regulations promote safe use of equipment for moving and handling, in work environments. They highlight the prevention and reduction of risks to injury for nurses and patients while using handling equipment. Both regulations specify the duties of the employer to ascertain that all work equipment is maintained in good functioning condition for the intended purposes. Training programmes must be established for employees to be competent to use the equipment safely and successfully without injury to all involved. LOLER covers lifting and lowering equipment such as beds, hoists and slings (including attachments used for anchoring, fixing or supporting) used at work and private homes as part of work. PUWER complements LOLER by covering all other handling equipment used within working environments e.g. sliding sheets, Zimmer frames, transfer boards and others.

Case study 11.3

Legal case 2 'Failure of the employer to provide training to ensure staff competence in use of equipment'

In 2006, South Downs NHS Trust was prosecuted by HSE, after a 77-year-old man fell from a sling being used to move him from his wheelchair to his bed. They were prosecuted because of a series of management failures including failing to train some staff in safe moving and handling and not undertaking a risk assessment on the gentleman in question. The Trust pleaded guilty to a breach of key health and safety legislation. See: www.gov-news.org/gov/uk/news/south_downs_nhs_trust_fined_16325000_after/59853.html

Human Rights Act (HRA) 1998

This Act is one of several laws within health and social care which aims to reinforce the need for healthcare professionals to engage in humane, dignified, respectful and morally upright practices to protect vulnerable people. The HRA stipulates comprehensive rights for all people, acknowledging that in care settings, nurses and patients' human rights are equally susceptible to being breached. Handling activities also present potential risks for injury to both groups. The Act has 16 rights which have an impact on people's social and work life (e.g. case study 11.4), and are applicable to moving and handling, e.g. handling techniques should not humiliate or embarrass the patient; promotion of physical safety and movement.

Case study 11.4

Legal case 'Private life aspect'

In *R (A, B, & X, Y) v East Sussex County Council* (2003) the High Court in England considered the application of the 'private life' aspect of Article 8 to disabled people (in particular that element of the right to respect private life which encompasses a right to establish and develop relationships with other human beings and the outside world). The case raised issues relating to the Council's operation of a manual handling policy which prohibited manual lifting.

Nurses need to engage in a careful consideration of some of these rights before and during moving and handling interventions to avoid unintentional offence or being construed to practise in a professionally disrespectful and demeaning manner.

Acts and Regulations provide guidelines and state responsibilities, of workers and employers to ensure safety at work. Nurses are expected to comply with laws, the employers' systems of work for safety and policies. It is paramount that nurses know laws related to handling people and apply them to practice.

The future of the Human Rights Act within the UK is currently being debated at the time of publication.

Summary

Moving and handling are essential parts of patient care and require as much attention as any other aspect of nursing practice. Regulations bound in the law and policy aim to eliminate manual handling from all but exceptional or life-threatening situations of care. There is an increasing focus on employers investing in equipment to encourage minimal lifting by employees. This is most certainly the case in the health and social care sector within the UK. It is imperative for nurses to have a grounded knowledge of the law and employers' safe systems of work, to practise safely. Complacency can result in injuries that are entirely preventable. Nurses should apply the evidence-based knowledge, biomechanical principles and personal risk assessment to their daily practice. They should engage and encourage patients to participate in decisions that avoid manual lifting and use suitable equipment competently. Communication, with mutual respect, fosters a good working relationship between the nurse and their patient. It is the pivot of compassionate and dignified care and is particularly applicable to the moving and handling of patients.

References

Alexander, P. and Johnson, C. (2011) *Manual Handling of Children*. Professional Series, vol. 2. National Back Exchange UK.

Brooks, A. and Orchards, S. (2011) Core person handling skills. In J. Smith (ed.) *The Guide to Handling of People*, 6th edn. Middlesex: BackCare.

Dimond, B (2011) *Legal Aspects of Health and Safety*. London: Quay Books.

Disability Discrimination Act 2005 c13.

HASWA Health and Safety at Work Act 1974 c22.

Hignett, S., Wolf, L., Taylor, E. and Griffiths, P. (2015) Fire fighting to innovation: using human factors and ergonomics to tackle slip, trip, and fall risks in hospitals. *Human Factors: The Journal of the Human Factors and Ergonomics Society*, 57(7): 1195–1207.

HSE (Health and Safety Executive) (1998b) Lifting Operations and lifting Equipment Regulations (LOLER).

HSE (Health and Safety Executive) (2001) *Handling Home Care*. Norwich: HMSO.

HSE (Health and Safety Executive) (2004) *Manual Handling: Manual Handling Operations Regulations (1992) Guidance on Regulations*, 3rd edn, Sudbury: HSE Books.

HSE (Health and Safety Executive) (2010a) *Health and Safety Executive and Safety Statistics 2008/9*. Sudbury: HSE Books.

HSE (Health and Safety Executive) (2010b) Electric profiling beds in residential and nursing homes: manual handling and service user benefits. HSE UK.

HSE (Health and Safety Executive) (2011) Getting to grips with hoisting people. HSE health services information sheet no. 3.

Human Rights Act 1998. Available at: www.legislation.gov.uk/ukga/1998/42/contents

Management of Health and Safety at Work Regulations 1999 no. 342.

Mental Capacity Act 2005 c9.

NMC (Nursing and Midwifery Council) (2015) *The Code: Professional Standards of Practice and Behaviour for Nurses and Midwives.* London: NMC.

Polak, F. (2011) Mechanics and human movement, in J. Smith (ed.) *The Guide to Handling of People.* Middlesex: BackCare UK.

PUWER (Provision and Use of Work Equipment Regulations) 1998b (2306).

RIDDOR (Reporting of Injuries, Diseases and Dangerous Occurrences Regulations 2013.

Chapter 12

Wound management

Jane Preece

The overall aim of wound management is to promote wound healing. Wound management is a vast topic with an ever expanding and developing knowledge base. Good wound care and management are paramount for positive wound healing and patient experience. Despite the rise in technology, evidence and wound care products, wounds continue to be an area of care that nurses face regularly. Many wounds can be prevented with good quality nursing care but others are unavoidable. Inappropriate assessment and care and management can lead to delayed healing, infection, pain, overall reduced quality of life and distress for the affected patient and their family.

Key concepts

Wound healing	Principles of wound management
Wound assessment	Pressure ulcer prevention
Aseptic technique	Sutures or clips

Learning outcomes

By the end of this chapter you will be able to:

- Discuss the wound healing processes and factors which affect a patient's ability to heal
- Demonstrate how to undertake a wound assessment and develop a management plan
- Discuss the reason for choice of wound care products
- Take effective measures to prevent pressure ulcers and recognise the significance of international and national policies
- Demonstrate when and how to undertake an aseptic technique
- Demonstrate how to remove sutures and clips.

Introduction

Wounds can cause pain, distress, social isolation, increased dependency on healthcare resources and can lead to death. Treating wounds is costly and it is said that in the UK £2.3 to £3.1 billion per annum, 3 per cent of total expenditure on healthcare (Prosnett and Franks 2008), is spent on healing chronic wounds. It must be remembered that not all wounds will heal despite medical and nursing care, the aim in these instances will be to enable the individual to function as independently as possible, providing optimal treatments and management to enhance quality of life.

As well as aiding healing wounds, preventing tissue breakdown is an essential role of all healthcare providers. Pressure ulcers are seen as a cause of harm to patients and in 80–95 per cent of cases are said to be avoidable (www.nhs.stopthepressure 2013). Nurses need to understand how pressure ulcers develop in order to implement preventative plans. A wound may be described in many ways; by its cause, anatomical location, by whether it is acute or chronic, by the method of closure, by its presenting symptoms or indeed by the appearance of the predominant tissue types in the wound bed. All definitions serve a critical purpose in the assessment and appropriate management of the wound through to symptom resolution or, if at all possible, healing.

Wound healing

Wound healing is the collective term for the physiological process that repairs and restores damage to the skin. It is a complex process reliant on a number of inter-related factors. The same basic cellular and biochemical processes are involved in the healing process of all wounds independent of type.

Definition of a wound

A wound by definition is a breakdown in the protective function of the skin; the loss of continuity of epithelium, with or without loss of underlying connective tissue (i.e. muscle, bone, nerves). This may follow injury to the skin or underlying tissues caused by surgery, a cut, chemicals, heat/cold, friction shearing forces, pressure or as a result of disease, such as leg ulcers or tumours. Thus, overall any damage associated with a break in the skin can be called a wound.

Types of wounds

Acute   Burns, surgical or intentional, lacerations, traumatic
Chronic   Pressure ulcer, leg ulcer, diabetic foot ulcer, non-healing surgical wound.

You may have considered acute to be examples such as knife injury, surgical cuts or incisions, traumatic injuries and falls. Chronic wounds might include pressure ulcers or diabetic ulcers, these will be discussed later.

Activity 12.1

In your field you will see specific wounds, insert in the table the type of wound you might come across in practice.

Acute wounds	Chronic wounds

The wound healing process

The wound healing process is a series of events that start when injury occurs and end with complete closure and successful scar tissue. Wounds heal in three ways and this is dependent on their cause, location or amount of damage to the tissues:

- *Primary intention*: Clean surgical wound or laceration, the edges can be held together with sutures, glue, tape
- *Secondary intention*: Open wounds with significant tissue loss
- *Delayed primary closure*: Wounds left open, e.g. open abdominal wound and closed using sutures at a later date.

Do revisit the structure of skin and the underlying tissues to enhance your understanding of the skills in wound assessment and management. Brief processes will be outlined here only. The wound healing process has four stages:

1 Vascular/haemostasis
2 Inflammation
3 Proliferation
4 Maturation.

These processes do overlap and wounds can be at various and several stages at any one time.

Vascular/haemostasis

Any trauma to the skin that penetrates the dermis will cause bleeding. The first response of the body is to stop bleeding. Damaged blood vessels immediately vasoconstrict to reduce blood flow and release plasma protein, resulting in platelet aggregation and formation of a fibrin clot. As this dries, it becomes a scab.

Inflammation

This is a non-specific local reaction to tissue damage (Box 12.1).

Box 12.1 Signs and symptoms of inflammation (first stage in healing)

Redness	Vasodilation increases blood to the area
Heat	Metabolic reaction
Swelling	Vasodilation and leakage of fluid into the wound and surrounding tissue
Pain	

Inflammatory mediators such as prostaglandins and histamine are stimulated by the vascular response. Vasodilation and increased permeability occur as a result. There is an increase in exudate which contains plasma protein, antibodies, erythrocytes, leucocytes and platelets. This is sometimes referred to as 'inflammatory exudate' (Dealey, 2012).

Clinical significance

High levels of exudate at this stage require both energy and nutritional resources. In large wounds the requirement may be considerable (Dealey, 2012).

The two main inflammatory cells are neutrophils and macrophages. Neutrophils have a short life span and after three days without infection their numbers reduce rapidly. Macrophages arrive 2–3 days after injury followed by lymphocytes which also destroy bacteria by the process of phagocytosis. They are a rich source of biological regulators, including cytokines and growth factors which are essential for wound healing and are important elements to destroy bacteria.

Proliferation

The proliferation stage usually begins at 3 days and lasts for weeks. This phase is characterised by the development of granulation tissue. Proliferation of endothelial cells, fibroblasts, collagen synthesis and hyaluronic acid forms an extracellular matrix which is seen as granulation tissue. Macrophages produce fibroblast growth factors attracting them to the wound which stimulate them to divide, later producing collagen fibres. These growth factors start the angiogenesis process. Fibroblast activity is dependent on local oxygen supply, if tissue oxygen perfusion is poor, the wound will not heal. Healthy granulation tissue is 'pinky-red'. It is highly vascular and very vulnerable to damage.

Watch out

Granulation tissue that is dark or dusky is a signal that the wound is ischaemic or infected.

Undamaged capillaries grow towards the surface of the wound and form a network supplying oxygen and nutrients. As the wound fills with new tissue and the capillary network develops, macrophages and fibroblasts decrease. Wound contraction occurs following connective tissue production, fibroblasts congregate around the wound margin and the edges pull together. Do note this only occurs in wounds healing by secondary intention.

Epithelialisation is the final stage of proliferation and takes place when macrophages release epidermal growth factors. The epithelial cells migrate from the wound margin or hair follicle in the dermis and grow over the surface of the wound. When they meet, this process stops. New epithelial cells are translucent and whitish-pink in appearance. In sutured wounds, epithelial cells migrate along the suture line. These either gradually disappear or pull out with the suture.

Don't forget!

Epithelial cells only move over viable tissue and require a moist environment, so non-viable tissue, necrosis or slough need to be removed from the wound bed.

Maturation

This is the final stage of healing. At this stage the wound becomes less vascular as the need to bring new cells to the wound site decreases. The collagen fibres are re organised, lying at right angles to the wound margins. Scar tissue forms, initially it is raised and reddish in colour, as it gradually remodels and matures, the blood supply decreases and it becomes flatter, paler and tensile strength increases. This can take up to a year in closed wounds and longer in open wounds.

Factors which delay healing

Some wounds do not heal without complications or delay. There are many factors which can affect healing (Table 12.1). Holistic assessment it very important so factors which may affect healing can be identified.

General principles of wound management

There are several general principles to bear in mind for successful wound management (Table 12.2).

Patient assessment

The ability to undertake a comprehensive holistic assessment is the most important component of wound management and essential nursing skill. The key is to observe, document and report. Assessment includes these aspects:

Table 12.1 Factors which delay healing

Local factors at the wound site	Pathophysiological factors	Psychosocial/ lifestyle factors	Other therapies	Inappropriate wound management
Poor blood supply, local hypoxia	Infection Malnutrition Ageing	Smoking	Radiotherapy	Failure to assess the wound and address causal factors
Non-viable tissue Necrosis, slough	Cardiovascular disorders	Non-prescription drugs	Chemotherapy	Application of inappropriate topical products
Excessive exudate	Immune disorders	Who is the person caring for the wound?	Prolonged steroids	Poor wound care technique
Infection	Endocrine and metabolic disorders Diabetes mellitus	Stress		
Recurrent trauma		Immobility Poor sensation		

Table 12.2 General principles of wound management

General principle	Example/Consideration
Holistic patient assessment	General patient assessment Wound bed characteristics Psychological and social needs
Identifying and treating the cause	If the wound is a pressure ulcer – then remove the pressure Leg ulcer – establish the aetiology, venous, arterial, mixed. Requires specialist intervention and investigation Ankle Brachial Pressure Index (ABPI) Diabetic foot ulcer – Diabetes control, pressure relief, determining aetiology
Setting realistic objectives and aim of treatment	Be realistic what you can achieve in your care setting **Adult:** in secondary care: perhaps to debride the wound, treat infection and control pain. If in primary care areas, then perhaps reduce lower leg oedema **Children:** to enhance granulation tissue and healing, without pain.
Provide wound management	Wound cleansing method Appropriate wound care products including primary and secondary
Plan treatment and care with the patient	Does the wound need debridement? Will dressings be enough or do we need specialist referral e.g. tissue viability specialist, surgical intervention Leg ulcer – Is it arterial? Do we need referral to vascular specialist How often do we need to do the wound care? Who is going to undertake the wound management? How is the wound affecting the patient and their family?

1   General holistic assessment of the patient to determine factors which can delay or impede wound healing:
   a   Patient's history, such as medical status and history, considering the presenting symptoms, the results of any investigations, as well as the indicators for the success or failure of treatment
   b   Psychological well-being to elicit patients' perceptions of their condition or wound and to involve them in their care
   c   Social environment to give clues as to lifestyle, income and support to aid healing
   d   Lifestyle and behaviours such as smoking, drinking or drug use (not only prescription medications or not) which may impact on healing or self-care
   e   Physical state, i.e. nutrition (over- or under-weight), pain, mobility, hygiene.
2   Wound assessment including:
   a   Wound history
   b   Type of wound, wound classification
   c   Wound bed appearance and characteristics.

Clinical significance

Patients vary, so age and general well-being will all influence wounds, either development or the healing process! You may want to watch this online video to help with understanding this: www.youtube.com/watch?v=zZpMQ_7qiRg

Wound assessment

It is important to determine how long the wound has been present, and any factors that may have contributed to the wound's development, e.g. surgery, trauma, poor mobility, inadequate pressure care, infection or general poor health. Inadequate wound assessment can lead to incorrect, inadequate or inappropriate treatment, with potentially serious consequences. Local assessment of the wound provides information relevant to three areas: (1) type of wound (classification); (2) location and wound bed characteristics; and (3) healing stage or increase or decrease in wound size.

Wounds and injecting drug users

Wounds assessment and management can be challenging in long-term drug users, particularly those who inject regularly. Long-term injecting of drugs can lead to vascular damage as a result of sclerosis and thrombosis of superficial veins and formation of hard lumps known as granulomas or sterile abscesses. Injecting drug users are at risk of chronic venous hypertension, leg ulceration and lower limb cellulitis (Powell, 2011). Individuals might inject drugs into the femoral veins in the groin and the veins in the legs because the upper body veins have collapsed. Nerve and muscle damage may also occur, which can lead to pain and may adversely affect mobility, consequently worsening chronic venous hypertension and ulcers. Patients in this category often do not comply with treatment for a number of reasons and need careful assessment and communication. Treatment may be complicated in this patient group, because individuals may be homeless and medical records may be incomplete, with patients being removed from GP lists if they do not attend appointments. It is important to establish a trusting nurse–patient relationship to promote patient adherence to treatment and consider:

- The degree to which the patient wishes to be involved in their care, including the adoption of a realistic self-care regimen
- Wellness, nutrition and general health
- The correct choice and application of dressing or therapy
- Avoid blaming the patient for any lack of progress in wound healing
- Provide verbal and written information for patients.

Wound classification

- *Chronic wound* – is defined as a wound which fails to progress to heal in a timely and orderly fashion (Baronski and Ayello, 2012). This is frequently referred to a wound that has failed to heal or shown signs of healing after six weeks, e.g. pressure ulcer, leg ulcers
- *Acute wounds* – these may be due to traumatic injuries, e.g. lacerations, burns, cuts, abrasion. These wounds normally respond rapidly to treatment
- *Post-operative wounds* – these wounds heal by primary intention, whereby the wound edges are pulled together and secured using suture or glue. Donor or graft sites are also an intentional wound.

Location of the wound

The location of the wound should be documented using the correct terminology, e.g. right greater trochanter not right hip. The use of a body map to document the location is useful. The location can be an indicator of potential problems which could affect wound healing and consideration in planning care, such as contamination in wounds at the sacral area, or mobility problems if the wound is on the foot.

Wound bed characteristics

There are five main wound bed tissue types. The type of tissue present is an indication of the stage of healing or any complications present. These may include necrotic, sloughy, granulation, epithelial and hypergranulation tissue. A wound may have a variety of these tissues present at any one time. Understanding tissue type is important in documentation and the development of a management plan.

- *Necrotic*: Appearance – black, brown or grey. The area of tissue becomes ischaemic and dies as it is devitalised, avascular tissue. As it becomes dry, it may present as thick leathery hard eschar (scab). Necrotic tissue hides the extent of tissue damage and the size of the wound is not apparent on assessment. This has implications for practice as to perform an accurate assessment and to promote healing, devitalised tissue may need to be removed

Watch out

Necrotic tissue is an ideal medium for bacteria proliferation leading to infection and will inhibit healing.

■ *Sloughy wounds*: This is a particular description of a specific appearance – yellow, white stringy devitalised tissue. It may be dry or slimy in nature and is attached to the wound base and may appear in patches. Slough is dead cells which have accumulated in exudate

■ *Granulation*: The formation of new tissue which takes place during the proliferation stage of healing. The appearance is red and granular. Granulation tissue forms at the base of the wound and consists of new capillary loops and cells. The capillary loops cause the wound to look granular and red in appearance. Granulation tissue can easily be damaged as the capillary loops are very thin, this can lead to bleeding if inappropriate wound cleansing or wound products are used

■ *Epithelialisation*: This occurs at the final stage of proliferation. The appearance is pinky-white. Epithelial cells migrate across the surface of the wound. In large shallow wounds, islets of epithelialisation may be seen. It eventually covers the granulation tissue and is the final visual sign of healing.

Documentation of wound appearance

When documenting wound appearance, you need to write what you see. Wounds may contain more then one tissue type, which can be recorded as percentages, e.g. 75% necrosis (black), 15% slough (yellow), 10% granulation (red).

Activity 12.2

Think of practice settings where you have had your placements, reflect on the tissue types that you have seen.

Infected wounds

All wounds are colonised with bacteria as the skin contains natural flora and organisms. This does not mean the wound is infected. If a wound is infected, then there should be clinical signs of infection.

The amount of bacteria on a wound bed can be defined as:

Contaminated   Presence of bacteria with no multiplication
Colonisation   Multiplication of bacteria with no host reaction
Infection   Multiplication of bacteria in the tissue with an associated host reaction.

Clinical signs and symptoms of infection

Surgical and acute wounds:

- Heat
- Redness
- Swelling
- Pus or purulent discharge
- Pain
- Pyrexia.

Chronic wounds:

- Heat
- Redness
- Swelling
- Increased exudate
- Increased or change in pain
- Odour
- Change in appearance of the wound bed
- Pyrexia.

Critical colonisation

Critical colonisation is described as the multiplication of organisations without invasion but interfering with wound healing. This is commonly associated with chronic wounds healing by secondary intention.

Signs of critical colonisation include:

- The wound fails to heal or progress even with appropriate treatment
- Increased serous or purulent exudate
- Malodour
- Increased pain
- Dusky red granulation tissue
- Granulation tissue may bleed easily.

Clinical significance

Wound infection is not diagnosed by a wound swab, a wound swab informs the practitioner of the types of bacteria present in the wound. Diagnosis should not be made on wound swab microbiology alone, but in combination with clinical signs and symptoms.

Procedure for taking a wound swab

This is a frequently practised task and needs to be done correctly to obtain the right answer to the question of types of bacteria present.

1   Prepare the required equipment (swabs, dressing packs (if needed), gloves, apron etc.).
2   Inform the patient of the need for a swab and obtain their consent.
3   Maintain hand hygiene.
4   Always clean the wound first, to remove excess exudate.
5   Using the correct sterile microbiology swab, holding it with thumb and finger, rotate the swab in a zig-zag direction across the wound bed.
6   Insert into the medium.
7   Label correctly with all patients' details and wound location, send to the laboratory.
8   Document in the patients' nursing notes.
9   Remember to tell doctor or nurse in charge immediately so the result can be acted on as appropriate.

Case study 12.1

'Ace' is a 43-year-old man with a five-month history of forearm ulcers resulting from heroin injection, who came along to a drop-in clinic for drug users. He has been an intravenous drug user for 20 years and has been on a methadone maintenance programme. 'Ace' admitted to ('skin popping'), injecting into the skin so the drug is absorbed subcutaneously and he had a subsequent abscess formation, infection and scarring.

1   What will you assess?
2   What particular problems are there for 'Ace'?
3   'Ace's' care plan included coming to clinic every two weeks for dressings and assessment and in between to do the dressing himself at home. How could you encourage 'Ace' to comply with this and aid wound healing?

Wound photography

Wound photography is used in some clinical situations to record wounds and is a useful aid to wound assessment (Box 12.2). It provides a visual record of the wound appearance and surrounding skin. Placing a ruler at the wound edge enables the size of the wound to be visualised. Sequential photographs should be taken from the same aspect as the original, which will allow for more meaningful comparisons.

Wound size and measurement

There are many ways to measure a wound, however, some are not appropriate in the clinical setting. The simplest and cheapest method is to calculate the wound surface area by measuring linear dimensions with a tape measure and not other objects such as coins (Fette, 2006). The purpose of wound measurement is to monitor wound progression and healing. In the early stages when necrosis or slough is present in the wound, the wound

Box 12.2 Taking a wound photograph: dos and don'ts

Do

1 Get patient consent, written consent is always required for photographs being used for teaching or research. Refer to local organisation policy on consent for photos, as some organisations accept verbal consent only.
2 Always position patient in the same way.
3 Label the photo with patient's medical record number, date of birth, initials.
4 Consider patient confidentiality.
5 Store the photo on a secure site.
6 Medical photography departments will provide the best quality photographs.

Don't

1 Use personal smartphones or iPhone or iPad.
2 Share with others who are not involved in the patient care.

may increase in size as the devitalised tissue is debrided. The full extent of tissue damage is identified.

All wounds require a two-dimensional assessment of the wound opening and a three-dimensional assessment of any cavity or tracking:

■ Two-dimensional measures – use a paper tape to measure the length and width in millimetres. The circumference of the wound is traced if the wound edges are not even – often required for chronic wounds. (You may also consider photography)
■ Three-dimensional measures – the wound depth is measured using a dampened cotton tip applicator.

Don't forget!

Wounds may appear angry and increasing but this does not mean the wound is deteriorating – keep assessing.

Linear measurement

■ Measure greatest length – head to toe
■ Greatest width – side to side
■ Depth if appropriate.

Use a cotton tip applicator or probe, e.g. microbiology swab. Place the probe into the deepest point, keep probe vertical to the wound bed. Hold the probe with thumb and finger at the point the probe exits the wound. Remove it and measure against a ruler.

Using the 'Clock system' with 12 o'clock being the head and 6 o'clock being the feet is helpful when documenting and measuring undermining, sinus tract and tunnelling (Figure 12.1). Undermining, sinus tract or tunnelling can complicate healing.

■ Sinus tract/tunnelling – this is a channel that extends from any part of the wound and passes through subcutaneous tissue and muscle. There is a dead space which can lead to abscess formation.
■ Undermining – this is tissue destruction which occurs around the perimeter of the wound, underlying intact skin.

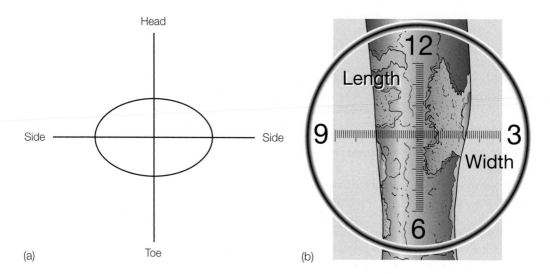

Figure 12.1 **Measuring wounds using the 'Clock Method'**

How to measure

■ Tunnelling/sinus tract – as for measuring depth, use a cotton probe, insert into the tunnel and grasp at the wound edge and measure (Morgan, 2014)
■ Undermining – using the cotton probe, insert into the undermining area, progressing in a clockwise direction document and measure the deepest point working along the wound perimeter (ibid.)
■ Periwound measurement – document the amount of erythema or cellulitis around the wound, working from the wound margin
■ Wound tracing – using a grid film or sterile transparent film, place directly onto the wound and trace around the wound margin. Repeat at frequent intervals and compare the shape and size of the wound. Wound tracing does not provide information on the depth of the wound.

Frequency of measurement

This depends on the wound type and local organisational policy and guidance. Acute wounds should be measured at each dressing change/assessment as it is expected for the size and shape of the wound to change more rapidly than chronic wounds. Chronic wounds should be measured at 2–4 week intervals as changes are unlikely to be seen if more frequent.

> **Don't forget!**
>
> Wounds should be measured using cm and mm, not objects such as coins.

Exudate

Exudate is accumulated fluids which contain serum, cellular debris, bacteria and leukocytes. Assessment of level and type of wound exudate is important as it is an indicator of wound progression and in wound dressing selection. In a normal healing wound there is a large amount of exudate during the inflammatory stage and very little at epithelialisation. Copious amount of exudate may indicate wound inflammation or infection (WUWHS, 2007). Exudate assessment should include amount, type, consistency and colour.

Odour

A wound may have an odour and this could be due to a variety of reasons. Odour from a wound may be non-existent, non-offensive, present or offensive. Odour from a wound can have a huge psychological effect on a patient and their quality of life. If devitalised tissue is involved, wound debridement and removal of excess exudate and toxic material (pus, dead cells and bacteria) may be needed. However, this may not always be possible in patients with fungating lesions. Odour can be controlled by a variety of dressings, e.g. carbon-impregnated dressings. Prior to assessing for malodour, always cleanse the wound, e.g. a leg ulcer which has been bandaged for a week can have an odour. Once cleansed, this may go away.

However, some micro-organisms such as Pseudomonas aeruginosa will cause an odour which would indicate wound infection. Necrosis and gangrene can also smell so odour is an important indicator that something is not right.

Pain

Pain is common in patients with chronic wounds, generally associated with wound dressing procedures. Pain assessment should be undertaken as part of assessment, focusing on type, severity, location, constant, temporary or intermittent pain. Pain at the wound is frequently underestimated and thought given to providing pain relief prior to procedures may be needed (Chapter 5).

Peri wound

Skin changes at the perimeter or 'peri' wound area, the area around the wound, will occur. There may be warmth, erythema, which could indicate inflammation, or infection. Blistering or pustules where the dressing has been may indicate an allergic reaction to the dressing. Maceration which would indicate increased exudate requires a review of the dressing regime or product and may be an indication of colonisation or infection. Induration (hard to the touch), fluctuance (bubbly) could indicate abnormal fluid accumulation and that probable further tissue damage is occurring. The edge of a wound can be advancing (getting smaller) or non-advancing and/or getting bigger. There may be undermining at the edge of the wound with cavities, tracts or sinus present. The edges of the wound can be cliff-edged, sloping, rolled, regular, irregular, elevated, with changing shapes as the wound moves through the healing process. It is important to monitor and record the wound edges as they can be an indicator of healing or non-healing.

The acronym T.I.M.E has been used to trigger assessment steps:

T – Tissue
I – Infection
M – Margins
E – Edges of wound.

Wound cleansing

The primary objective of wound cleansing is to remove debris from the wound, to allow for accurate assessment before application of a wound dressing, and to maintain an optimum environment for wound healing. Wound exudate contains anti-microbial substances that clean the wound bed, routine cleaning of granulating wounds should be avoided.

Rationale for wound cleansing

- Removal of debris, such as foreign bodies, dressing residue and devitalised tissue
- To keep the surrounding skin clean and free from excessive moisture and exudate
- To facilitate wound assessment
- To minimise wound trauma when removing adherent dressings
- To promote patient comfort and psychological well-being.

Methods of wound cleansing

- Wound irrigation – this can be performed using a variety of methods including 30 ml syringe, spray cleansers.
- Shower – as well as cleansing the wound, this can be of psychological benefit to the patient. Wounds to the sacral, perineal, pilonidal sinus or rectal abscess would benefit from showering. Always clean the shower before and after use in accordance with local infection control policies.
- Limb immersion – this is an ideal method for those with chronic leg ulcers. It allows

for excess scale and exudate to be removed. Immerse both legs in a clean bucket (for this one patient only) of warm tap water, for a maximum of 10 minutes. The use of bath emollients can be beneficial.

Don't forget!

When using a syringe or spray cleansers, caution is required to prevent splash back and needlestick injury.

Watch out

Do not immerse patients with dry necrotic diabetic foot ulceration or gangrene. The sensation is impaired and this can lead to further damage.

Use a method appropriate to the care environment, location and type of wound, e.g. when caring for someone with a chronic leg ulcer limb, immersion would be a method of choice and an aseptic technique is not required.

Cleansing agents

- Tap water is an acceptable wound cleansing agent. It should be warm to minimise wound cooling. There is no evidence that there is an increased risk of infection with using tap water. Always consult your infection prevention team and local policies. Some microbiologists recommend that the tap is run for a few minutes
- Normal saline (0.9% sodium chloride) is often the cleansing agent of choice for wounds and it should be used at room temperature. Sterile normal saline is available in sachets, pods, canisters and 0.5 litre and 1 litre bags for larger wounds
- Antiseptic solutions such as hypochlorites, chlorhexidine and betadine iodine should not be used for routine wound cleansing because they cause pain and reduce the proliferation of macrophages and lymphocytes which are essential to the wound healing process
- Prontosan solution is a wound irrigation containing Betaine which penetrates, disturbs and removes biofilm, the bacteria that adhere to surfaces in some forms of watery environment and begin to excrete a slimy, glue-like substance. The irrigation thus helps control bacterial levels on the wound (Cowan, 2014), and it is becoming an increasingly popular wound cleansing agent. It has been shown to be an effective wound cleanser for both chronic and acute wounds.

Aseptic technique

There is a high risk of cross-infection while carrying out invasive procedures, wound management and caring for intravenous devices. It is with this in mind that a clean or sterile process is required. The term 'aseptic' refers to free from living pathogenic organisms or sterile. Thus, the technique involves tasks which avoid moving or contaminating with bacteria or micro-organisms and is also known aby the term aseptic non-touch technique (ANTT). Central to this is hand hygeine.

Procedure for performing an aseptic technique (ANTT) for wound management

The need to carry out wound management using an aseptic technique will be determined by the wound type and generally it is used when caring for acute and surgical wounds the rationale is to reduce the risk of surgical site infections. ANTT is a process where 'key parts' e.g. sterile gloves or dressings remain sterile and do not touch the wound so as to maintain sterility and avoid any contamination or transfer. The key is to identify and protect 'key parts' and keep them sterile.

Equipment needed at the bedside

- Sterile procedure pack which contains gloves
- Cleansing agent
- Sterile scissors
- Wound dressing product
- Non-sterile gloves and apron
- Tapes
- Bandages
- Alcohol hand gel
- Syringe.

1 Explain the procedure to patient, gain their consent and cooperation. Remember to assess their pain and give analgesia prior to the dressing if needed.
2 Position the patient comfortably.
3 Wash hands with warm water and soap.
4 Clean the trolley, tray or flat surface, see Chapter 15 on infection control.
5 Gather all the equipment together before commencement of the procedure and place on the bottom of the trolley or near to hand on a cleaned surface.
6 Take to the patient's bedside, maintaining privacy and dignity.
7 Wash hands with soap and water and dry thoroughly.
8 Put on apron and non-sterile gloves, loosen old dressing, remove bandages if applicable.
9 Remove non-sterile gloves and wash hands with soap and water.
10 The outer pack should be peeled open and the wrapped contents dropped onto the trolley top/tray/surface.
11 Decontaminate hands using alcohol rub.
12 The sterile pack should be opened by holding only the corners of the pack.
13 Place your hand inside the yellow/white clinical waste bag and arrange the sterile field.
14 Remove the old dressing with the yellow/white clinical waste bag, turning it inside out and place lower than the sterile field secure to the work surface.

15 Decontaminate hands with alcohol rub.
16 Open all remaining packs and place onto the sterile field. Open the saline solution and pour into sterile receiver (gallipot).
17 Decontaminate hands with alcohol rub.
18 Put on the sterile gloves without touching the sterile field (key part).
19 Arrange the remainder of the equipment protecting the 'key parts' maintain sterility.
20 Clean the wound if necessary by irrigating with normal saline, ensure neither syringe nor gauze touches the wound (these are clean parts).
21 Clean the surrounding skin only with gauze. Using each gauze once only.
22 Redress the wound with the appropriate wound product.
23 Decontaminate hands. Make the patient comfortable.
24 Make patient comfortable.
25 Clean trolley, tray, work surface and dispose of waste.
26 Wash hands with soap and water.
27 Complete all relevant documentation.

Choosing a wound dressing

There are many dressings available on the market today, many of which have different properties and modes of action. The most frequently used dressing types will be discussed as it is not possible to discuss all ranges within the chapter. More information can be found in texts such as the *Wound Care Handbook* by Cowan (2014).

The practitioner's decision on product will be determined following a comprehensive assessment, taking into account the type of wound, wound bed characteristics, exudate level, objective of treatment, patient group and patient choice.

Before using any wound care product for the first time, always read the manufacturer's information for contraindications, precautions and warnings. There will be instructions on when and how to use the product.

Don't forget!

Always remember to check the expiry date – DRESSINGS DO EXPIRE!
Most organisations have locally developed wound management formularies or lists of dressings to be used.

Dressing types and classification

Most dressings have been classified according to their properties and mode of action and the rationale for choice depends on the type of wound and mode of healing. For generic wound care groups the following are useful for consideration:

- *Alginates* are made from alginic acid, which is found in certain species of brown seaweed and are designed to absorb wound exudate, form a gel and maintain moisture at the wound surface. Alginate dressings can absorb 15–20 times their weight in fluid so are indicated for wounds with high levels of exudate. Alginates should not be used on wounds with little or no exudate or those with hard necrotic tissue. Alginates are manufactured in the form of flat sheets, ropes and ribbons

  ■ Indication for use: Moderate to highly exudating wound.

■ *Foams* are available as either polyurethane or silicone and used to absorb exudate. Foams have often been perceived as highly absorbent, however, in clinical practice this is not always the case. They are therefore more suited to low to moderate levels of exudate. They are available with and without adhesive borders and can be used as primary or secondary dressings

  ■ Indication for use: Low to moderate exudate, granulation and epithelialized wounds. Should not be used on dry wounds with a scab (eschar).

■ *Hydrocolloids* are occlusive (closed) dressings primarily composed of carboxy-methyl cellulose. On contact with wound exudate, the hydrocolloid matrix swells and liquefies to form a moist gel, which softens devitalised and sloughy tissue, maintains moisture and promotes granulation. It is generally not suitable for heavily exuding wounds. Usually worn up to 3–5 days (Cowan, 2014)

  ■ Indication for use: Superficial sloughy, necrotic wounds with low to moderate exudate.

■ *Hydrogels* are mostly made up of carboxymethylcellulose or starch polymer and up to 96 per cent water (Cowan, 2014). They are available in the form of sheets or unshaped gels and are used to promote debridement by re-hydrating dry, necrotic or sloughy tissue. The term 'debridement' refers to the removal of dead, devitalised, or contaminated tissue, and any foreign material from a wound

  ■ Indications for use: Dry wounds, assist with debridement of devitalised tissue. Should not be used on moderate to highly exudating wounds as increased moisture may contribute to maceration of the surrounding skin.

■ *Odour-absorbent and deodorising dressings* are low adherent dressings that have been impregnated with activated charcoal or silver. It should be remembered that while these products may reduce the odour, they will not remove devitalised tissue, which can harbour bacteria causing the odour

■ *Anti-microbial dressings* such as honey, Iodine, silver and PHMB (polyhexamth-ylene biguanide) are designed to kill or prevent the formation of wound bacteria. Anti-microbial dressings are to be used as a primary dressing, however, some may require being cut to fit the size of the wound.

If the infection is not contained within the wound bed, then the use of anti-microbial dressings does NOT replace the need for antibiotics.

Table 12.3 gives some examples of generic wound product choice in certain situations.

Wound drains

A wound drain is used to prevent accumulation of fluid in a wound bed, which may delay healing and predispose the wound to infection. Indications for use include:

■ To redirect body fluids to allow time for a new suture line to heal
■ To drain collections of pus from the body cavities

Table 12.3 Decisions for certain wound care products

Removing dead tissue – necrosis or slough	If the necrosis is dry and hard, then rehydration is required Other forms of debridement may be required, e.g. larvae therapy, sharp debridement
Infection	Use of topical antimicrobials as an adjunct to systemic antibiotics
Exudate management	Assess underlying pathology such has congestive cardiac failure. Infection Use an alginate as primary dressing and superabsorbent dressing. Protect the surrounding skin
Malodour	Identify the cause and treat it Odour controlling dressing will only control but will not get rid of it
Warm, moist environment for healing – protection of new granulation and epithelised tissue.	Depending on the amount of exudate, depth of the wound, then a foam or hydrocolloid may be considered.

- To drain collections of fluid post-operatively
- When haemostasis has not been achieved during surgery.

The most common types of surgical wound drains include:

- *Suction drainage*: An active (vacuum) drain works by gentle suction, e.g. redivac (Figure 12.2). The colour and amount of the fluid can be seen, which is important for the surgeon. As the area heals, the amount of drainage collected lessens until it is low enough for the drain to be removed
- *Passive drainage*: This relies on gravity to take fluid away without additional suction (Figure 12.3). Once the drain output is less than 30 mls in 24 hours and the surgical team is happy, the drain is removed. As the area heals, the amount of drainage collected lessens until it is low enough for the drain to be removed.

Prior to any of the following procedures it is important to consider analgesia. This will minimise pain, distress and trauma. Drains when in position should be emptied frequently to reduce the strain on the suture line and ensure maximum suction. The following principles apply:

- Tubing should also be kept free of kinks and twists
- Redivac bottles are not emptied but replaced when full
- All nursing procedures must be documented, including analgesia administered, the length of drain in situ (if shortened) and the number of the drain removed (if more than one)

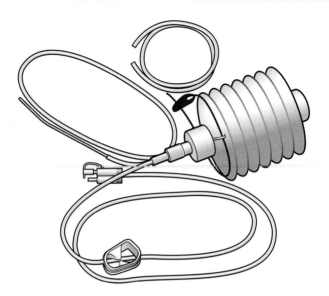

Figure 12.2 An active vacuum drain

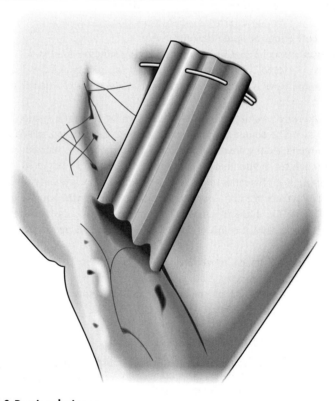

Figure 12.3 Passive drainage

■ Contents of the drain must be documented on the fluid balance chart.

Procedure for dressing a drain site

This is done using ANTT.

Equipment needed at the bedside

■ Trolley or tray
■ Sterile dressing pack,
■ Non-sterile gloves
■ Sterile gloves and apron
■ Cleansing solution (sterile sodium chloride 0.9%)
■ Alcohol swab
■ Sterile dry dressing of choice
■ Hypo-allergenic tape
■ Pair of sterile scissors.

1   Explain to the patient what you are about to do and, where possible, gain their consent.
2   Ensure privacy for the procedure.
3   Apply the non-sterile gloves and remove the dressing.
4   Dispose of gloves and dressing as appropriate.
5   Clean hands. Apply a pair of sterile gloves.
6   Follow steps 10 to 19 of ANTT. Apply a sterile protective field under drainage site.
7   If exudate is present, clean around the wound site using saline and gauze swabs. Check for any wound drainage perforations (if appropriate). Also ensure tubing is not bent or kinked.
8   Check that the skin suture (if used) is intact.
9   If the skin around the drain site is becoming sore or broken, protect with an adhesive dressing/no-sting barrier film.
10 Cover the drain site with a sterile dressing. This may be a prepared to look like a 'keyhole' by using sterile scissors. Secure this with tape.
11 If the drain is a vacuum one – ensure the vacuum is present.
12 Make the patient comfortable.
13 Clean the trolley, tray, work surfaces and dispose of waste appropriately.
14 Wash hands.
15 Complete all the relevant documentation.

Top tip

Wound/drain site swabs should only be taken if infection is suspected. Signs of infection include pain, inflammation at wound margins, oedema, pyrexia and purulent exudates. Any wounds that show signs of infection should be reported to the medical staff.

Procedure for changing a vacuum pump drain

This is a clean procedure. Ensure you explain the process clearly to the patient to gain their cooperation and consent. Collect all the necessary equipment, this will include: a new drainage system (previously 'vacuum' ready), non-sterile gloves, artery forceps/clamp. This is generally done by registered nurses but students will observe and assist.

1   Explain the procedure and where possible gain patient's consent.
2   Ensure privacy.
3   Put on gloves.
4   Clamp the tubing of the existing drainage bottle above and below the point of disconnection. Remove drainage bottle. Ensure protection of 'key parts'.
5   Attach new, already vacuumed drainage bottle to the drainage tubing.
6   Release clamps or artery forceps and the clamp on the bottle.
7   Ensure new drainage bottle remains vacuumed.
8   If vacuum is being lost, remove the dressing around drain entry site and examine. If this does not appear to improve, notify the medical staff *immediately*. Monitor the patient for signs of distress, alterations at the wound site, vital signs and report these.
9   Measure and record the contents of the old drainage bottle by either:
    - Redivac-type (disposable) – use the markings on the bottle. Dispose of bottle and contents
    - Pump-type (disposable) – empty contents into measuring jug and then dispose of into the sluice.
10 Dispose of the bottle and the contents appropriately (nurses may need to previously consult the local clinical waste disposal policy).
11 Ensure the patient is comfortable.
12 Wash hands.
13 Complete all the relevant documentation.

Procedure for the removal of a drain

A drain should only be removed following either specific instructions from medical staff or according to local protocol, i.e. if exudate or secretion drainage falls below a specific amount. Medical notes should be checked prior to any procedure to ensure the correct procedure, i.e. that the correct drain is removed. This is not something students may have the opportunity to do but they may observe or assist.

Equipment needed at the bedside

- Non-sterile gloves and sterile gloves
- Sterile dressing pack
- Cleansing solution (e.g. sterile sodium chloride 0.9%)
- Alcohol swab
- Sterile stitch cutter
- Sterile dry dressing

▨   Hypo-allergenic tape
▨   Sterile scissors
▨   Sterile universal specimen container (if tubing tip is required for culture)
▨   Sharps box
▨   Measuring jug (if required).

1   Check the medical notes to do a final check to ensure removal of the drain is
    required; if there is more than one drain, then the correct one is identified and
    documented.
2   Explain the procedure to the patient and gain consent.
3   Offer analgesia if necessary prior to procedure and wait the appropriate amount of
    time for this to work.
4   Ensure privacy.
5   Clean hands and apply the disposable gloves and remove the dressing.
6   Dispose of the gloves and dressing, as appropriate.
7   If this is a vacuum drain, clamp the tube to discontinue suction and stop drainage.
8   Clean hands and apply a second pair of gloves. Place a sterile protective field under
    drainage site. Using the principles and equipment for ANTT, continue with the
    following.
9   If exudate is present, clean the wound using saline and gauze.
10 If the drain is sutured in place, remove the suture (see below).
11 Holding the tubing with gloves or gauze gently, but firmly, withdraw the drain
    while applying gentle counter-pressure around the drain site, using a gauze
    square. Protect the 'key parts'.
12 If the tip of the tubing is requested for microscopy or culture, then cut off the tip
    (approximately 2 cm) using the sterile scissors and place into a pre-labelled sterile
    specimen container.
13 If exudate is present then irrigate the wound using saline.
14 Cover the drain site with a sterile dressing and secure with tape.
15 Measure the contents and dispose of the drainage bottle as outlined within the local
    policy.
16 Ensure the patient is comfortable.
17 Wash hands.
18 Complete all the relevant documentation and, if requested, send the specimen to the
    laboratory.

Removal of clips or sutures

The time to remove clips, staples and sutures will depend on location and type of
the wound and type of surgery and instruction from the patient's medical or surgical
consultant. As patients' stay in hospital is reduced, this will often take place within a
community setting.

   Since removing sutures leaves a breach in the skin or integument, this is the rationale
for employing a sterile approach (aseptic non-touch technique).

Procedure for removal of sutures

1   Prepare the necessary equipment and take this to the patient's location: suture removal pack, non-sterile gloves and apron, sharps box. Use principles of ANTT.
2   Explain procedure to patient, where possible, gain their consent and cooperation.
3   Hold the knot of the suture with forceps, gently lift upwards and out to ensure it is clear of skin.
4   Cut one side of the suture with the stitch cutter or scissors as close to the skin as possible.
5   Gently but firmly pull the suture out from the opposite side – DO NOT cut both sides of the knot – this will leave the suture under the skin which is potentially dangerous! Afterwards, ensure the patient is comfortable.

Procedure for removal of clips

1   Prepare the necessary equipment as above.
2   Explain procedure to patient, where possible gain their consent and co-operation.
3   Gently place the lower two prongs of clip remover under the staple or clip (Figure 12.4).
4   Squeeze the handles to lift the edges of the clip.
5   Lift one side, then the other and ease out of the skin. Afterwards, ensure patient is comfortable.

Top tip

Do search the internet, there are useful videos especially YouTube to help with these skills!

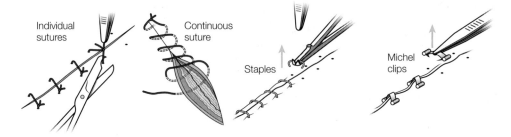

Figure 12.4 Removal of sutures and clips

Pressure ulcers

A pressure ulcer is a localised injury to the skin and/or underlying tissue usually over a bony prominence as a result of pressure or pressure in combination with shearing.

(NPUAP/EPUAP, 2014). Pressure ulcers are also known as bed sores, pressure sores, or decubitus ulcers.

Pressure ulcers are preventable in 80–95% of cases (nhs.Stopthepressure 2013). It is said that 700,000 people are affected by pressure ulcers every year (ibid.). With each pressure ulcer putting an additional cost of £4,000.00 per occurrence (ibid.). This has a huge impact on healthcare providers and causes harm to patients.

There is a great interest in pressure ulcer prevention with local commissioners setting targets to reduce the prevalence of pressure ulcers across communities, hospitals and wider populations. This forms part of the NHS commissioning for quality and innovative (CQUIN) payment framework 2008. Pressure ulcer prevention is a key skill for all healthcare practitioners, however, it is an important skill for all nurses.

Causes of pressure ulcers

Pressure ulcers occur predominately over bony prominence and are caused by a combination of intrinsic and extrinsic factors (Figure 12.5). In adults, the highest incidence is the sacrum and the heels. In infants and children, the occipital and the ears (Jones *et al.*, 2001).

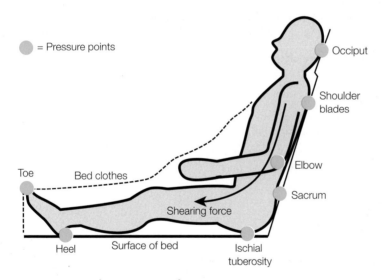

Figure 12.5 **Locations where pressure ulcers can occur**

Extrinsic factors

▪ Pressure – localised direct pressure causes distortion of the skin and underlying tissues when the soft tissue is compressed between the bone and hard surface, e.g. bed, chair. The blood cannot circulate, causing a lack of oxygen, and localised ischemia. Death of the cells occurs. This prolonged pressure causes distortion and destruction of the tissue closest to the bone. It is referred to as a cone shape ulcer with the widest part near the bone (Figure 12.6)

■ Shear – disturbs local blood supply by gliding of internal tissues, causing blood vessels to kink and stretch. This occurs if the patient slides down the bed or chair and if incorrect moving and handling techniques are used, e.g. if slide sheets are not used to move a patient in the bed.

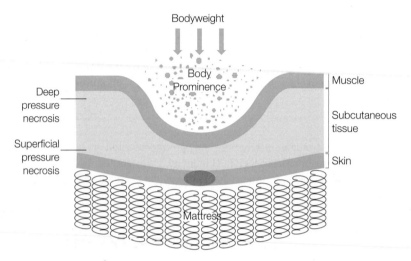

Figure 12.6 **Pressure ulcer creation**

Watch out

Friction itself does not cause pressure ulcers but it contributes to shear forces which can be exacerbated by moisture (Dealey, 2012).

Intrinsic factors

■ Reduced mobility is consistently shown to be independently predictive of pressure ulcer development (NPUAP/EPUAP, 2014). May be due to age, medications such as hypnotics, antidepressants, opioid analgesia, major surgery, considering length of time on the table, anaesthetic, pain and restricted movement due to drains
■ Reduced nutrition impairs elasticity of the skin. Can lead to anaemia and reduced tissue oxygenation
■ Age, as people get older, the skin becomes thinner and has decreased elasticity due to reduced collagen
■ General health, the acutely ill are particularly vulnerable. Some medical conditions associated with pressure ulcer are stroke, diabetes mellitus, lung disease, heart failure, hip fracture, limb paralysis, peripheral vascular disease, and rheumatoid arthritis

■ Neurological conditions where there is sensory deficit. The patient is unaware of the pressure

■ Skin moisture caused by incontinence, sweat, wound exudate. Moisture will increase friction and shear forces.

Pressure ulcer prevention

The key to prevention is identifying those patients at risk and then implementing an individualised preventative plan. Five key practical steps in pressure ulcer prevention will be discussed using the SSKIN developed by NHS Midland and East, now adopted by NHS England: (1) skin assessment; (2) support surface – beds, mattresses, cushions; (3) keep moving – mobility and repositioning; (4) be aware of incontinence and moisture; and (5) nutrition. Further information is available at: www.stopthepressure.co.uk.

Pressure ulcer risk assessment tools

There are many risk assessment tools available (Norton, 1975; Waterlow, 1985; Braden, 1985) to name a few. In the UK, Waterlow (1985) is the most widely used tool (Dealey, 2012). Risk assessment tools are made up of factors known to contribute to the development of pressure ulceration. Risk assessment tools should not be used in isolation, they should be used in conjunction with a comprehensive skin inspection, assessment and clinical judgement.

In NPUAP/EPUAP (2014) it is suggested that all patients should be assessed within 8 hours of admission to hospital or on the first visit in a community setting. Patients should be reassessed regularly, determined by the healthcare setting and patient condition.

Don't forget!

Always refer to local organisational policy.

Case study 12.2

Mrs Yarrow is a 76-year-old lady, who lives alone and normally walks with a stick. She recently had a fall and has now lost her confidence, has pain in her leg, and so has taken to sitting in her chair. A neighbour has been helping by doing some shopping and cooking some meals, however, her appetite is poor and she is now incontinent. She has type 2 diabetes and hypertension.

Using a risk assessment tool used in your practice area, what is her risk of pressure ulcer development?

Skin assessment

Assessing the skin for early signs of pressure damage is very important. In dark pigmented skin it is more difficult to identify early skin damage, such as erythema, therefore you must assess for other signs, such as heat, swelling and indents (induration). This is when the finger pressure method should be used to assess for Category 1 pressure damage. A finger is pressed onto the erythema for 3 seconds, then blanching is assessed following removal.

Pain is also an early indicator of pressure damage, so pain assessment must be undertaken.

Watch out

Always consider bed-bound or chairfast patients of ANY age as 'at risk' (NPUAP/EPUAP, 2014).

Support surface – beds, mattresses, cushions

There is a wide range of pressure-redistributing equipment available. Choosing a product will depend on patient assessment, comfort, cost, where the individual is being cared for, treatment and rehabilitation objective.

NPUAP/EPUAP (2014) suggest high specification foam mattresses are suitable for patients identified as being 'at risk' and active support surfaces for those deemed at higher risk:

- Low tech devices: constant low pressure such as high specification foam
- High tech devices: dynamic systems, including highly sophisticated beds used in critical care units.

Cushions should be considered when patients are sitting out, but there is limited evidence to promote one cushion over another. When considering using a cushion as an addition, the chair must be assessed to ensure it is the right size for the patient so they are able still to place their feet on the floor.

Heels are the second highest location where pressure ulcers develop. Use of additional heel protection devices, e.g. foam cushions lift heels clear of the bed. The device should be placed along the calf and avoid pressure on the Achilles' tendon (NPUAP/EPUAP, 2014).

Keep moving – mobility and repositioning

Repositioning is the main strategy to relieve pressure. Reduced mobility has consistently been shown to be independently predictive of pressure ulcer development (NPUAP/EPUAP, 2014). Traditionally repositioning every 2 hours is the suggested frequency of moving a patient. However, the evidence to support this is limited and the frequency will be dependent on the location of the patient, and healthcare setting, e.g. hospital, care home. It has been suggested that depending on how you position the patient affects the frequency of turning. Some suggest that using the 30 degree tilt is more comfortable and the length in between repositioning can be extended.

Clinical significance

Avoid positioning the patient on an area of erythema (NPUAP/EPUAP, 2014) as this may damage the area even further and it will not be seen. It might also be painful for the patient!

Always use correct positioning and repositioning techniques using appropriate methods and manual handling devices and local manual handling policy Chapter 11. The frequency of repositioning should be documented on the individual plan and a repositioning chart is useful to record position changes. (NPUAP/EPUAP, 2014).

Incontinence or moisture

Moisture on the skin surface caused by sweat, incontinence, or wound exudate makes the skin more vulnerable to pressure ulceration. Moisture affects collagen in the dermis and softens the stratum corneum, resulting in breakdown often termed 'maceration' (Clark *et al.*, 2010). The cause of the moisture should be identified and treated.

Nutrition

Reduced nutrition impairs the elasticity of the skin. It can also lead to anaemia and reduced oxygen to the tissues. Malnutrition is strongly linked to severe pressure ulcers. A nutritional assessment using a recognised tool, e.g. MUST, should be undertaken on admission and repeated regularly. Observation at meal times and recording of nutritional intake helps with providing advice on nutritional support and when referral to nutritionist or dietician is required.

Pressure ulcer classification system

Pressure ulcers should be classified using the NPUAP/EPUAP (2014) categorisation. Only pressure ulcers are categorised or staged (Figure 12.7).

Incontinence-associated dermatitis or moisture lesions should not be mistaken for pressure ulcers. The precise location of the skin damage should be documented and if the skin damage is not over a bony prominence, then it is more likely to be a moisture lesion.

Compression bandaging for leg ulcers

Alongside appropriate wound management for leg ulcers, compression therapy is often used. Compression therapy supports leg veins and valves to push venous blood up the legs towards the heart, thereby reducing congestion and oedema in lower limbs. This increases the blood velocity and contributes to improving skin condition and aiding

Category i Non blanching erythema

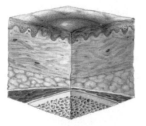

There is intact skin with non-blanching redness. Its colour may differ from the surrounding area. It may be painful, firm, soft, warmer or cooler as compared to adjacent tissue.

Stage 1

Category ii Partial thickness skin loss

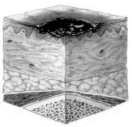

This indicates partial thickness loss of dermis presenting as a shallow open ulcer with red pink wound bed, without slough.

Stage 2

Category iii Full thickness skin loss

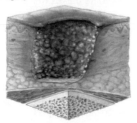

This indicates full thickness tissue loss. Subcutaneous fat may be visible but bone, tendon or muscle are not exposed. Slough may be present but does not obscure the depth of tissue loss. May include undermining and tunnelling.

Stage 3

Category iv Full thickness tissue loss

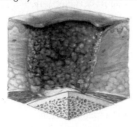

Full thickness tissue loss with exposed bone, tendon or muscle. Slough or scab/eschar may be present on some parts of the wound bed. Often includes undermining and tunnelling and extends into muscle and/or supporting structures making osteomyelitis possible.

Stage 4 Unstageable: Depth unknown. Stable (dry, adherent, intact without erythema or fluctuance) eschar.

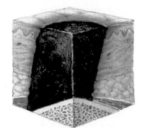

Full thickness tissue loss means the base of the ulcer is covered by slough, (yellow, grey, green or brown) and/or eschar (tan, brown or black) in the wound bed. Until enough slough and/or eschar is removed to expose the base of the wound, the true depth, and therefore Category/Stage, cannot be determined.

Unstageable

Deep tissue injury may be difficult to detect in individuals with dark skin tones.

Figure 12.7 Modified from International NPUAP/EPUAP pressure ulcer classification system (2014)

healing and reducing dryness and improving elasticity. Compression bandaging can take a number of forms and is a skilled process which needs to be undertaken by a qualified nurse following careful assessment and measurements (e.g. ABPI), thus student nurses should watch out for it in practice. The rationale for this skill is so that compression is applied so that the pressure at the ankle is higher than the pressure at the knee in a graduated manner. The various forms of compression include:

- Elastic bandages (may be multi-layer or long)
- Non-elastic bandages (short stretch)
- Intermittent compression (wave-like motion in boots)
- Compression hosiery (stockings).

Activity 12.3

Using Case study 12.2, develop a pressure ulcer prevention care plan for Mrs Yarrow.

Activity 12.4

Go to www.stopthepressure.com and complete the Stop the Pressure Game (SSKIN). What is your high score? Can you improve upon this score?

Summary

An understanding of wound types, assessment and care is essential for all nurses. Some wounds are preventable (i.e. pressure ulcers) while others are a consequence of procedures. Yet all need skilled nursing care to ensure optimal healing. This includes observing, cleaning and dressing wounds, attending to dressing types or removal of sutures aseptically as well as addressing the wider patient ability to heal.

References

Baronski, S. and Ayello, E.A (2012) *Wound Care Essentials: Practice Principles*, 3rd edn. Philadelphia, PA: Wolters Kluwer.

Clark, M., Romanelli, R., Reger, S.I., *et al*. (2010) Microclimate in context. In *Pressure Ulcer Prevention: Pressure, Shear, Friction and Microclimate in Context*. Wounds International. Available at: www.woundsinternational.com/consensus-documents/view/international-review-pressure-ulcer-prevention-pressure-shear-friction-and-microclimate-in-context-1

Cowan, T. (2014) *Wound Care Handbook 2015*, 7th edn. London: Mark Allen healthcare.

Dealey, C. (2012) *The Care of Wounds: A Guide for Nurses*, 4th edn. Oxford: Wiley-Blackwell.

Fette, A.M. (2006) A linimetric analysis of wound measurement tools. Available at: www.worldwidewounds.com/2006/january/Fette/Clinimetric-Analysis-Wound-Measurement-Tools.html (accessed 10 September 2015).

Jones, I., Tweed, C. and Marron, M. (2001) Pressure area care in infants and children: Nimbus Paediatric System. *British Journal of Nursing,* 10(12): 789–795.

Morgan, N. (2014) Linear wound measurements basics. Wound care advisor. Available at: http://woundcareadvisor.com/linear-wound-measurement-basics-vol3-no6/ (accessed 10 September 2015).

National Pressure Ulcer Advisory Panel, European Pressure Ulcer Advisory Panel and Pan Pacific Pressure Injury Alliance (NPUAP/EPUAP) (2014) Prevention and treatment of pressure ulcers: quick reference guide. Available at: www.npuap.org/wp-content/uploads/2014/08/Updated-10-16-14-Quick-Reference-Guide-DIGITAL-NPUAP-EPUAP-PPPIA-16Oct2014.pdf (accessed 10 September 2015).

NHS stopthepressure (2013) HYPERLINK www.stopthepressure.com

Powell, G. (2011) Wound care for injecting drug users *Nursing Standard* 25(46): 51–56

Prosnett, J. and Franks, P.J. (2008) The burden of chronic wounds in the UK. *Nursing Times,* 104(3): 44–45.

WUWHS (A World Union of Wound Healing Societies' Initiative) (2007) Principles of best practice: wound exudate and the role of dressings: consensus. Available at: www.woundsinternational.com/media/issues/82/files/content_42.pdf (accessed 10th September 2015).

Chapter 13

Pre-operative and post-operative care

Jenny Phillips and Carolyn Perriman

Historically, during surgical procedures the patient was put to lie on a wooden table with an anaesthetist and a room of people holding them down. There was no infection control and most of the patients died from sepsis and infections compared to those who survived. Today, surgical procedures are more complex, sometimes lasting for hours. There has been the emergence of keyhole surgery. It is interesting to note that paediatric surgery was not considered a specialised area until the early twentieth century, although other specialist areas were recognised.

Key concepts

Pre and post-operative care
Pre- and post-operative fasting (nil by mouth)
Consent

Assessment
Observations
Pain
Discharge

Learning outcomes

By the end of the chapter you will be able to:

- Identify reasons why infants/children/young people/adults and older people need surgery
- Identify different types of surgery
- Demonstrate an understanding of the principles of pre-operative and post-operative care
- Recognise the importance and role of the family/carer
- Recognise and identify post-operative complications
- Demonstrate knowledge and awareness of the discharge process.

Introduction

There are four classifications for surgery outlined by NCEPOD (2004):

- *Immediate*: normally surgery is within minutes of the decision to operate, this could occur at any time of day or night. The patient's condition is life-threatening. So, the intervention is to save a life, organ or limb. Types of emergencies include: ruptured aortic aneurysm; major trauma to the abdomen or thorax; bone fracture(s) with major neurovascular deficit/insult.
- *Urgent*: this is a surgical intervention for an acute onset of the problem or in the case of clinical deterioration of potentially life-threatening conditions. Normally surgery is within hours of the decision to operate. Types of cases would include those conditions that may threaten the survival of limb or organ (e.g. perforating eye injury); compound fractures; acute abdomen with peritonitis (e.g. perforated appendicitis); critical organ or limb ischaemia (e.g. bowel obstruction); acute coronary syndromes (ACS); patients who develop complications post-operatively ('returns to theatre').
- *Expedited*: this occurs in the case of patients who require early treatment BUT the condition is not immediately life-threatening or the patient is at risk of losing a limb or use of an organ. This intervention normally occurs within days of a decision to operate. Examples would include tendon and nerve injuries; patients who are in a stable condition but require surgery; retinal detachment; accidental injuries; non-accidental injuries, repair of fractured hips.
- *Elective:* this is planned surgery (all conditions that are not classified as immediate, urgent or expedited). Therefore, the intervention has been planned or booked in advance of a routine admission to hospital. Normally timings should suit the patient and hospital. These would include insertion of grommets; adenoidectomy; tonsillectomy; dental restorations and extractions; hernia repair; circumcision; correction of congenital abnormalities – the list is endless.

Within these four classifications, surgery can be either major or minor, depending upon the degree of risk. With major surgery there is a higher risk and the length of surgery may be long or complicated procedure (or indeed both). There is a high risk of post-operative complications, compared to minor surgery where the risks of post-operative complications are less and there is little risk attached to the surgical procedure.

Watch out

The top three greatest concerns for those undergoing elective musculoskeletal surgery were potential complications (20 per cent), effectiveness (15 per cent) and recovery time (15 per cent) of surgery (Ghandi *et al.*, 2011). Ensure you plan for this when preparing patients for surgery.

Risk factors

These additional complications do not change the surgery itself but will have an impact on the styles and methods used to prepare and care for these patients before, during and after the procedure. These include:

■ *Time* – for patients who are aware of their pending surgery they have time to prepare themselves for the procedure both mentally and physically, and may well have the opportunity to go through the pre-surgical procedures and therefore get to know the ward environment and the people prior to admission (but this is not always the case). For patients who undergo emergency surgery there is no or very little time for preparation and this process adds anxiety and stress to an already anxious, stressed, patient in pain and their relatives.

Because of the underlying causes of their condition, patients requiring emergency surgical interventions and management are among the sickest patients treated as they are already physiologically compromised. In order to minimise morbidity and mortality, these patients require efficient and effective emergency surgical intervention and management.

■ *Age* (from premature babies to the older person – both ends of this spectrum being most vulnerable).

■ *General health* – malnutrition delays wound healing and patients are at risk of developing infection. Reduced energy will also lead to reduced mobility during the post-operative period leading to complications.

■ *Obesity* – with most procedures the risk is greater in terms of the procedure itself and post-operative recovery.

■ *Uncontrolled diabetes, cardiac problems, coagulation problems* (increased risk of bleeding post-operatively) all increase intra-operative and post-operative complications.

■ *Mental health, learning disability* – surgery produces physiological stress reactions (neuroendocrine responses) and psychological stress reactions (anxiety and fear) and possible social stressors (family adaptation to temporary or permanent role changes). Any pre-existing problems causing anxiety and affecting cognitive judgement may heighten post-operatively and may influence patient compliance.

There are three phases to the patient's experience during the process of surgery. These are: (1) the pre-operative phase; (2) the intra-operative phase; and (3) the post-operative phase.

1 *Pre-operative*: this involves activities before the patient reaches the operation room: a thorough assessment and interventions to minimise the intra-operative and post-operative risks. For example, controlling blood glucose levels, cleansing the bowel (colonic washouts) before bowel surgery.

2 *Intra-operative*: this occurs in the operating room. Careful monitoring of the patient's physiological status and identifying actual (intra-operative) and potential (post-operative) problems with timely interventions are key during this phase.

3 *Post-operative*: this time period is from recovery until healing has taken place

(which may happen in the community). The patient is in the rehabilitation phase. Monitoring and care are managed in relation to the specific procedure.

Activity 13.1

Imagine you are in pain, and have potentially been so for a period of time. You now find yourself in a strange bed in a strange environment, surrounded by people you don't know and who use words to explain things that you have never heard before. You know what is ultimately going to happen to you, but you are unaware of the processes that are going to take place and what that involves. You are unsure of what to do and when and also find yourself anxiously waiting to see if the time you were given for the big moment is the actual time for action or if for some reason the time has been moved.

Write down your immediate thoughts.

When caring for these patients, no matter the reason for the surgery or the age, it is important to remember how your patient may be feeling at this time and to care for them accordingly.

Pre-operative phase

Nursing assessment and pre-procedure preparation (physical and psychological) are a very important part of the surgical process as this ensures that the relevant and important information is obtained before the procedure and that the patient is properly and safely prepared beforehand. This is the phase where investigations and tests may be performed to assess the functioning of the relevant body systems. Physical preparation will be dependent upon the type of surgery intended.

Psychological preparation

Any decision relating to surgery is a big one by anyone's standards and is never taken lightly. There are many factors that need to be taken into account, even if the surgery is a minor one that is undertaken regularly. There is the physical impact of the surgery to start with and this relates to bodily image, 'What will I look like after the procedure?', 'How long will I look like that?' There are also the possible physical limitations after the procedure, especially if mobility is reduced or the activities of daily living will be impacted. Questions then arise around the issues of how I will manage to wash/bathe, cook, clean, shop. All of these issues will need to be addressed before consent can be given. There is also the issue of the patient's emotional stress level and their understanding of what is to happen along with possible coping mechanisms or support they can implement or call on which will ultimately affect any decision they make.

Ensuring procedures minimise anxiety for the patient and family is not only considered good practice on the nurses' part but also makes the whole surgical experience easier on all those involved. Heightened blood pressure, heart rate and respiratory rates can ultimately affect the decision to operate if their impact is severe enough, as will the impact of lack of sleep due to the patient worrying. Anxiety also has an impact on patient behaviour, making them short-tempered, snappy, and abrasive when speaking and could possibly even make them act out and display behaviour unusual to their normal demeanour. All this in turn has an effect on their loved ones, who then worry for their relative, becoming stressed and worried and acting in a similar manner.

If a patient's anxiety level can be reduced it should ensure that the physical impact is minimised and a relatively calm and healthy patient is transferred to the theatre ready for their surgery. It also helps reduce their overall emotional response to stress and fear. It will aid and facilitate patient cooperation in all aspects of their surgical journey. It will allow and support the patient to feel that have some control over a situation where control has been taken away from them. If the patient feels as though they are being heard and respected in regards to their thoughts and opinions and have their questions answered in a friendly, open and honest way, this ensures good working staff–patient relationships.

If the patient is calm also, they are more likely to have a speedier and timelier discharge due to better and speedier healing, with lack of stress and anxiety, leaving the body to concentrate more energy on the healing of surgery. Some ideas to consider when working with patients and families who are awaiting surgery to facilitate anxiety reduction.

Pre-operative care

Pre-operative teaching is a vital aspect of care. Not only does it involve giving patients information about the surgery and what to expect but also teaching patients ways to improve their recovery, e.g. deep breathing exercises, how to splint incisions to ease the pain, how to move (up and down/in and out of bed) post-operatively, how to cough, leg exercises to prevent deep vein thrombosis.

Hospital wards and departments have check lists and specific paperwork with regards to pre-surgical preparation and these need to be completed as required and filed in the patient notes for all staff concerned to see. It also ensures that all required information, procedures and interventions are undertaken and accounted for.

There are different standard documents for surgery for all different patient categories (child and adult). These are updated as new procedures become available; research highlights the need for changes in the procedures or the delivery or method of care, to ensure safe surgical provision and the best possible care is provided, and meets the needs of the patient. Therefore, it is paramount that nurses keep up to date with the changes to standards, policies and guidelines which will impact their care provision and delivery.

The World Health Organisation (WHO) produced a surgical safety check list in 2009 (Figure 13.1). 'Safe surgery saves lives' is the initiative which aims to reduce the number of surgical deaths around the world. The aim of the initiative is to strengthen the commitment of clinical staff to address safety issues within the clinical setting in relation to surgery (anaesthesia, operating room, recovery). This idea also includes improving safety practices within the areas of:

- Ensuring correct site surgery
- Avoiding surgical site infections
- Improving communication within the team.

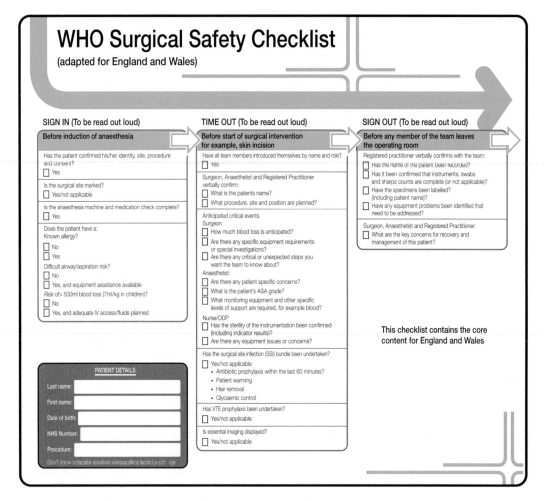

Figure 13.1 The WHO pre-operative check list

Table 13.1 gives an example of the minimum components of pre-operative geriatric assessment specific to anaesthesia.

Standards for pre-operative check list

The pre-operative check list should include the following:

- *Demographic details* including home address, phone numbers, date of birth, contact details of next of kin (parents, spouse, significant others), GP, social worker, other professionals involved with the patient/family
- *Baseline observations* are of paramount importance, as these are used for comparison with observations taken from the patient during the recovery process, including temperature, pulse, respiration rate, blood pressure, and any other surgical-specific

Table 13.1 Minimum components of pre-operative assessment specific to anaesthesia of the older person

Domain	Items to be assessed	Appropriate assessment tools
Medical: Musculoskeletal	Co-morbidity/severity: ■ Cardiovascular ■ Respiratory ■ Haematological ■ Renal ■ Nutritional ■ Previous anaesthesia Anaesthesia-specific ■ Alcohol intake ■ Pain intensity	■ Vital signs, ECG ■ Oxygen saturations, (pulmonary function tests) ■ Full blood count ■ Urea and electrolytes, estimated glomerular filtration rate ■ Weight, body mass index, albumin (liver function tests) ■ Enquiry after (age-related) problems ■ Airway assessment ■ CAGE questionnaire for alcoholism ■ Visual analogue pain score
Medication	Medication review Anti-coagulant therapy	Relevant allergies Coagulation screen
Cognitive	■ Mental capacity ■ Decision-making capacity ■ Communication ■ Risk factors for post-operative delirium	Mental test score Alert for alterations in vision, hearing speech Ask if they have alterations in their memory
Mobility	■ Gait ■ Assess aids to mobilise	Observe mobility Ask about getting into/out of bed or going to the toilet Frailty assessment
Other aids to support daily functions	■ Vision ■ Hearing ■ Eating/drinking	Assess for glasses, hearing aids, dentures

Source: adapted from AAGBI (2014).

observations need to be taken and accurately documented on the appropriate chart, dated, timed and signed. Influencing factors such as anxiety or stress should be taken into consideration as this may cause false results

■ Patient's *weight* is taken before surgery and accurately charted. This weight is used to calculate medications required pre-/post-operatively, for anaesthesia and for indications of fluid retention after the surgical procedure

■ The intended procedure is accurately *documented*, including details of the surgery being prepared for, the position of the surgical intervention site highlighting the specific area, i.e. LEFT ear, and this is normally documented in both writing and pictorially on a diagram

■ Patient's *medical and anaesthetic history* should be taken and documented comprehensively and given in detail, as all past medical interventions must be reviewed, no matter how much significance. This is anything that could have an impact on the surgery presently being considered. Current and past medication should be recorded along with the name of the drug, doses and frequency taken where possible. If the medication has been stopped, this should be documented and the reason provided or the planned duration of use (where applicable) as well as the route the medication has been/is given. It is also good practice to document any issues for the patient in regards to the method of drug administration, i.e. 'patient is unable to swallow tablets'

- *Allergies* need to be highlighted and recorded in BOLD CLEAR writing, giving clear details of the type of allergy and reaction type that manifests in the patient. Red identification bands need to be made and put on the patient, along with a signature, date and time that this happened

- *Recording of immunisation status* (especially important in infant/child/young person), details should be given as to what immunisations have been given and any that have been missed (with reasons why they were missed). All this information can be obtained from the child's red child health record book that all parents are provided with

- A decision regarding *Nil By Mouth (NBM) status* will be made and is guided by the time the patient is due to go down to theatre for their surgery. Guidelines exist from the Royal College of Nursing (2005) who recommend that for an adult under-going general anaesthetic (providing there are no complicating factors, e.g. bowel obstruction), they can have water, clear tea and black coffee (both without milk) up to two hours before surgery and food up to six hours before. These fasting times are based on well patients. For those who have already existing medical conditions where these times could have a greater impact on the patients' health, such as diabetes, the surgical and anaesthetic team would need to be consulted and a plan of fasting care developed and implemented as instructed.

In the case of children, providing there are no contraindications, the RCN (2005) recommend the following fasting guidance:

- 2 hours for clear fluids
- 4 hours for breast milk
- 6 hours for cow's milk, formula and food (including sweets)
- Chewing gum should not be allowed.

Care should be organised with this requirement taken into consideration as to when the patient's last food intake can be, and they should be offered something shortly before that time.

The anaesthetic team should also consider further investigation if the patient has a greater risk of regurgitation and aspiration.

- It is important that *regular prescribed medication* taken orally should be continued pre-operatively unless there is advice to the contrary. Up to 0.5 ml/kg (up to 30 ml) of water may be given orally to help children take their medication

- *Psychological preparation* will depend upon the type of surgery and the individual patient. None-the-less, this is paramount for all patients of all ages and abilities. Doctors, surgeons and anaesthetists need to come and speak to the patient (family, next of kin where required) to explain what the possible complications are, the procedure which is being prepared for, including both the positive and negative aspects and possible outcomes. Nurses should check that the patient fully understands what they have been told and have all the information to make an informed decision. Advice for this includes:

- Appropriate environment to ensure privacy and dignity
- Language and communication methods used need to be appropriate for the patient, so easier simpler words and explanations for children and adults with learning difficulties, pictures, interpreters where needed
- Patients should be encouraged to ask any questions and, where possible, written information should be given
- For children, there is also the provision of play specialists to work through their understanding of what is going to happen, along with the emotions that accompany this process
- Any intervention needs to be clearly documented along with any concerns about the patient's understanding of what is happening. Should a concern arise in relation to patient understanding, it needs to be communicated to the relevant senior people and actions implemented and addressed.

Consent involves explaining to the patient the procedure, site, the risks and benefits. It needs to be obtained from the patient or correctly identified other, i.e. parent. In the case of adults with mental health problems and learning difficulties, these family members could be their advocates and hold power of attorney over decisions, if it is felt they are unable to understand what is happening and are unable to provide full informed consent. In addition, this process is undertaken by the surgeon and needs to be signed by them. This intervention also needs to be documented in the patient notes along with details of the conversation, date, time and signature.

Consent has to be obtained for all surgical procedures and most importantly needs to be informed consent. This is obtained by the doctor and the surgical team talking through the patient's problem and the resulting surgical intervention. The team have to inform the patient/relevant person of both the positive and negative aspects of the procedure. They are also required to detail any possible complications that could occur later after the procedure, even if they may not happen or have an impact in future years. Without this information, consent is not deemed as informed consent and is also considered poor practice. Patients should not be under the influence of any medication that will interfere with their decision-making processes when seeking to obtain consent. An authorised legally recognised signature is required for the surgery to take place.

In the case of children, staff should work in accordance with the Fraser Guidelines, where it is recognised that:

- The child or young person should be involved in their own care and contribute to decisions according to their understanding and competence
- In general, hospitals should follow Department of Health guidance on consent and Trust policies should specifically address young people and their families who need accurate information appropriate to their level of their understanding before deciding to consent to treatment.

Confidentiality needs to have been maintained throughout the whole process, both in terms of all conversations had between patient and doctor and where necessary referral to other medical professionals as patient condition and requirements as dictated. Confidentiality also relates to the patients' notes being handled and dealt with in a sensitive and law-abiding way adhering to data protection legislation.

The decision to operate by the medical team relies on the provision of necessary information and documentation. If at any point any information is absent or incomplete, there is a very good chance that the surgery will not go ahead as planned unless the problems can be rectified in a timely manner, still ensuring that all the necessary requirements are fulfilled, not just to the doctor's requirements but also meeting the requirements of the hospital and the law.

Other pre-operative considerations are:

- *Make-up and nail polish* need to be removed before going down to surgery and explanations need to be given to the patient as to why this is a requirement. They should be informed of the need to be able to observe their skin colour and any changes to this during or after the procedure (cyanosis, pallor).
- *Jewellery, piercings and hair grips* all need to be removed before going for the procedure, again along with explanations as to why this is done. Wedding bands can be covered with tape
- *Glasses and contact lenses* need to be left or brought back to the ward while surgery is being undertaken. They can be found upon return to the ward or given in the recovery room for children by their parent when they go down to see them
- Any *loose teeth* need to be documented in case of oral surgery or emergency intubation so that medical staff can be aware of possible complications should they come out during the procedure
- *Drug charts* need to be checked after the surgeon and an anaesthetist have visited to see if any pre-operation medication has been prescribed. If medication has been prescribed, a note of the time should be taken and the drug should be administered as prescribed at the appropriate time. The provision of the drug should not only be signed on the drug chart, but should also be documented in the patient's notes. It is also paramount that the patient's drug chart accompanies the patient to theatre, so that doctors and theatre/recovery staff are able to see what has been administered, when, by which route and the dosages. This is in case further medication is required or there is a reaction to anything given
- *Identity bands* need to be applied. This also includes the red allergy bands. If the patient is allergic to something, ensure that the patient has two bands on and that the bands hold the correct information. They should not be damaged in any way and should be read easily. If the band is damaged, unclear or holds incorrect information, it should be rectified and new ones applied
- Ensure the *operation site* is clearly marked in the right place on the patient and corresponds to both the verbal and written information in the patient's notes. If there is a discrepancy, then the surgeon and other relevant Health care professionals need to be informed before the patient is taken down to theatre
- The *anaesthetic record* needs to be completed by the anaesthetist and this needs to be filed within the patient's notes, all of which will accompany them to theatre.

■   *Blood results* should to be checked by the relevant doctors and, where needed, action taken in case of deteriorated results. All interventions will then need to be documented. If no action is required, the results need to be dated and signed after review and filed in the notes

■   Allow patients *to wear their own clothes* for as long as possible and if possible allow them to change down in the theatre area. This allows the patient to feel more comfortable and secure in an environment that is scary and ever changing. Their own clothes afford them some control over their situation and allow them to retain their identity in an environment where it can be easily lost

■   *Care plans* should be made in advance of the procedure, and equipment/resources should be identified and obtained ready for the patient's return. The required equipment can be set up and put in place while the patient is in surgery, so it is ready for use upon their return

■   When nursing any patient, it is important to remember that they are more than likely to have *friends and family*. For the child patient, they come with parents/carers who are the child's advocates/legal guardians and consent givers. They could also possibly have siblings who also need care and support. For adult patients there could husbands/ wives/partners and children, all of whom will also need care and support.

Transferring to theatre or intra-operative care

Care continues from the ward or clinic environment all the way through the escort to and from the operating theatre. This is an anxious time for patients. Imaginative modes of transportation to and from the theatre can be used for children. This can also be adapted for adult patients where they are allowed to walk to the department or be pushed in a wheelchair where possible and deemed safe to do so. This allows the patient to have more freedom and control for a longer period of time and feel less like a helpless patient.

Safety is paramount when transferring patients to theatre for their surgical procedure. The RCN have outlined guidance for transferring to and from theatre (Box 13.1).

Documentation for transfer

All documentation should be completed in a clear and concise way. It should be dated and signed at the time the intervention took place. This is an integral part when transferring a patient to theatre (NMC, 2015). Most hospital guidance will only allow students to transfer patients when they are in their second year of training and once they have been assessed as competent in this procedure.

The documentation should include the following data:

■   Patient details
■   Consent
■   Baseline observations
■   Record of allergies
■   Pre-operative fasting information
■   Risk assessment
■   Pre-operative safety check list.

Box 13.1 Check lists for transfer to theatre and return to ward

Transfer to theatre check list

- Ensure the patient is in a stable condition
- A preoperative checklist is completed (WHO, 2009)
- A consent form must be signed. In infants/children and young people, this must be signed by a person with parental responsibility, unless the individual is deemed competent to give their own consent (Fraser Guidelines). Trust policies should specifically address young people and their families who need accurate information appropriate to their level of their understanding before deciding to consent to treatment
- The patient has had choice in the method of transport and clothing to wear, where appropriate
- Ensure the patient identity is clear (name band, patient notes)
- A baseline set of observations are available
- Prostheses are removed if there are any and documented
- Surgical site is marked
- A member of staff with appropriate skills has been identified to accompany the patient
- Appropriate equipment has been identified
- Handover to theatre staff with the appropriate documentation, i.e. reports, X-rays, investigations, results as available.

Transfer to ward checklist

- Ensure the patient is in a stable condition
- Transfer back to the ward on a bed, with oxygen and suction
- A registered nurse must accompany the patient back from recovery
- Clear handover of the patient should include clear post-operative instructions.

Documentation following a surgical procedure should include:

- A summary of the operation, signed and dated by surgeon who performed the procedure, including any unforeseen actions
- Clear post-operative instructions
- Prescription chart with appropriate analgesia
- Fluid management
- Oxygen prescription
- A record of observations taken in the recovery room.

Preparation for day case surgery

Patients may have elective procedures as a day case, depending on the type of procedure, physical capacity for surgery and prior assessment of suitability and local resources or availability of the day case approach. The preparation and care will depend on the type of surgery performed and whether under a local or a general anaesthetic. Often a pre-operative assessment is carried out by a nurse approximately two weeks prior to surgery to determine fitness and readiness for surgery. Regardless of the surgery, the following principles and procedures are undertaken.

Procedure for preparing for surgery before leaving home

1   Take usual medication unless otherwise advised.
2   Patients should take a bath or shower and clean teeth as usual.
3   Arrive at appointed time – this is not the time of their procedure but of awaiting their procedure – may be up to two hours beforehand.
4   Bring the following items:
    ▪ Dressing gown and slippers
    ▪ Small bag for belongings
    ▪ Equipment and aids needed, i.e. glasses, hearing aids
    ▪ Books or something to occupy them when waiting
    ▪ Any medicines and cards, i.e. warfarin or steroid cards.
5   Ensure they leave valuables at home – minimum possessions, i.e. money, jewellery, mobile telephones to be switched off.

Procedure for preparing for day surgery

1   Fasting:
    ▪ No food for 6 hours prior to arrival time (includes sweets or chewing gum)
    ▪ Water can be drunk up to one hour prior to arrival on day surgery ward.
2   Patient puts on gown and locks away belongings.
3   Explanations of the procedure are given again; time allowed for questions and consent form will be signed or double checked if it was done at the pre-operative assessment appointment.
4   Ensure the patient is informed of what is happening at all stages. Aim to minimise medical jargon.
5   Circulation: encourage the patient to walk around before surgery.

After the procedure:

▪ The same as above in Box 13.1
▪ Patients will be allowed home when stable and have recovered from the procedure
▪ If patients have a general anaesthetic, they are allowed to go home accompanied by a relative or friend when they are sufficiently alert and awake
▪ Information on follow-up and contacts for concerns if there are post-operative pain, swelling, bleeding or other unexpected features is also provided.

Top tip

Accompany doctors when they speak to patients as often the department or ward is noisy and the patients may ask for explanations or clarity or have the need to reinforce some aspects of their procedure or processes if possible in written form.

Clinical significance

Emergency patients require the same information but it might be rushed, so be prepared to repeat and re-explain.

Post-operative phase

The patient needs to be cared for in a safe environment; this means an area with working oxygen and suction (with appropriate-sized mask, suction catheters – including yankauer), and an appropriate-sized bed with bed sides (where indicated). The bed space should also hold any other equipment required by the patient upon their return. This equipment should be in safe working order and clean, ready for use. In addition, the space around the bed should be clear, to enable easy access to the safety equipment, should an emergency situation arise.

Immediately when the patient returns back to the ward and when their condition allows, the patient's vital signs (heart rate; respiratory rate; blood pressure; temperature; oxygen saturation; capillary refill; level of consciousness – but remember this will be impaired in patients who have had recent sedation or are receiving opioid analgesia) should be taken and recorded (Box 13.2). The National Early Warning Score (NEWS) was developed by a Working Party to provide a national standard for assessing, monitoring and tracking acutely and critically ill patients (not for use with children under 16 years or in pregnancy); the intention was that Trusts would use it to replace their locally adapted early warning systems (Royal College of Physicians, 2012). Like other early warning systems, NEWS has six physiological parameters which students who assist registered nurses will become familiar with:

- Respiratory rate
- Oxygen saturation
- Temperature
- Systolic blood pressure
- Pulse rate
- Level of consciousness (this will be impaired in patients who have had recent sedation or are receiving opioid analgesia, which should be taken into consideration in assessment).

Box 13.2 Recommended observation times

Post-operative observations in adults

- 30 minutes for 1 hour
- Hourly for the next 2 hours
- Then every 4 hours dependent on patient's condition.

Post-operative observations in children (RCN, 2013)

- 30 minutes for 2 hours
- Hourly for 2–4 hours, until child is fully awake, eating and drinking.

Post removal of tonsils and adenoids

- Every 30 minutes for 4 hours, or more if there are signs of bleeding.

Complex procedures

- Longer than 6 hours in surgery
- Significant fluid loss
- Under 1 year of age
- Physiological instability pre-operative
- Physiological instability during the recovery period
- Patients must have pulse oximetry and continuous cardio-respiratory monitoring for 4 hours.

NB: these are ONLY guidelines – if the patient's condition is unstable – more frequent observations are indicated.

Level of consciousness

Post-operative patients should respond to verbal stimulation, be able to answer questions and be aware of their surroundings before being transferred back to the ward and throughout the post-operative period.

Any change in the individual's conscious level could be a sign of shock and should be escalated immediately. When it has been identified that an individual's condition is deteriorating, this information can be exchanged verbally by using the Situation, Background, Assessment, and Recommendation (SBAR) (Box 13.3). This tool is advocated by the NHS Institute for Innovation and Improvement (2008).

All observations need to be documented on the appropriate charts to the local area. This includes:

Box 13.3 The SBAR tool (see Chapter 2)

Situation

- Identify where you are calling from
- Identify the patient and reason for the report
- Identify what you are concerned about.

Background

- Significant medical history
- Information from charts, notes.

Assessment

- Vital signs
- Concerns.

Recommendation

- Explain what you need
- Clarify expectations.

- *Neurological observations*: neurological observations are recorded to determine deterioration or improvement in a patient's condition. These should be recorded and interpreted in conjunction with systematic observations, including paediatric early warning score (PEWS), to obtain an overall clinical picture (Chapman *et al.*, 2010)
- *Neurovascular observations*: neurovascular observations need to be performed, to assess if an individual has adequate blood circulation and nerve function. It is essential to perform this assessment if an individual has the following:
  - Had pre- and post-orthopaedic surgery
  - Had plastic surgery
  - Are in traction/plaster
  - Have an infection
  - Suffered bony or muscular trauma
  - Burns, snake bites, crush syndrome
  - Application of an orthotic device.
- *Fluid balance (strict input and output)*: the monitoring of a patient's fluid balance in order to prevent dehydration or over-hydration. This includes recording:
  - Oral intake
  - IV fluids (IV fluids and IV medications)
  - Urine output: catheter urine measurements should not be less than 0.5 ml/kg/hour

- ▦ Nausea and vomiting
- ▦ Oral care
- ▦ Nasogastric tube drainage
- ▦ Colour and amount of wound drainage
- ▦ Colour of stoma (where appropriate) and whether there is any bleeding
- ▦ Faeces output.
- ▦ *Wound assessment chart*: wound observations need to be undertaken ensuring the site is regularly observed for infection or other complications, colour, smell, ooze, drainage amounts.
- ▦ *Pain assessment charts*: a pain assessment tool is used to assess the level of pain an individual is experiencing. In children, young people, patients with special needs, it is essential to use a tool that is appropriate for the individual, their age and stage of development (see Chapter 5).

Observations should be recorded appropriately, clearly and acted on in a timely, safe and effective manner in accordance with guidelines for record keeping.' (NMC, 2015)

The correct amount of oxygen should be given as prescribed on the medication chart (Chapter 9). Close monitoring of the patient's oxygen saturation levels in comparison to the percentage of inspired oxygen should be made. Any decrease in oxygen saturation levels should be brought to the attention of the doctor as soon as possible. Should a patient return to the ward in air and then upon return require oxygen the doctors should also be informed immediately.

Pain

The patient's pain level should be closely assessed and evaluated. At no point should any patient be left in pain for any reason, and this is relevant to ALL patient types regardless of age, reason for admission, mental or physical ability. Pain is very subjective and every patient will feel it in varying degrees. Nurses are unable to feel another person's pain and should believe their patient when they say they are in pain. Pain can be potentially inflicted on patients every day of their stay. Not just through the more obvious routes of surgical procedures, but also through less intrusive interventions such as venepuncture, cannulation, injections to name but a few. Due to the subjective nature of pain manifestation, nurses need to regularly consult with their patients to monitor their pain. This can be made more complex with patients who have limited articulation skills (children), with limited understanding and communication skills (patients with disabilities and special needs), or those who are confused, disorientated and fearful. Chapter 5 has more details on pain scales and medications.

While the World Health Organisation has developed the pain ladder for the effective treatment of pain, this is often inverted in post-operative management, that is, the stronger opioid analgesia are used initially, reducing in strength as the patient recovers.

Alternative methods can also be implemented for lesser degrees of pain and also in more severe degrees of pain. If pain management is undertaken correctly recovery should be achieved in a quicker time span, is a more comfortable process and will ensure that the patient's surgical journey is a more satisfied one.

Clinical significance

Seminal work appeared in the 1970s which has implications for the twenty-first-century post-operative patient and pain experience. Hayward (1975) researched post-operative pain experiences in patients. He theorised that giving patients pre-operative information lessened their anxiety and thus lessened their experience of pain post-operatively. This is an important message to aid successful recovery and a supportive surgical experience for patients.

It is important the patients and their families receive appropriate information about their care at all stages of the care pathway. Facilities should be provided to ensure the patient and their family are as comfortable as possible throughout their care. Patient information leaflets should be given to the patient/family when deemed appropriate. Additional support services can be used as required. These include:

- Translation
- Advocacy advice and support
- Play therapy
- Health visitors and liaison officers
- Social care
- Networks
- Nurses
- Interfaith.

Upon their return from surgery, the patient should be kept hydrated with the correct type of fluid and at the correct amount. Any fluids which were started in the theatre or recovery room will have been prescribed on the patient's prescription chart and should be checked upon return to the ward, along with the hourly amount being received. Any discrepancies need to be investigated and reviewed by the medical staff immediately. Any changes to fluids or infusion amounts need to be undertaken and documented in the notes.

Provided the patient is awake and alert, and it has been deemed safe and agreed, patients should be offered water/juice in small quantities to start and as the patient tolerates. If tolerated, the patient could possibly eat and drink as normal. Observe post-operative recommendations from the hospital Trust and surgical care guidelines and policy. For some patients the decision will be made after bowel sounds have been heard (particularly in the case of abdominal surgery). For patients undergoing gastric and bowel surgery, introducing fluids and diet may be a slower process.

Complications of surgery

Each procedure will carry its own potential complications, however, there are several that are common or can be generalised to all surgical procedures following a general anaesthetic:

1   *Post-operative nausea and vomiting (PONV)*: this may be a reaction to the anaesthetic, analgesia, gastric or other changes following surgery. Some people are more

at risk of this than others, e.g., the very young or very aged, patients excessively starved pre-operatively, patients with a history of PONV or motion sickness or highly anxious patients. The management of this involves:

■ Withholding food or fluids initially
■ Removing the cause if possible
■ Placing in recovery position to avoid aspiration
■ Administering antiemetics as prescribed
■ Providing privacy if vomiting, offering sufficient vomit bowls, tissues and mouthwash.

2   *Haemorrhage*: there are three main types of potential haemorrhage post-operatively:

■ Primary – occurring at the time of surgery
■ Reactionary – occurring soon after surgery as blood pressure and the circulation improves
■ Secondary – due to infection or other damage often days after the surgery.

If this occurs the key actions are to do the following:

■ Observe for haemorrhage and, if in hospital, monitor pulse and blood pressure to determine the progress of the bleeding
■ Observe the location of the blood loss – if the wound is still intact, if not, report immediately
■ Record the amount of blood loss – may require weighing dressings
■ Report the blood loss to the medical or surgical staff
■ Reassure the patient they are being monitored and closely observed
■ If bleeding persists – this may require either resuturing, taking back to theatre or another invasive procedure. Initial care will be application of pressure through a pressure bandage and close monitoring
■ At all times explain what is happening to the patient and offer support and attention.

3   *Deep vein thrombosis*: this is a serious problem. It occurs in the deep veins located in the dorsal region of the lower leg (calf) but can occur in the pelvis or thigh. This is often due to a mix of poor blood flow, impeding blood flow (as in some orthopaedic procedures), dehydration or poor venous return or a history of clotting problems or heart attacks. The signs of this occurring are evident several days post-operatively and include: a swollen painful calf area which is hot and tender to the touch, this worsens on walking and may cause a colour change in the affected limb. Early mobilisation post-operatively improves circulation, encouraging fluid intake improves hydrations which reduces the risks. Patients may have anticoagulant medication and this ought to be given as prescribed.

4   *Constipation*: this may occur due to reduced peristalsis which can persist post-operatively especially in patients who have had gastric surgery. This is further complicated by immobility, dehydration and opioid medications. The key action is to improve mobility and hydration as soon as possible. Going to the toilet might be painful if the patient has an abdominal wound but should not be avoided and strategies such as holding onto the wound site (with a pillow) may help the feeling of pain. Straining must be avoided to minimise damage to the wound.

5   *Chest infection*: some patients are reluctant to cough or breathe deeply post-operatively as it may be painful. Adequate analgesia ought to be given and then

encouragement to breathe deeply and, if needed, to cough to release secretions built up during the procedure. Lack of deep breathing may lead to basal consolidation and infection setting in. Vulnerable groups include: smokers, patients with chronic lung conditions, asthmatics, and underweight or weak individuals. Physiotherapists are often on surgical wards to assist in addressing this problem. Nurses ought to observe for signs of infection which include:

- Elevated temperature
- Flushed skin
- Shallow rapid breathing
- Chest rattle or sounds suggestive of sputum in the airways
- Bubbly cough
- Reduced oxygen saturations
- Tachycardia.

6   *Confusion or disorientation*: acute confusion may affect elderly people or those with other organic or mental health problems or those feeling psychologically vulnerable or a reaction to anaesthetic. This may occur in people with no history of confusion. This can be manifest in a number of ways:

- Impaired attention
- Altered activity (reduced or excessive)
- Memory impairment
- Thought impairment
- Disorientation – location, time, reason for being in hospital
- Altered sleep/wake cycle
- Delusions/agitation
- Psychotic ideas are common but of short duration especially in elderly patients.

If this occurs, monitoring the individual is recommended:

- Observations: for signs of physical problems – temperature, pulse and blood pressure
- Monitor oxygen saturations
- Neurological assessment. If no cause is found, then awaiting recovery from anaesthetic is advised, otherwise mental state assessment, environmental and medical management, i.e. medication.

Other measures include:

- Clear communication
- Reminders of the day, time, location and identification of surrounding persons
- Have a clock available
- Have familiar objects from home around patients, especially glasses, walking aids and hearing aids
- Staff consistency – both doctors and nurses
- Relaxation, e.g. watch television
- Involve the family and carers
- Avoid sensory extremes (over- or under-stimulation)
- Adequate space and sleep.

This list is not exhaustive just a start to approaches and procedures.

7   *Wound infection and wound care*: following surgery, wounds are observed for their progress in healing and any changes, e.g., bleeding or swelling. Wounds may need

cleaning or sutures may need removing. This will be indicated by the surgical team. Sutures are often removed approximately 7–10 days post operation. This is addressed in Chapter 12 on wound care.

Post-operative fasting

Box 13.4 shows the rules for post-operative fasting for children and adults.

Box 13.4 Post-operative fasting

Children (0–18 years) routine surgery

- Oral fluids can be offered when the patient is fully awake following anaesthesia, providing there are no medical, surgical or nursing contraindications
- Consider clear fluids or breast milk first to gauge tolerance to drinking
- If fluids are tolerated, then normalise the patient as tolerance dictates and encourage solids
- It is not required that a patient drinks before discharge, but they have to pass urine before discharge.

Adults

- When the patient is fully awake following anaesthesia, providing there are no complications oral fluids should be encouraged
- Consider clear fluids first to gauge tolerance
- If fluids are tolerated, then normalise the patient as tolerance dictates and encourage solids.

If a patient's condition has been identified as deteriorating at any time, this information must be passed verbally to appropriate health professionals immediately and relevant interventions undertaken till the team come to review and make new plans of care.

Good communication and multidisciplinary team working facilitate minimising waiting times and aid delivery of timely, safe, effective care that is cost-effective and in the patients' best interests. A timely return to the ward allows the patient to be reunited with their loved ones, return to surroundings and people that are more familiar and the mental reassurance that they are on the journey to recovery and home.

Recovery areas generally have a physical separation between children and adults, allowing them their own appropriate space and environment to aid their recovery without impacting or having a negative effect on each other.

Additional areas to think about when caring for infants/children/young person/adults/older people

- Parents/carers are able to be present with their child when they wake up
- As soon as possible post-surgery a member of the medical/nursing team updates the patient/family/carer of the outcome of surgery
- Patients and families are given clear information on discharge from the service and are able to make contact with a healthcare professional for advice and support following discharge
- The service has mechanisms to receive feedback from patients and carers.

Discharge from hospital

Planning for discharge with clear dates and times (NHS Institute for Innovation and Improvement, 2008) reduces:

- Patients' length of stay
- Emergency readmissions
- Pressure on hospital beds.

The discharge process should ideally start before admission to hospital (Box 13.5). This can happen with elective surgery, but is not possible in emergency cases.

Box 13.5 The discharge process

DISCHARGE PROCESS – On admission

- Assess: Issues that will affect hospital and home care
- Inform: What to expect in hospital and after discharge
- Key Contacts: In hospital and community
- IDENTIFY DISCHARGE TYPE AND DISCHARGE PLANNING PARTNERS.

DISCHARGE PROCESS – During hospital stay

- Assess: Needs and identify emerging care issues
- Plan: Discharge and homecare in partnership
- Educate, Train and Support: Child, family, other carers
- Anticipate: Discharge day – timely discharge decision, supplies, pharmacy, etc.

DISCHARGE PROCESS –Departure day

- Inform: Follow-up, discharge letter, aftercare, normal activities
- Medicines and supplies
- Home safely: *Verify who the patient is going home with and inform key contacts*
- Complete and sign Discharge Checklist
- HOME.

Hospital discharge can be very challenging for the health professions, the patients, the family and carers. While the majority of patients go home with no further complications or ongoing care needs, other patients may need some support or a comprehensive care package delivered by a number of different healthcare professionals.

Early on, health professionals need to identify whether it will likely be a simple or complex discharge. An adult going to theatre for an MUA (manipulation under anaesthesia for a fractured radius and ulna) will likely be a straightforward discharge, whereas an older person admitted for a hip replacement might be a complex discharge process if there are concerns with mobility and caring for themselves when returning home.

As nurses and health professionals it is essential that we assess an individual's circumstances and look at any issues that might cause additional concerns when looking at the discharge process. For example:

- Does the patient have complex medical needs/additional needs?
- Does the patient live at home/in a care home/assisted living/hospice?
- The type of accommodation, e.g. a patient may have had complex leg surgery, and through the assessment you find out that they live on the 6th floor of a block of flats, that has no lifts. Additional planning will need to be completed within the discharge process, to ensure patient safety
- Is there is someone who can support and care for the patient when they are discharged?

Case study 13.1

Ben Kembu, 42 years old, is admitted for day surgery for hernia repair. He admits he is worrying constantly about losing his job and being unable to provide for his children. This worry has been troubling him for the past 8 months. Despite his best efforts, he hasn't been able to shake the negative thoughts. Ever since the worry started, Ben has found himself feeling restless, tired, and tense. He's had several embarrassing moments in meetings where he has lost track of what he was trying to say. When he goes to bed at night, it's as if his brain won't shut off. He finds himself mentally rehearsing all the worst-case scenarios regarding losing his job, now not waking up from the anaesthetic and leaving his children homeless. He is diagnosed with Generalised Anxiety Disorder.

1   Ben has not disclosed his problem, you find it in his notes – why do you think that might be?
2   Ben is taking medication (Selective serotonin reuptake inhibitors (SSRIs)), what specific advice do you give him about his medication during his preparation for surgery?
3   What other approaches can you take to manage Ben's anxiety at this time?

It is important that the discharge process is discussed with the patient/family/carer at the earliest opportunity, so that any concerns can be raised and a plan of action can be devised. Patients/families/carers should be informed clearly on what to expect when discharged from hospital.

- Patients may need to take medications home with them
- Wounds may need dressing
- May have a follow-up outpatient appointments, e.g. physiotherapy, occupational therapy
- They may have to wait for equipment to be delivered
- Equipment may need to be put in the home before discharge for the patients safety, i.e. hand rails
- The discharge process should be discussed at all stages so patients/families/carers have an input and therefore can plan, alleviating undue stress and anxiety.

Summary

This chapter has discussed the nursing skills and considerations for the patient undergoing a surgical procedure. The primary goal of the nurse during this time is to maintain patient safety, ensure patients understand what is happening, prepare and support the patient throughout the surgical procedure until discharge home. Patients will have different needs and concerns depending on their surgery. There may be complications which vary depending on the type of surgery, the patient's presenting problem and any other specific needs to the patient (i.e. age, mental well-being, long-term prognosis) and the nurse is in a good position to advise and minimise complications.

References

Association of Anaesthetists of Great Britain & Ireland (AAGBI) (2014) *Peri-operative Care of the Elderly*. London: AAGBI.

Chapman, S.M., Grocott, M.P. and Franck, L.S. (2010) Systematic review of paediatric alert criteria for identifying hospital children at risk of critical deterioration, *Intensive Care Medicine*, 36: 600–611.

Ghandi, R., Rampersaud, N., Mahomed, R., *et al.* (2011) Patient concerns about undergoing elective musculoskeletal surgery. *Orthopaedic Proceedings*. Available at: www.bjjprocs.boneandjoint.org.uk/content/93-B/SUPP_IV/561.4 (accessed 10 January 2016).

Hayward, J. (1975) Information: a prescription against pain. *The Study of Nursing Care Project* Series 2 No. 5. London: Royal College of Nursing.

NCEPOD (2004) *Scoping Our Practice: National Confidential Enquiry into Patient Outcome and Death*. London: NCEPOD.

NHS Institiute for Innovation and Improvement (2008) *A Portrait of Progress: Annual Report and Accounts of the NHS Institute for Innovation and Improvement 2008–2009*. London: The Stationery Office.

Nursing and Midwifery Council (2015a) *The Code: Professional standards of practice and behaviour for nurses and midwives*. London: NMC.

RCN (Royal College of Nursing) (2005) *Peri-operative Fasting in Adults and Children. An RCN Guideline for the Multidisciplinary Team*. London: RCN.

RCN (Royal College of Nursing) (2013*) Guideline 3: Day Surgery Information*. London: RCN.

Royal College of Physicians (2012) *National Early Warning Score (NEWS): Standardising the Assessment of Acute-Illness Severity in the NHS. Report of a Working Party*. London: RCP.

WHO (World Health Organisation (2009) WHO Surgical skills checklist. Available at: www.who.int/patientsafety/safesurgery/tools_resources/SSSL_Checklist_finalJun08.pdf (accessed 24 March 2016).

Chapter 14

Tracheostomy care

Tina Moore

This surgical procedure can be traced back to Egyptian times. It is also written that Alexander the Great was supposed to have used his sword to relieve a soldier's upper airway obstruction. Hippocrates (a Greek physician) had also warned against the procedure, because of the risk of life-threatening haemorrhage from damage to the carotid arteries.

Key concepts

Tracheostomy

Suctioning

Tracheostomy tubes

Complications of tracheostomy

Learning outcomes

By the end of this chapter you will be able to:

▪ Demonstrate knowledge and understanding of a tracheostomy
▪ Identify reasons for this procedure
▪ Recognise and understand the use of different types of tracheostomy tubes
▪ Develop a plan of nursing care for a patient with a temporary tracheostomy
▪ Use the correct techniques to provide safe and appropriate tracheostomy care
▪ Detect possible complications and know the appropriate interventions for prevention.

Introduction

Anecdotal evidence suggests that nurses lack adequate knowledge and skill regarding this type of care. Indeed, reports conclude that there is still a lot of developmental work to be done to ensure that patients with tracheostomies are managed effectively, efficiently and safely. Practice settings receiving this patient group must ensure that staff have the appropriate knowledge and skill to manage such patients. This includes additional training and assessment of competence. While national competencies do exist, they do not appear to be fully integrated into mandatory training programmes for all healthcare professionals (ICS, 2014).

This chapter will discuss the principles of tracheostomy care as dictated by national guidelines. Readers should follow individual local guidelines on aspects such as humidification, cuff pressure, monitoring and cleaning of inner cannulae.

The trachea

The trachea (Figure 14.1) is the first part of the upper airway and stretches between the larynx and the carnia. It is D-shaped, with incomplete cartilaginous rings that are designed to protect the trachea. The main function of the trachea is to provide a clear airway for the passage of air to and from the lungs. The epithelial lining produces mucus that traps dust and other toxins, preventing it from reaching the lungs. Cilia on the surface of the epithelial cells move the mucus superiorly toward the pharynx where it can be swallowed and digested in the gastrointestinal tract.

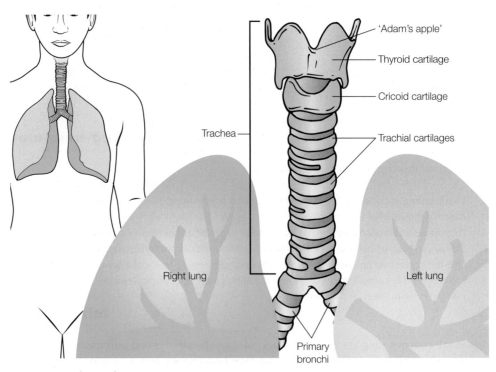

Figure 14.1 **The trachea**

Tracheostomy

A tracheostomy is an artificial opening in the trachea, created by a surgical procedure at the level of the 2nd and 3rd cartilaginous rings and it is kept open by the insertion of a tracheostomy tube.

In most cases (except in an absolute emergency), tracheostomies are performed with the patient under general anaesthesia, intubated, and paralysed. Performing a tracheostomy is difficult in children, because a child's neck is anatomically different from that of an adult. This is due to a number of reasons:

■ The neck is short (significantly less working space and all structures are close together, including carotid arteries)
■ The trachea is pliable and sometimes difficult to palpate
■ The cricoid can also be injured if it is not correctly identified (Mathur, 2014).

Types of tracheostomies

■ *Cricothyroidotomy* (also known as a mini-tracheostomy) provides an opening in the cricoid membrane (the cricoid space/area between the thyroid cartridge and the cricoid cartilage) allowing access to the airway below the glottis. It is lower than the conventional tracheostomy (i.e. between the tracheal rings). The tracheostomy tube is cuff-less and may be the quickest, easiest, safest and most effective way to obtain an airway for emergency intubation/difficult intubations. A cricothyroidotomy can also be used for an oxygenation and suctioning purposes. This procedure is more difficult in the child as their cricoid is the narrowest part of the airway (Mathur, 2014)
■ *Percutaneous tracheostomy* is more common. It is easier, safer and faster to perform than a surgical procedure. This approach uses a dilator system which reduces the incidence of complications (namely, bleeding). This tracheostomy is usually a horizontal 1.5–2 cm incision where dissections of the subcutaneous and deeper tissues are performed. The trachea is identified, then a cannula or needle is inserted into the trachea (usually at the level of the 2nd and 3rd cartilaginous rings) to aspirate air. Next, the trachea is dilated and tracheostomy tube inserted. This procedure is usually performed locally in ICU or theatres
■ *Translaryngeal tracheostomy* is a technique where a cannula or needle is inserted into the tracheal lumen. The guidewire is directed upwards and out through the mouth via direct visualisation. The existing tube is temporarily replaced with a narrower ventilation tube for the remainder of the procedure. The tracheostomy device is then drawn back through to the oral cavity, oropharynx, larynx, trachea and out into the surface of the neck (stoma). This technique may lead to lower rates of bleeding, trauma and infection of the tissues surrounding the insertion area compared with surgical techniques (NICE, 2013).

Indications for a tracheostomy

■ *To reduce the work of breathing*. Any condition causing the patient to struggle to breathe can lead to respiratory failure with dangerous levels of hypoxaemia and hypercapnia. No exchange of gas occurs until the alveoli. This is known as the anatomical 'dead space' (from the nose to the terminal bronchioles). A tracheostomy reduces this dead space by up to 50 per cent.

Endotracheal intubation lasting more than two weeks can result in tracheal stenosis. To aid more efficient gas exchange, a tracheostomy may also be performed in patients who are to be artificially ventilated for more than two weeks (reducing the anatomical dead space)

■ *To bypass a severe acute upper airway obstruction.* These include a foreign body that cannot be dislodged with abdominal thrusts or chest compressions; severe infections of the structures of the upper airway; laryngeal inflammation caused by burns to the mouth/neck; tumours, congenital abnormalities, vocal cord paralysis; facial fractures; facial/tongue swelling; oedema following head/neck surgery/ anaphylaxis and severe subcutaneous emphysema

■ *To remove excessive bronchial secretions.* Patients who have copious sputum and/or cannot cough adequately (due to pain or weakness) will require frequent suctioning, this may be more comfortable for the patient via a cricothyroidotomy.

Pre-operative care

Having a tracheostomy may cause the patient a lot of anxiety. To minimise this, the patient should be given as much information as possible about the procedure and after care (e.g. where the incision will be; type of tracheostomy tube; need for possible suctioning; altered body image; inability to talk, drink or breathe properly).

Alternative modes of communication should also be discussed and agreed. e.g. pen, paper, picture boards. Pre-operative education should occur as early as possible to give the patient adequate time to adjust. This will not be possible for emergency procedures.

Careful monitoring of the patient is required in patients who have coagulation problems; active bleeding in the neck; infection of the soft tissue of the neck (surgical site); gross distortion of the neck anatomy due to haematoma; tumour or scarring or obesity. Nurses need to be aware of these complications and these will influence their monitoring and clinical decision-making post operatively.

Types of trachoeostomy tubes

Tracheostomy tubes are made from medical grade polyurethane, polyvinyl chloride or silicone. These may mould themselves to the shape of the patient's airway. They should be rigid enough to maintain an airway but flexible enough to limit tissue damage and maximise patient comfort.

They are angled to allow the correct entry angle into the trachea and reduce the risk of trauma to the tracheal wall. The length of the tracheostomy tube is a critical variable, especially in neonates and infants, ranging from 2.5–5.5 mm in internal diameter and has lengths ranging from 30–36 mm for neonates and 39–56 mm for a child. A tube that is too short may result in accidental decannulation, the formation of a false passage or it may touch the posterior tracheal wall, causing obstruction and ulceration. Equally, a tube that is too long curves forward and can erode the anterior tracheal wall, which can be dangerously close to the innominate artery, causing possible haemorrhage.

If the tube is too big, the end may rub against the carina or lie within the right main bronchus, thereby occluding the left bronchus. Nurses must be aware of the type and size of the tube inserted.

Cuffed tracheostomy

These tubes are mainly used in critical care areas but are sometimes used post operatively. Cuffed tubes (Figure 14.2) allow positive pressure ventilation and help to prevent aspiration. If the cuff is not necessary for those reasons, it should not be used as it can irritate the trachea and can cause damage to the tracheal wall if over-inflated.

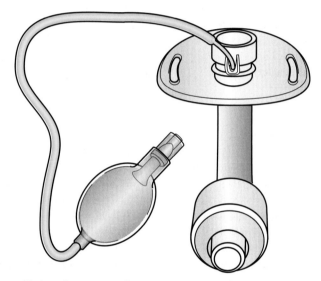

Figure 14.2 Cuffed tracheostomy tube

Cuffed tubes allow the trachea to be sealed off from the oesophagus and prevent reflux of contents, avoiding aspiration into the lungs. Therefore, eating and drinking are not advisable until assessed as able to do so. Ideally the tracheostomy tube should be changed to an uncuffed one, but if this is not possible, the balloon should be deflated. The patient should be able to produce sound. If there is a risk of aspiration, the cuff should be kept inflated.

Due to the delicate developing tracheal tissue and the narrow cricoid ring, cuffed tubes are not recommended and rarely required in children (although small cuffed adult tracheostomy tubes are sometimes used in large children and adolescents). An over-inflated cuff can cause trauma to the endothelial lining of the trachea, causing inflammation and fibrosis, leading to narrowing of the trachea, resulting in possible difficulty with future intubations.

The pressure within the cuff should be maintained between 20 and 25 cm H_2O. (ICS, 2014) and assessed/recorded a minimum of once per 8-hour shift with a pressure manometer (Figure 14.3). An over-inflated cuff can cause ischaemia to the tracheal mucosa causing ulceration or pressure necrosis.

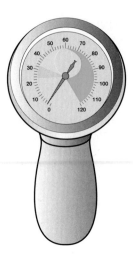

Figure 14.3 **Manometer**

Clinical significance

Particular attention should be paid to patients who have low perfusion, i.e. they are in shock as the epithelial wall can very quickly break down.

If an air leak occurs, check the cuff pressure and inflate the cuff when indicated. If the cuff pressure is at the maximum recommended and there is still an air leak, the tracheostomy may have become displaced and may require changing.

Ideally, the cuff should be deflated as soon as the patient is able to cough/swallow and the risk of aspiration is reduced. If the patient is at risk of aspiration, the cuff should be kept inflated.

Uncuffed tubes: non-fenestrated (tubes without windows)

Single-lumen tubes contain only the outer cannula. Today, most tracheostomy tubes used also have an inner tube (which is removable) (Figure 14.4). The outer cannula is the main body of the tube that passes into the trachea. The size of the tube usually refers to the inner diameter of the outer cannula. The inner cannula has the standard 15 mm attachment to connect to a breathing circuit (ICS, 2014). Failure to properly lock the inner tube in place can unlock the inner cannula in some devices, resulting in disconnection of the breathing circuit, in circumstances where it is connected to this rather than the outer cannula.

The first outer tube (and cuffed tube) are usually changed around 5–7 days postoperatively to allow for the stoma formation. The change is performed by a surgeon or anaesthetist. In the long term, it should be changed at least every 30 days or as per manufacturer's guidance.

The inner tube enables the maintenance of an open airway from occlusion caused by mucus and plugs. Removing just the inner tube may be enough to clear secretions

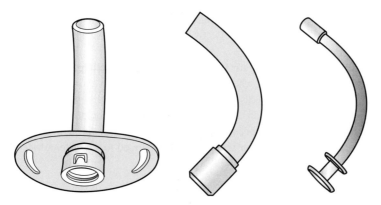

Figure 14.4 **Outer and inner tracheostomy tubes**

and can provide immediate relief of life-threatening airway obstruction in the event of blockage of a tracheostomy tube with clotted blood or encrusted secretions. Nurses need to be aware of the risk of blockage despite the use of an inner cannula and consider additional actions to unblock the tube. Maximum intervals for removing and cleaning inner tubes are recommended as four hourly for patients with a productive cough and eight hourly for other patients (ICS, 2014).

The inner tube should not be cleaned with tap water as evidence highlights the risk of contamination from legionella disease (Public Health England, 2010). Instead use sterile water or 0.9% saline.

Fenestrated tubes (tubes with windows)

Some tubes have single or multiple fenestrations on the superior curvature of the shaft (Figure 14.5). Fenestrations permit an airflow, which, in addition to air leaking around

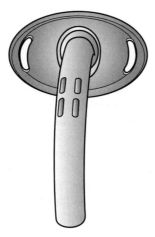

Figure 14.5 **Fenestrated tube**

the tube, allows the patient to produce sound (by air passing around the tube and through the vocal cords) and to cough more effectively. Patients must sit upright to minimise the risk of aspiration.

Cuffed fenestrated tubes (Figure 14.6) are particularly used in patients who are being weaned off their tracheostomy when a period of cuff inflation and deflation is required. Uncuffed fenestrated tubes are used in patients who no longer depend on a cuffed tube and are not at risk of aspiration. Under no circumstances should a suction catheter be passed through a fenestrated tube, as the catheter can be passed through the fenestrations and damage the trachea, the inner tube should be changed to a non-fenestrated tube for suctioning.

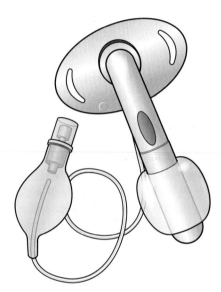

Figure 14.6 **Cuffed fenestrated tube**

Dressing

The risk of tube displacement is extremely high during the first few days. Generally it takes 7–10 days for percutaneous stoma to be established. Normally sutures are not used to anchor the tube, as this can be problematic during emergency decannulation. Instead the tube is kept in place by cotton tapes or a tracheostomy tube holder (Figure 14.7) through the neck plate (Figure 14.8). For safety reasons, changing of the tracheostomy dressing and tapes requires two people – one securing the position of the tracheostomy tube and the other performing the dressing. Any movement of the tube may cause irritation and stimulate the patient to cough and risk displacing the tube.

The original dressing should not be touched for the first 48 hours following surgery, this helps to prevent re-bleeding, infection and displacement of tube. If the dressing is soiled, it should be changed. The stoma site should be kept clean and dry to minimise infection. Wet dressings can cause infection and irritate the skin. If there is a collection

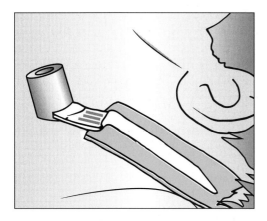
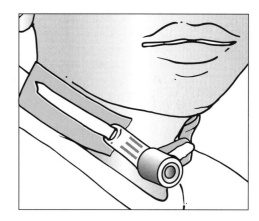

Figure 14.7 Tracheostomy tube tapes

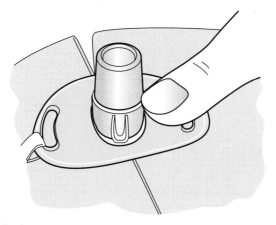

Figure 14.8 Neck plate

of secretions around the stoma, this should be cleaned with 0.9% saline at least once every 24 hours using aseptic technique, to prevent colonisation of bacteria. If the stoma becomes sore or red, a swab should be taken for microbiology.

A dressing is usually applied behind the flanges (Figure 14.9) to protect the skin. The dressing should be changed regularly. Some creams cannot be safely applied to the neck area near the stoma, so please check with your nurse specialist before applying.

Humidification

As the tracheostomy tube bypasses the normal processes of warming, moistening and filtering air, inadequate humidification of respiratory gases may lead to life-threatening blockage of the tracheostomy with tenacious sputum, keratinisation and ulceration of the tracheal mucosa, sputum retention, atelectasis, impaired gas exchange and secondary

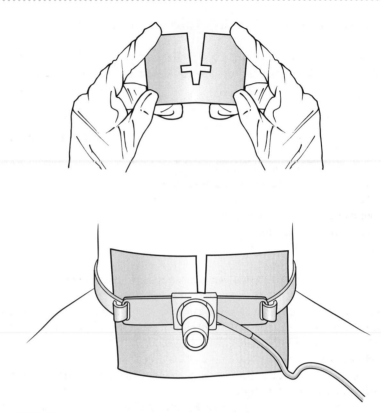

Figure 14.9 Flange

infection. Humidified oxygen helps prevent a build-up of secretions in the tube from becoming viscous.

The level of humidification required by patients will change depending on their clinical state, level of respiratory support required and their degree of hydration (ICS, 2014).

Humidification should be complemented by physiotherapy, early patient mobilisation, adequate hydration, appropriate suctioning, prompt treatment of infection and mucolytics in certain circumstances.

Suctioning

Suctioning must occur when the patient requires it, not as a matter of routine. This procedure should be performed under aseptic conditions with the patient sitting upright, when possible. Suctioning should be performed with a non-fenestrated inner tube as the suction catheter can pass through the holes of the tube and cause trauma to the tracheal tissue.

In order to prevent hypoxaemia occurring during suction, the size of the catheter selected should NOT occlude more than half of the diameter of the tracheostomy tube (ICS, 2014) i.e. the suction catheter should have a diameter no greater than half the internal diameter of the tracheostomy tube. The sizing formula is as follows:

Suction catheter size (Fg) = 2 × (size of tracheostomy tube – 2)

So, a size 8 tracheostomy tube would require a size 12 Fg (8 – 2 = 6; 2 × 6 = 12).
The lowest possible vacuum pressure should be used to minimise atelectasis.

Procedure for suctioning

Equipment needed at the bedside

- Suction machine (wall-mounted or portable)
- Suction catheter (a selection of appropriate sizes)
- Sterile water for irrigation
- Disposable plastic gloves and apron
- Sterile disposable container
- Bactericidal alcohol hand rub
- Tissues
- Goggles – nurses should consult their Trust's infection control policy.

1   Explain the procedure and gain consent if able. This may be a very traumatic procedure for children, so gain the cooperation of the parents. Possibly use play.
2   Wash and dry hands before and after the procedure.
3   Check that the suction machine is on and working.
4   Set at appropriate negative suction pressure (adult: 100–120 mmHg, child: 80–100 mmHg, infants: 60–80 mmHg).
5   Calculate the appropriate catheter size. For endotracheal and tracheostomy tubes the catheter size should not be larger than one half of the tube diameter.
6   Some patients may require hyperoxygenation and hyperinflation prior to suctioning (increasing their oxygen intake and encouraging the patient to take five deep breaths – this will need to be repeated post suctioning). Any increase in oxygen should be prescribed by the doctor.
7   If possible, the patient should be sitting upright with head and neck supported with a pillow.
8   Clean hands with alcohol rubs.
9   Use a clean disposable glove on one hand.
10 Withdraw catheter from sleeve without contaminating it.
11 Insert the suction catheter. Do not apply negative pressure on insertion.
12 On withdrawing the catheter, slowly apply suction pressure (by placing the thumb over the suction port control).
13 Withdraw catheter gently. Multiple-eyed catheters have holes around their diameters making the rotating method unnecessary. The whole procedure (insertion and withdrawal should not take longer than 10–15 seconds).
14 Monitor oxygen saturation levels and heart rate levels for any decrease indicating hypoxemia throughout the procedure.
15 On completion, wrap the catheter around the gloved hand, then pull back glove over soiled catheter and discard safely.

16 Rinse connection by dipping its end in the jug of sterile water and discard other glove.
17 Clean hands with bactericidal alcohol hand rub.
18 If further suctioning is required, start the procedure again with another catheter and glove. Cross-infection can become a problem if nurses do not adhere to the correct procedure for suctioning and as a result hands become contaminated. Patients who require suctioning are usually very ill and are often debilitated and susceptible to colonisation by the hands of staff during suctioning.
19 Repeat until the airway is clear (auscultate post suctioning). However, no more than a total of three suction passes are suggested (Glass and Grap, 1995). The patient must be allowed to rest between each suction pass.
20 Reconnect oxygen as soon as possible.
21 Evaluate effectiveness by conducting a comprehensive post-suctioning procedure – respiratory assessment.
22 Clean patient's oral cavity.
23 Ensure patient is left as comfortable as possible.
24 Document findings (NMC, 2015).

Post-suctioning assessment should include the type, tenacity, consistency and amount of secretions. Normal secretions (if produced, as most are swallowed) are white and mucoid (Box 14.1).

Clinical significance

Any difficulty in passing the suction catheter should lead to consideration that the tube may be partially blocked, badly orientated or misplaced and requires immediate attention.

Box 14.1 Complications of tracheal suctioning

- Hypoxaemia
- Infection
- Mucosal trauma
- Bradycardia and hypotension
- Prolonged coughing
- Haemorrhage
- Atelectasis
- Paroxysmal coughing
- Obstruction.

Speaking

Phonation is an important process that should be encouraged as soon as the patient's condition allows. Fenestrated tubes allow the air to go to the vocal cords and therefore produce sound. For patients with a cuffed tube, they should be able to tolerate the passive closure of the tracheostomy and as soon as the cuff can be deflated, a speaking valve (Figure 14.10) can be used to enable to patient to speak and eat. This is a one-way valve that fits at the end of the tracheostomy tube.

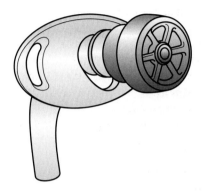

Figure 14.10 Speaking valve

Speaking valves will allow the patient to breathe in through the tracheostomy, but not out. The airflow has to go up through the larynx and out of the mouth, which allows the patient to talk, but it can be tiring for the patient due to increased resistance to airflow. Please note: because air cannot flow out through the tracheostomy, these valves can be extremely dangerous. Speaking valves should ideally only be used with an uncuffed and fenestrated tube (with fenestrated inner cannula).

If the patient has a cuffed tube, a speaking valve can be used with the cuff deflated; this is potentially dangerous and should only be used by staff with the experience and the necessary infrastructure to recognise and immediately manage any resulting complications (ICS, 2014).

Watch out

With the speaking valve in place, the cuff must ALWAYS be deflated otherwise the patient cannot exhale and will asphyxiate, suffer barotrauma or lose cardiac output as the intra-thoracic pressure rises.

A child's speech and language development should be addressed. And with early speech and language therapy intervention, their understanding of spoken language and production of speech will not be compromised. The speech and language therapist should be involved in their care as soon as possible to discuss communication options. This is particularly important in children as alternative ways of communication and ways to develop speech and language skills are required.

A baby (under six months) with a tracheostomy tube will communicate by using facial expressions such as smiles and frowns. Even though they are unlikely to be able to make a voice at this stage, it is important to continue to talk to them in a natural and enjoyable way and to respond to their communications.

Case study 14.1

Tomeka, 26 years old, was admitted to the Intensive Care Unit following a ruptured appendix. Post-operatively, she developed a wound infection and became ill. She was diagnosed with sepsis. She spent a total of 25 days in the intensive care unit – 15 of which she required mechanical ventilation. On day five of her stay in ICU, the decision was made to insert a tracheostomy. Her condition is now stable and she is on a general surgical ward.

- Think about how Tomeka might feel in relation to her altered body image.
- Think about any potential problems that may occur with the tracheostomy and formulate a plan of care to prevent them occurring.

Swallowing

Although oral intake may be difficult, it is possible. All patients should have an assessment performed for the risk of aspiration. If there is a problem or potential problem, e.g. those with neurological/mechanical causes of dysphagia, patients should be referred to the Speech and Language Therapy (SLT). SLT teams specialise in speech and swallow functions and can recommend if it is safe for the patient to start fluids/diet.

Sips of water should be started first and, providing the patient shows no signs of respiratory distress (coughing, desaturation, increased tracheal secretions, increased respiratory rate), gradually increased to free fluids and then a soft diet. The patient should be warned that initially they may feel discomfort on swallowing.

Monitoring of the patient's fluid intake, output and overall balance is essential as dehydration can cause the sputum to become thick and tenacious, leading to possible airway obstruction.

If the patient is unable to swallow or cannot tolerate fluids/diet and therefore is unable to maintain adequate nutritional hydration, alternative routes for nutrition and fluid should be administered, e.g. IV fluids, enteral feeding (see Chapter 17).

Complications

NCEPOD (2014) reported that half of all airway-related deaths and cases of brain damage in critical care of the airway problem were attributed to tracheostomy complications. Therefore nurses should be aware of these and take steps to minimise them. Some complications have already been discussed earlier in the chapter and Box 14.2 describes management of a blocked tracheostomy tube.

The following emergency equipment should be kept at the bedside at all times and checked at least once per shift:

- Tracheal dilators
- Suction machine/appropriate size catheters
- Disposable plastic gloves and apron
- Goggles (follow Trust policy)
- Oxygen with tracheostomy mask
- 10 ml syringe (if cuffed)
- Scissors
- Stitch cutter (if tube is stitched in)
- Non-rebreathing bag and tubing or bag-valve mask with reservoir and tubing
- Spare tracheostomy tubes – one same size and one size smaller (the stoma reduces in size due to the healing process).

Box 14.2 Management of a blocked tracheostomy tube

Signs and symptoms of a blocked tracheotomy tube

- Increase in respiratory and heart rate
- Agitation
- Cyanosis
- Patient may attempt to cough
- Secretions in the airway
- Wheeze
- Coarse breath sounds
- Change in pattern of breathing
- Absence of breath sounds
- Deterioration in oxygen saturations
- Coma and ultimately death.

This is an emergency situation!

- Assess urgency – contact anaesthetist immediately
- If possible, encourage the patient to cough
- Suction tracheostomy tube and oral pharynx
- Alter position
- Remove inner tube, if present
- If cuff is inflated – deflate it and suction again by deflating the tube – this can also allow some air to get into the lungs
- Remove tube and replace with spare tube
- Give 100% oxygen
- Monitor patient's respiratory status
- Cardiac arrest call if patient has stopped breathing.

Airway occlusion: blocked tracheostomy tube

- This is the most serious complication and is a life-threatening emergency. Changing and cleaning the inner tube should help minimise this. Nurses must remember that this can interfere with the promotion of sleep and rest. Care for these patients should be done at the same time where possible in order to create adequate time in between for resting/sleep
- In order to avoid complications, the main priorities are humidification, ensuring the cleanliness and patency of the inner tube, secure the fixation of the tube and pay attention to the cuff pressure (ICS, 2014).

Displaced tube

- Although dislodgment of the tracheostomy tube may occur at any time after tracheostomy placement, this complication is most problematic in the immediate post-operative period before the tracheostomy tract has developed – i.e. the first four days. Caution should be undertaken when moving, handling and caring for the patient to avoid any displacement. This can also occur through excessive suctioning, vigorous coughing, and inadequately secured tapes
- Tracheostomy tube dislodgement should be suspected when a patient is able to speak immediately after tracheostomy placement, the airway becomes obstructed, or respiratory distress develops.

Haemorrhage

- Early bleeding is usually the result of increased blood pressure as the patient emerges from anaesthesia (and relative hypotension) and begins to cough. Very close monitoring during the immediate post-operative period is imperative
- Massive bleeding is a life-threatening situation and will indicate rupture of the great vessels (i.e. the carotid arteries, the internal jugular veins). This is a risk in children or obese patients
- The thyroid gland lies anteriorly to the trachea with a lobe on both sides and the isthmus. This crosses the trachea at approximately the level of the second and third tracheal rings. This tissue is extremely vascular and could be at risk of accidental penetration.

Surgical emphysema

- Subcutaneous emphysema (air in the subcutaneous tissue) can potentially be dangerous as it may cause pressure on the organs of the upper airway.

Infection

- Nurses need to monitor the patient very carefully for signs of infection
- Tracheitis may be present. Humidification or saline nebulisers may help to moisten and warm the air, preventing drying out of the trachea. The patient also requires adequate hydration to help minimise the problem of thick sputum

■ Impaired cough reflex – an effective cough relies on the closure of the glottis. The tracheostomy tube prevents this closure. Suctioning may be required. If there is thick, tenacious fluid – a large bore – possibly a size 12 tube may be required.

Removal of tracheostomy (decannulation)

The tracheostomy tube should be removed as soon as is feasible. This allows the patient to resume breathing through the upper airway and reduces dependence (psychological and otherwise) on the lesser resistance of the tracheostomy tube.

Within the ward setting, this procedure will be performed by one of the medical team/anaesthetist and someone who can reinsert the tracheostomy tube (cannulation) should the patient develop problems immediately post decannulation – never by a nurse.

The recommended time for this procedure is early morning as the patient should be rested, and very close monitoring can be performed during the day for signs of deterioration of their respiratory status. Once the tracheostomy tube has been removed, the stoma should be covered with a semi-permeable dressing. The stoma should be dressed daily until the stoma is closed and the stoma site fully healed.

If the patient requires oxygen therapy, this should be administered via face mask or nasal specs. The patient should be instructed to apply gentle pressure with their fingers over the site when coughing.

Summary

Caring for a patient with a tracheostomy tube can be a daunting experience for student nurses. They should never be in a situation where they are left to care for the patient unsupervised. Care management requires a higher level of knowledge and understanding together with psychomotor skills. Often, when a patient has a high level of care demand to meet their physical requirements, this is often to the detriment of psychological needs. Nurses must pay attention to the effects that this procedure has on the way patients perceive themselves in relation to altered body image.

References

Glass, C. and Grap, M. (1995) Ten tips for safe suctioning. *American Journal of Nursing*, 5(5): 51–53.

Intensive Care Society (2014) *Standards for the Care of Adult Patients with a Temporary Tracheostomy*. London: Intensive Care Society.

Mathur, N. (2014) Pediatric tracheostomy, emedicine. Available at: http://emedicine.medscape.com/article/873805-overview (accessed 18 May 2016).

National Confidential Enquiry into Patient Outcome and Death (2014) On the Right Trach? A review of the care received by patients who underwent a tracheostomy, NCEPOD, London.

NICE (National Institute for Clinical Excellence) (2013) *Interventional Procedure Guidance: Translaryngeal Tracheostomy*, IPG 462. London: NICE.

NMC (Nursing and Midwifery Council) (2015) *The Code: Professional Standards of Practice and Behaviour for Nurses and Midwives*. London: NMC.

Numa, A.H. and Newth, C.J. (1996) Anatomic dead space in infants and children. *Journal of Applied Physiology*, 80(5): 1485–1489.

Public Health England (2010) *Guidance: Notifiable Diseases and Causative Organisms: How to Report*. London: Department of Health.

Part IV

Safety and protection

Chapter 15

Infection control

Sheila Cunningham

The control of infections is a serious problem in the UK in all settings (hospitals and community areas) and the reduction of infection risk which affects patients, carers and healthcare professionals is a priority (DoH, 2010, 2013). Consequently practices and skills which reduce or eliminate sources of infection help to protect clients and healthcare professionals from disease and illness.

Key concepts

Infection cycle

Standard precautions

Isolation procedures

Hospital-acquired infection (HCAI)

Personal protection/hand washing

Environment and waste disposal

Learning outcomes

By the end of this chapter you will be able to:

- Discuss the transmission of infection, the risks and potential consequences to the patients and the use of Standard Precautions in the prevention of hospital acquired infections (HCAIs)
- Take effective measures to prevent and control infection
- Demonstrate familiarity with the processes and purpose of environment hygiene and appropriate waste disposal or management to minimise overall risk
- Demonstrate knowledge and practice of effective practice in hand hygiene
- Explain the principles and procedures of standard isolation techniques for patients with infectious disease or who are immune-compromised and vulnerable to infectious disease and the risk of Exposure Prone Procedures.

Introduction

The news and the media often report on problems with infection and the consequences of it to human health. Examples include food-borne illnesses, influenza and of course 'superbugs' (like MRSA). Healthcare professionals and particularly nurses are often exposed to numerous micro-organisms, many of which can cause serious or even lethal infections (Efstathiou *et al.*, 2011). Infectious micro-organisms occur naturally in the environment potentially causing harm but can also be introduced to patients and clients though healthcare professionals performing caring practices and encounters. Termed 'healthcare associated infections' (HCAIs), they can cause unnecessary pain and suffering to patients and cause a range of symptoms from minor discomfort to serious disability and in some cases even death (NICE, 2014) and HCAIs cost the NHS approximately £1 billion per year (DoH, 2013). HCAIs are infections that develop as a direct result of medical or surgical treatment or contact in a healthcare setting. As health professionals we critically need to ensure we practise high quality caring skills to avoid such infections. There are regulations and frameworks to guide us and emphasise this responsibility including: the Health and Social Care Act (Regulation 12), Care Quality Commission (Outcome 8: The Hygiene Code), Essential Skills Cluster (Numbers 21–29: Infection Prevention and Control), NMC Standards (2010) as well as Health and Safety legislation (i.e. the HSAW Act, 1997) and the newer epic3 guidelines (Loveday *et al.*, 2014).

Activity 15.1

Choose an internet search engine and enter the term: 'Infection'. There will be over 200 MILLION UK 'hits' alone. There are options for a variety of information (type of infection, definitions, advice from NHS Choices and news and media reports). Select one or two of these choices and read them to familiarise yourself with some information on infection. You might be interested in the historical account of 'Typhoid Mary' and her work as a cook or the rise of 'Superbugs' like MRSA. Briefly reflect on these points:

■ How infection could affect you as a person (type of infection, prevention, risks)
■ How this might affect you as a nurse (in an elderly ward, for example)
■ List three or four ways in which an infection is passed on from person to person.

Rationale for prevention and control of infection

HCAI is a catch-all term for a wide range of infections. The best-known HCAIs include those caused by Multi-Resistant *Staphylococcus aureus* (MRSA), Methicillin-Sensitive *Staphylococcus aureus* (MSSA), *Clostridium difficile* (*C. difficile*) and *Escherichia coli*

Case study 15.1

1   Miss Freda Stolya, aged 79 years. Admitted to the elderly care ward after having a stroke and has severe weakness in her right arm and leg. She has osteoarthritis and finds mobilising difficult and painful and is almost immobile despite the nurses' and physiotherapist's attempts to help her regain some mobility. She has recently had a urinary catheter inserted for urine retention.

2   Freddie Shah is 4 years old. After coming home from nursery school today he complained of an itching eye and 'crying' a lot. His family doctor says he has conjunctivitis and gave him some eye drops.

3   Jim Murphy, aged 69 years, was admitted to the orthopaedic ward a week ago for a hip replacement for long-standing painful bursitis. His pre-operative assessment indicated he was a healthy gentleman and his swabs for MRSA were clear. After a successful recovery from his surgery he went back to his residential home. However, his wound is now angry and breaking down. The swabs taken by the district nurse indicate MRSA is isolated in the wound. The man in the next room to him (Mr Quinn) is small, frail, confused and has dementia. He is unsure where he is most of the time and tends to wander and can be occasionally incontinent. The residential home is busy and full of residents, there are very few en-suite rooms and residents often share bathroom and toilet facilities.

- What 'risks' of infection are there for Mrs Stolya, Freddie and Mr Murphy?
- How can you minimise these?

(*E. Coli*). Over four million people in the EU are estimated to acquire a healthcare-associated infection (HCAI) every year, some of whom die as a direct result of the infection. It has been estimated that 20–30 per cent of all such infections could be prevented by better infection prevention and control procedures (ECDPC, 2008). The prevalence of healthcare-associated infections (HCAI) was 6.4% in 2011 compared to 8.2% in 2006 and the the prevalence of antimicrobial use was 34.7%. (DoH, 2011). It therefore means that as nurses we need to be skilled at recognising the potential for and control of infections.

The four main infections of concern to patients are:

- Gastrointestinal (22 per cent)
- Urinary tract infections (19.7 per cent)
- Pneumonia (13.9 per cent)
- Surgical site infections (13.8 per cent).

The two most significant organisms causing infections in the UK with severe consequences are Methicillin Resistant *Staphylococcus Aureus* (MRSA) and *Clostridium*

Difficile (*C. Difficile*). In the majority of cases, cross-infection is *preventable* with attention to personal and environment hygiene, in particular, with simple tasks such as hand washing (Gould *et al.*, 2007; Huang *et al.*, 2012).

Transmission of infection and potential consequences to the patients

Every day people come into contact with huge numbers of micro-organisms. It is beyond the scope of this chapter to address these and how they may potentially cause harm and if you are unsure, read further in nursing texts focusing on microbiology or infections (Table 15.1). However, fundamentally understanding the principles of transmission of micro-organisms, informs the care practices intended to prevent the spread of these which may lead to infection. The transmission routes are important and this contributes to understanding the impact of infection on the patient.

Activity 15.2

Complete the following table on transmission routes using the information provided in the text (some have been given).

Route of transmission of micro-organism	Description	Care practices which may cause this
Person-to-person (or contact transmission)	Sneezing in enclosed space	
Food-borne	Organisms in food such as Salmonella in undercooked chicken	Not cooking thoroughly
Waterborne		
Airborne		
Insect-borne		

Table 15.1 Remind yourself of the following definitions

Viruses are ...	Bacteria are ...	Fungi are ...	MRSA is ...	Infection is ...
Small infectious agents that can reproduce only inside the living cells of organisms	Small simple primitive micro-organisms, single cells are capable of living and reproducing on their own	Simple plants that are parasitic on other plants and animals	A bacterium responsible for several difficult-to-treat infections in humans. It is also called Multidrug-Resistant Staphylococcus aureus (MRSA)	Invasion by and multiplication of pathogenic micro-organisms in a bodily part or tissue, which may produce tissue injury and progress disease

One of the basic infection control principles is the chain of infection. Transmission of infection in a care setting such as a hospital or residential home requires at least three elements: (1) a *source* of infecting *micro-organisms*; (2) a *susceptible host*; and (3) a *means of transmission* for bacteria and viruses.

The specific 'links' in the chain of infection are: reservoir, portal of entry, mode or means of transmission and portal of exit. Each link must be present and in a sequential order for an infection to occur. You might find it useful to refer to Figure 15.1.

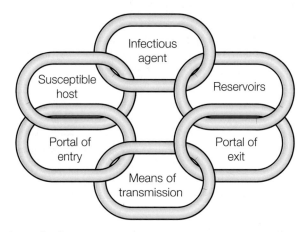

Figure 15.1 Chain of infection

Don't forget!

There are five main routes of transmission: person-to-person, airborne, waterborne (droplet), insect-borne and food-borne. Do note this categorisation varies a little in microbiological textbooks but not significantly so. The first three routes are critical to discussion of healthcare practice and control of infection.

Person-to-person (or contact) transmission

There are two key modes of contact transmission: direct contact and indirect contact. Direct contact transmission consists of direct contact from body surface to body surface and thus physical transfer of bacteria to a susceptible host from an infected or colonised individual. This may be through direct contact with body fluids, sexual contact or vertically from mother to baby. Bloodborne infections occur through sharp injuries or blood splashes, and the main concerns in healthcare settings are the direct transmission of HIV, Hepatitis B and C. Figure 15.2 shows human pathogen transmission.

Indirect contact transmission is the most significant route of transmission of micro-organisms. This involves contact of a susceptible host with an object contaminated by

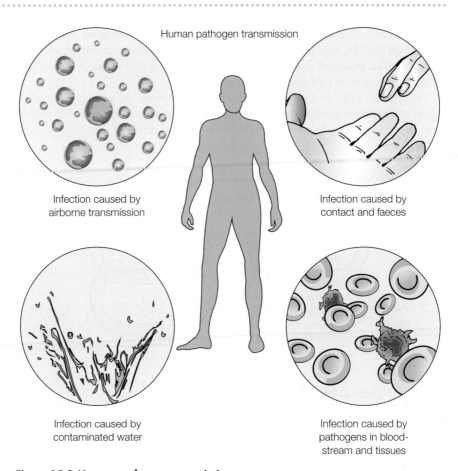

Human pathogen transmission

Infection caused by
airborne transmission

Infection caused by
contact and faeces

Infection caused by
contaminated water

Infection caused by
pathogens in blood-
stream and tissues

Figure 15.2 **Human pathogen transmission**

an infected individual, such as medical instruments, dressings, gloves or the hands of healthcare workers. Consider a community environment (a care home or nursery) with many staff equally busy with groups of people. If there are animals present, these also potentially present a source of microbes, a portal of exit and a route to transmission indirectly such as from the gastro-intestinal tract of animals passed on to humans e.g. *Escherichia coli*. This is also termed the 'faeco-oral' route of transmission.

Transmission can also be airborne or waterborne:

■ *Airborne*: this kind of transmission consists of dust particles containing bacteria or airborne droplet nuclei (small particle residues 5 mm or smaller in size) of evaporated droplets containing micro-organisms. Dust particles from bedclothes or ordinary clothing carry skin cells and can carry bacteria such as *Staphylococcus aureus* which can also be deposited to susceptible individuals

■ *Waterborne*: infectious droplets are generated during coughing, sneezing, talking or through procedures such as bronchoscopy and suctioning from infected individuals. Transmission occurs when these droplets are propelled a short distance through the air and deposited in a susceptible host's mouth, nasal mucosa, conjunctivae or inhaled. Droplet transmission is not to be confused with airborne transmission because droplets are larger and do not remain suspended in the air and special air handling and ventilation are not required.

It is important to appreciate that certain organisms can be transmitted through more than one of the above routes. Examples of organisms that can be spread by all of these routes are chickenpox (*Varicella zoster*) via airborne and direct contact or pneumonia (adenovirus) via droplet or direct contact.

Finally, the other routes only deserve a brief mention as they are not so frequently met but students should be aware of them. Food-borne transmission is via food stuffs. Insect-borne transmission involves insects such as fleas, lice, midges, mosquitoes and ticks.

The reservoir is the location where micro-organisms can be found. In healthcare settings this may include:

1   The environment, e.g. dust, bedding, equipment, furniture, carpets, sinks or washbowls, bedpans and surfaces.
2   Humans, including patients, staff and visitors, with sources especially from hands or clothing.

Susceptible host

The risk of an individual acquiring an infection is influenced by their susceptibility or vulnerability. The term 'host' is used to describe a welcoming (even reluctant) destination to harbour the organism. There are certain factors or characteristics which affect an individual's natural ability to fight against infection and these include:

1   *Physical and psychological well-being or presence of underlying disease*: diabetes mellitus, vascular disease, or malignancy may increase vulnerability by impairing the natural cellular or body defences.
2   *Immune status*: this will vary between individuals, especially those who are immune-suppressed. Immune-compromised statuses (due to HIV, chemotherapy treatment, steroid therapy) may also cause a weakness in the body's defences.
3   *Nutritional status*: if malnourished, this may impair the immune functioning.
4   *Age*: here susceptibility is greater in the extremes of age (the very young and the very old).
5   *Medical interventions or invasive techniques*: drug therapies such as antibiotics or steroids or procedures such as surgery, intravenous cannula, or indwelling urinary catheters all breach the body's natural defences and can be a source of susceptibility.

Points of entry into the body and portals of exit

These are required for micro-organisms to be transmitted from one individual to another. Pathogens gain entry into and exit the body in different ways (Figure 15.3), via:

- Natural orifices – openings such as mouth, nose, vagina, urethra, ear, rectum

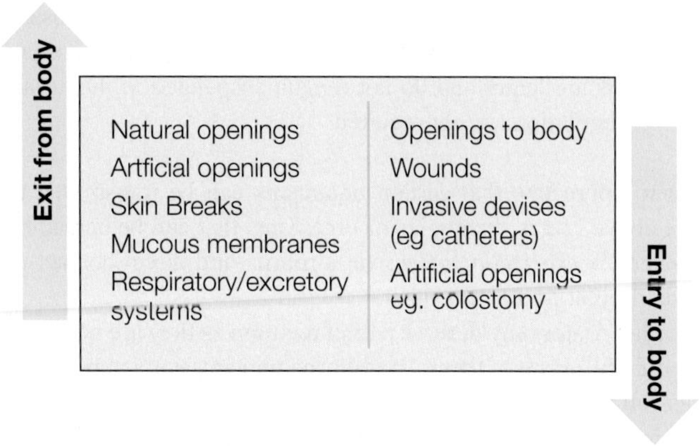

Exit from body	Entry to body
Natural openings	Openings to body
Artficial openings	Wounds
Skin Breaks	Invasive devises (eg catheters)
Mucous membranes	Artificial openings eg. colostomy
Respiratory/excretory systems	

Figure 15.3 **Entry and exit points to the body**

- Artificial orifices – breaching natural defences such as tracheostomy, ileostomy, colostomy
- Mucous membranes – which line most natural and artificial orifices, respiratory or excretory processes
- Skin breaks – either as a result of accidental damage or deliberate inoculation/incision
- Invasive devices, e.g. intravenous lines, urinary catheters, wound sites.

Essential measures should be taken by all health professionals to help prevent and control the chain of infection, including identifying and limiting reservoirs or sources, blocking routes of transmission, reducing portals of entry or exit and protecting vulnerable patients. Assessing these potential areas will help in formulating care practices to address this (Box 15.1).

Don't forget!

Recall the DH advertisement 'Catch it, Bin it, Kill it', what was being caught, how and why? Check out this site or find the video on YouTube: www.dh.gov. uk/en/Publicationsandstatistics/Publications/PublicationsPolicyAndGuidance/ DH_080839

Immunisation

This is often termed 'vaccination'. Immunisation is the process whereby a person is made immune or resistant to an infectious disease, typically by the administration of a vaccine. Vaccines stimulate the body's own immune system to protect the person against subsequent infection or disease. According to the WHO, immunisation is a proven 'tool'

Box 15.1 Sources of micro-organisms

Endogenous

Other sites on/in the host: example: *Escherichia coli* in the gut causes urinary tract infections.

Exogenous

Other people: examples: hands, coughs, sneezes.

Environmental

Contaminated equipment: examples: commodes, toilet handles/taps, patient contact, flat surfaces, dust, food and water.

for controlling and eliminating life-threatening infectious diseases. In the UK this is addressed through public health policies and schedules of immunisation which begin in the main in childhood but there are others: vaccinations (using manipulated organisms) for specific purposes such as when travelling to foreign countries or for vulnerable periods in people's lives, e.g., influenza vaccines for the elderly or immune-weakened individuals. The current DoH recommendations (2015) can be seen in Table 15.2.

Safe working practices: standard precautions

Safe working practice means making sure others are not put at unnecessary risk of acquiring or transmitting infection. For healthcare workers, breaking the chain of infection is very important (Figure 15.4). It is not always possible to identify who may have a transmissible infection and individuals may be unaware of the fact themselves (recall the extent of MRSA in the population). By relying on certain identification of infection or hosting infectious organisms, the healthcare worker may unknowingly expose themselves to potentially pathogenic micro-organisms. Safe practice involves:

- Effective hand hygiene
- Standard precautions (of blood and body fluids) to all individuals
- Effective cleaning, disinfection or sterilisation of reusable equipment, instruments or objects
- Aseptic technique
- Safe disposal of waste, non-reusable instruments, sharps and linen
- Isolation precautions when patients have known or suspected infection (or to protect from potential infection).

These aspects will be considered in the following sections.

To effectively prevent infections crossing between individuals and from environment

Table 15.2 Current 2015 UK vaccination schedules

Recommended age	Vaccine	Population
2 months	■ Diphtheria, tetanus, whooping cough (pertussis), polio ■ Haemophilus influenzae type B ■ Pneumococcal (PCV) ■ Rotavirus ■ Meningitis B	Children
3 months	■ Diphtheria, tetanus, whooping cough (pertussis), polio ■ Meningitis C ■ Rotavirus	Children
4 months	■ Diphtheria, tetanus, whooping cough (pertussis), polio ■ Pneumococcal (PCV) ■ *Meningitis B vaccine (infants born after May 2015)*	Children
12–13 months	■ Meningitis C ■ Hib ■ Measles, mumps and rubella (MMR) ■ Pneumococcal (PCV) ■ Meningitis B	Children
2–6 years old	■ Children's influenza vaccine (annual)	Children
3–4 years	■ Measles, mumps and rubella (MMR) ■ Diphtheria, tetanus, whooping cough (pertussis) and polio	Children
12–13 years (girls only)	■ Human Papilloma virus (HPV)	Young persons
13–14 years	■ Diphtheria, tetanus and polio ■ Men ACWY vaccine	Young persons
19–25 years (first-time students only)	■ Men ACWY vaccine	Young persons
65 and over	■ Influenza (every year) ■ Pneumococcal (PPV) vaccine	Older persons
70 years (and 78- and 79 year-olds as a catch-up)	■ Shingles	Older persons
Vaccines for special groups	Not routinely available, e.g. hepatitis B vaccination, TB vaccination and chickenpox vaccination	Risk groups, such as pregnant women, people with long-term health conditions and healthcare workers
Travel vaccines	Various: hepatitis A vaccine, the typhoid vaccine and the cholera vaccine Yellow fever	Travellers

Source: Adapted from DoH (2015).

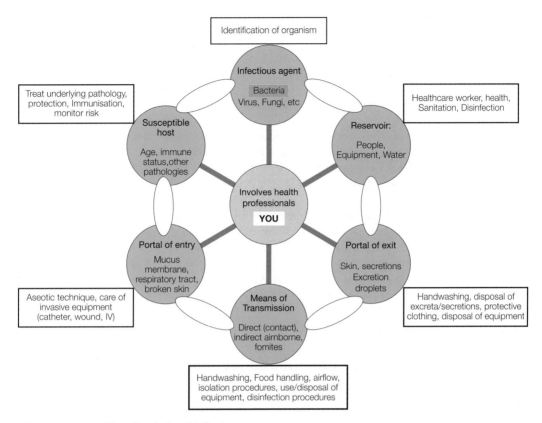

Figure 15.4 Breaking the chain of infection.

to individuals one 'breaks' the cycle of infection or transmission route. Standard (previously known as universal) precautions are the practices adopted by all healthcare workers when potentially coming into contact with hazardous body secretions, such as blood or body fluid. Some hospitals use the term universal infection control precautions (UICP) and others use the term standard precautions. The terms are now interchangeable. The key to this precaution is an assessment of risk of exposure to body fluids potentially infected by harmful viruses or bacteria, and the potential for staff to acquire or pass these organisms onto other individuals.

An example of the simplest chain of infection is an infected patient cared for by a healthcare worker who does not wash their hands before caring for another patient. The benefits of hand washing to avoid the spread of infection have been known for centuries. Cross-infection of organisms can be greatly reduced with simple precautions, including hand washing, asepsis and decontamination.

Clinical significance

Ask yourself – what precautions do I take? Assess the situation first.

Activity 15.3

Clinical significance

Sources of body fluids vary. Look back at Case study 15.1:

▪ What body fluids are potentially coming from these patients?
▪ What are the risks to you as a healthcare worker?
▪ What risks are there to the rest of the community (family, other patients, visitors, friends)?

Figure 15.5 shows your preliminary 'risk assessment' to consider the practices needed to prevent the spread of any infection.

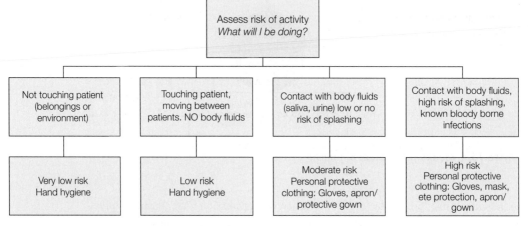

Figure 15.5 Safe working practices

Hand hygiene

Hands harbour millions of bacteria which can be passed on to equipment, the environment and other people. The number of bacteria (transient flora) on hands increases after routine actions, e.g. using the toilet, cleaning surfaces, opening doors. Thus the single most important task in controlling the spread of the bacteria is thorough hand washing (Gould *et al.*, 2007). Despite increased publicity and campaigns (Clean Your Hands, NPSA; 5 Moments, WHO), this procedure is still ineffective or insufficient in a number of practice settings, putting patients at risk. There are several terms used often interchangeably: hand hygiene, hand decontamination and hand washing. Hand washing is the key core skill. Hand decontamination refers to 'removal or physical removal of blood, body fluids and transient micro-organisms from the hands' (NICE, 2014), which can be achieved through hand washing or alcohol-based hand rubs. The

Watch out

Gloves are not a substitute for good hand hygiene. Hands still need to be washed before and after wearing gloves.

Don't forget!

The Clean Your Hands Campaign (2004) and the Catch it, Bin it, Kill it campaign (2011) emphasised when and how to perform hand hygiene. It is important to identify not only HOW to wash your hands but also WHEN. Additionally if there are grazes or breaks in the skin, these also need to be covered with a waterproof dressing.

type and availability of hand washing facilities influence how often and how adequately healthcare workers wash their hands (WHO, 2011).

The general guidelines are that hand hygiene should be performed:

- Before and immediately after each patient encounter or contact, especially if there is activity or contact that could potentially result in hands becoming contaminated
- If visibly soiled or contaminated with organic material then cleaned with soap and water
- At regular intervals if not visibly soiled with alcohol-based rub
- When in doubt – best to wash more often than not.

The WHO 5 Moments campaign identifies the points to think about hand washing as the need to perform hand hygiene at recommended moments as exactly where care delivery takes place. This requires that a hand hygiene product (e.g. alcohol-based hand rub, if available) should be easily accessible and as close as possible – within arm's reach of where patient care or treatment is taking place. Look at this site: www.who.int/gpsc/tools/Five_moments/en/. Point-of-care products should be accessible without having to leave the patient area.

WHO (2009a) identifies the concept of two virtual geographical areas: the patient zone and the healthcare area (or zone). The 'patient zone' relates to the patient and their immediate surroundings. Each patient has their own 'zone', so in a hospital ward situation, in a bay of four beds there are four 'patient zones'. This zone generally refers to a patient's person (body surface) and all inanimate surfaces that are touched by or in direct physical contact with the patient, such as the bed rails, bedside table, bed linen, utensils, clothing, infusion tubing and other medical equipment. It also refers to surfaces frequently touched by healthcare workers while caring for the patient, such as electronic machines, monitors, handles and buttons which could also be referred to in terms of 'high frequency' touch surfaces. The patient zone refers to all patients and the locations they generally are found in. In a clinical environment some patients may be in close contact with other patients (several zones nearby) or home care setting which is limited

Activity 15.4

Try one (or both) of these methods to see how effectively you wash your hands:

1   Obtain some glitter (any colour). Sprinkle this on your hands. Then wash your hands as you normally would with soap and water. In bright light can you see any remnant of glitter? If so, where? What areas did you neglect to wash effectively?

2   In your skills laboratory (or ask the Infection control team at your clinical area) for the 'germ' powder or gel. This is a substance which shows up under ultra violet (UV) light. Put a small blob onto your hands and rub it in like hand cream. Wash your hands as usual and then look under the UV light box to evaluate how effectively you washed your hands. What areas are missed? What steps did you miss when washing your hands?

to one patient zone. There are also 'critical sites' that encourage infection transmission in patients, which can be linked to the chain of infection: the patient as a reservoir of infection, or portals of exit or entry with the patient being a susceptible host. These critical sites may be natural or artificially created (intravenous cannula) as the source or potential vulnerable entry to micro-organisms.

The healthcare area contains all surfaces in the healthcare setting outside the patient zone (Figure 15.6). This area could be viewed as contaminated with micro-organisms that might be foreign and potentially harmful to a patient, either because they are multi-resistant or because their transmission might result in infection (HCAI). In the non-acute setting (residential homes, domiciliary areas), the choice of hand hygiene solution or procedure will depend on what is practically possible, the facilities available and what is appropriate for an episode of care. This is where an assessment of the risk is useful for the use of Personal Protective Equipment (PPE). It may be useful to carry some sort of alcohol gel rub until full hand hygiene is able to be performed.

Procedure to wash hands properly

The procedures for hand washing are simple: preparation, performing and drying. Best practice follows the guidance in Figure 15.7. Some areas of the hands are often missed when you wash your hands (HPA, 2011).

1   Ensure all the equipment you need is at hand (sink, soap, paper towels, bin).
2   Remove all jewellery.
3   Ensure water is at a comfortable temperature (ideally the sink will have elbow taps to adjust).
4   Follow the steps in Figure 15.8 (WHO, 2009b).
5   Use running water where possible.
6   If there are no elbow taps – use a paper towel to turn off taps and discard before drying your hands to avoid recontamination.

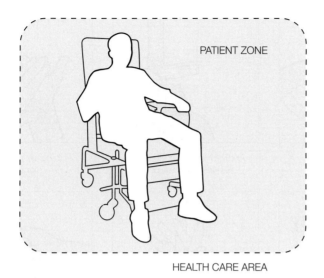

Figure 15.6 **The healthcare area**

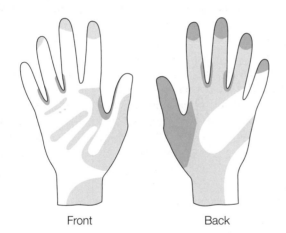

Front   Back

Figure 15.7 **Areas often missed when washing hands darker shade**

7   The stages of washing hands properly should take as long as singing 'Happy Birthday' twice (do not speed it up!).

In many skills laboratories you will be advised to perform this for a minimum of 30 seconds. However, the key is to attend to all the steps, being mindful of the potential 'missed areas'.

An alcohol gel rub

Alcohol hand rub is used for routine hand decontamination when hands are visibly clean. It should be applied in the same manner as hand washing outlined above but allow the

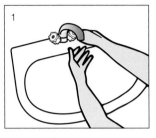

Wet hands with water

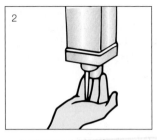

Apply enough soap to cover all hand surfaces (5 ml)

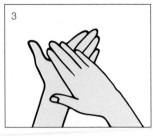

Rub hands palm to palm vigorously

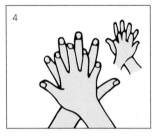

Right palm over left dorum with interlaced fingers and vice versa

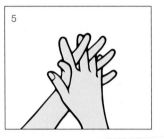

Palm to palm with fingers interlaced

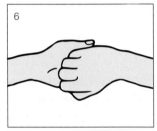

Backs of fingers to opposing palms with fingers interlocked

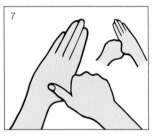

Rotational rubbing of left thumb clasped in right palm, not forgetting your wrists and vice versa

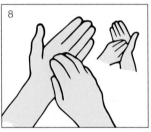

Rotational rubbing, backwards and forwards with clasped fingers of right hand in left palm and vice versa

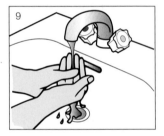

Rinse hands with water (downward direction)

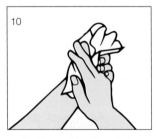

Dry thoroughly with a single use towel, use as many as required.

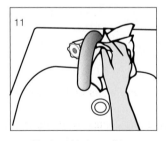

Use towel to turn off tap

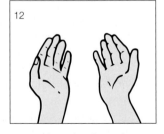

.... and your hands are clean.

Figure 15.8 **Hand washing for decontamination (adapted from WHO, 2009b)**

alcohol to evaporate from the hands. It should not be used when caring for patients experiencing vomiting and/or any diarrhoeal illnesses, e.g. Norovirus or *Clostridium difficile* spores and is not recommended in outbreak situations since it is not effective. Ultimately alcohol hand rub should not be relied on to replace hand washing with liquid soap and water. Remember the following:

- Cover cuts and abrasions with waterproof dressings
- Nails ought be short and avoid artificial nails or nail polish
- Emollient cream can be used to prevent hands from drying out. If hands develop problems, then advice ought be obtained from the local Occupational Health Department.

Don't forget!

It is important to know your glove size and ensure it is available and to keep your fingernails short and smooth. Gloves are single-use items and must be changed between patients or even between different procedures for the same patient. They also ought not be worn unnecessarily and special care is taken not to make the patient feel 'contaminated' with use of clear explanations of why they are being worn. In community settings, it is similarly important to remember that gloves are single use there too and performing tasks like writing in patient notes or answering the telephone are points at which gloves should be removed and hand hygiene performed.

Procedure to put on sterile gloves

1 Wash hands.
2 Check outer glove package for integrity and expiry date. Only open if intact and in date.
3 Sterile gloves are packaged pre-cuffed (the wrist part of the glove turned inside-out).
4 Set up your 'sterile field' before you begin in the middle of a clean dressing trolley, i.e. once you have opened the inner aspect of the first layer of packaging, this can be your sterile field (or a sterile towel).
5 Open the package and carefully empty the contents onto the sterile towel.
6 With dominant hand making sure you only touch the inner aspect of the cuff, ensure fingers of glove are face down to 'open'. Using the dominant hand to secure the glove, slide the non-dominant hand into the glove.
7 Put the second glove on, making sure you only touch the outer aspect of the glove with your sterile gloved hand (cup fingers under the cuff to only touch the sterile surface.
8 Sterile gloves should not come into contact with non-sterile surfaces or objects. If this does happen, then discard the gloves and start again.

See Figure 15.9 and watch this video: www.nottingham.ac.uk/nmp/sonet/rlos/placs/gloves/4.html

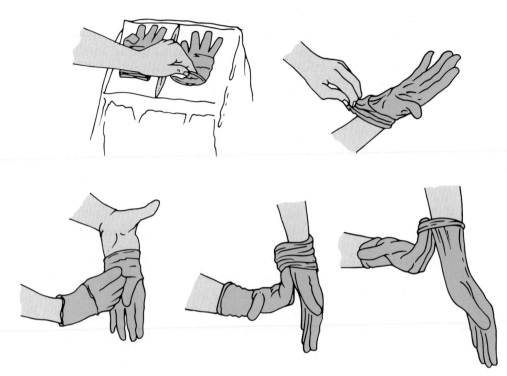

Figure 15.9 How to put on sterile gloves

Watch out

Other PPE includes face masks and eye protection. This will only briefly be touched on here. These are generally worn when there is a risk of blood or bodily fluids or organic matter splashing into the face, mucous membranes or eyes. Thus they would be more appropriate in areas where highly infected people are cared for or where there is increased risk such as surgical theatres and then a strict local policy of what and how the equipment is to be worn would be in place.

Personal protective equipment and clothing

Standard precautions also involve the use of personal and protective equipment (PPE) arising from the Personal Protective Equipment at Work Regulations 1992. This includes the use of gloves, aprons, gowns, face masks and eye protection (Figure 15.10). All disposable PPE is single use and should be changed between tasks, then discarded appropriately (e.g. clinical/hazardous waste if there is a collection system in place). Plastic aprons and gloves are most commonly used for protection. Uniforms are not regarded as Personal Protective Equipment. Different clinical areas use colour-coded aprons to distinguish use and purpose and are a visual reminder to healthcare workers. For example:

- White – where there is the risk of contamination from blood and body fluids
- Yellow – when caring for patients in isolation
- Green – when handling and serving food.

Gloves are worn for several types of care procedures but mainly for two main reasons:

- To protect the hands of the wearer from becoming contaminated with organic matter and micro-organisms
- To prevent the transfer of organisms already present on the skin and minimise cross-infection.

Gloves must be worn for invasive procedures, contact with sterile sites and mucous membranes. This also includes Health Care Professionals who have cuts or grazes (breaches in skin integrity); all activities that have been assessed as carrying a risk of exposure to blood, body fluids, secretions and excretions, and when handling sharps and contaminated instruments; gloves are not appropriate for routine care practices (e.g. assisting with meals, bathing.) and certainly not as a substitute for adequate hand hygiene. Some procedures may historically have required 'double gloving', particularly when punctures are likely to occur though this procedure will be evident in the local policy. This is not routinely advised especially if care risk has been assessed and good hand hygiene is performed.

Activity 15.5

Think about your current or last clinical placement.

- Where were the sinks for staff hand washing?
- How near to patients was it or did you have to walk a distance (more than a minute)?
- What were the taps like?
- What were the soap dispensers like?
- Were there instructions to aid the hand washing procedure?
- What hand drying facilities were there? Location of waste bins for the hand towels or wipes?

Were these HELPFUL or did they HINDER your own hand washing practice?

- Did you offer patients, relatives or visitors the opportunity to wash their hands?

Putting on Personal Protective Equipment (PPE)
· Perform hand hygiene before putting on PPE

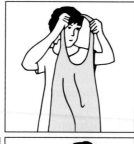

Apron
· Pull over head and fasten at back of waist

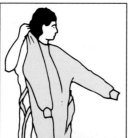 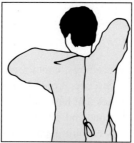

Gown, Fluid repellent cover
· Fully cover torso from neck to knees, arms to end of wrist and wraparound the back. Fasten at the back.

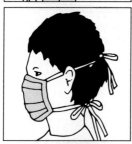 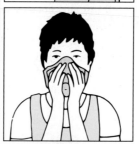

Surgical mask (or respirator)
· Secure ties or elastic bands at middle of head and neck
· Fit flexible band to nose bridge
· Fit snug to face and below chin
· Fit/check respirator if being wirn

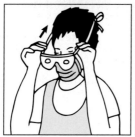 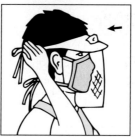

Eye protection (Goggles/Face shield)
· Place over face and eyes and adjust to fit

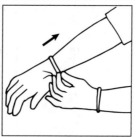

Gloves
· Select according to hand size
· Extend to cover wrist

Figure 15.10 (a) **Putting on Personal Protective Equipment**

Removing personal protective equipment (PPE)

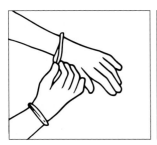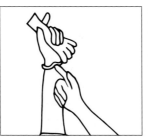

Gloves
- Outside of gloves are contaminated
- Grasp the outside of the glove with the opposite gloved hand, peel off
- Hold the removed glove in the gloved hand
- Slide the fingers of the ungloved hand under the remaining glove at the wrist
- Peel the second glove off over the first glove
- Discard into an appropriate lined waste bin

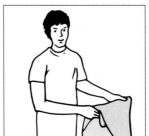

Apron
- Apron front is contaminated
- Unfasten or break ties
- Pull apron away from neck and shoulders lifting over head, touching inside only
- Fold or roll into a bundle
- Discard into an appropriate lined waste bin

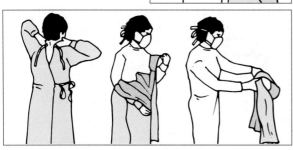

Gown fluid (repellent cover)
- Gown, Fluid repellent cover, front and sleeves are contaminated
- Unfasten neck, then waist ties
- Remove using a peeling motion, pull gown/fluid repellent cover from each shoulder toward the same hand
- Gown/fluid repellent coverall will turn inside out
- Hold removed gown/fuid repellent coverall away from body, roll into a bundle and discard into an appropriate lined waste bin or linen receptacle

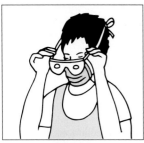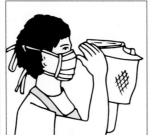

Eye protection (Goggles/Face shield)
- Outside of goggles or face shield are contaminated
- Handle only by the headband for reprocessing/decontamination or into an appropriate lined waste bin

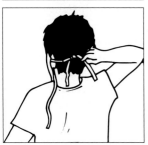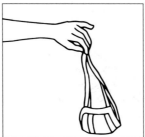

Surgical mask (or respirator))
- Front of mask/respirator is contaminated – do not touch
- Unfasten the ties – first the botoom, then the top
- Pull away from the face without touching front of mask/respirator
- Discard diposable items into an appropriate lined waste bin
- For reusable respirator place in designated receptacle for reprocessing/decontamination

Perform hand hygiene immediately on removal

Figure 15.10 (b) **Putting on and removal of Personal Protective Equipment**

Isolation procedures

This was formerly known as 'barrier nursing' and the term is still in use in some practice settings but the term 'isolation' will be used here to adhere to the NMC (2010) Essential Skills Cluster use as a specific skill. Healthcare providers need to demonstrate they are providing adequate isolation facilities for the prevention and control of infections (The Health and Social Care Act 2008). The Department of Health (DoH, 2010) suggests isolation of patients with suspected or confirmed infection is effective in reducing transmission. Isolation nursing is the use of infection control practices aimed at controlling the spread of, and eradicating, pathogenic organisms. Isolation nursing is undertaken in the patient's own room or home. There are two reasons for isolation nursing patients for infection prevention and control purposes:

■ To prevent transfer of infection from the patient to others (source isolation)
■ To prevent transfer of infection to another susceptible person (protective isolation).

In either situation, understanding of infection transmission, the use of standard precautions, PPE, hand hygiene, and waste disposal are key.

Activity 15.6

Draw up a care plan for a person entering isolation in a single room.

■ What are the key preparations for physical needs, emotional needs and psychological needs?
■ What advice would you give to visitors and family?

Clinical significance

Florence Nightingale was not a fan of 'germ theory' and challenged Pasteur's theory. However, she did believe infection was a self-perpetuating illness and best addressed with cleanliness and keeping the infected persons separate.

There is a move away from standard categories of isolation precautions (Gould *et al.*, 2007) to one of care tailored to meet the needs of the individual. However, there are times when the nature of the infection is not known and blanket measures must be implemented and standard principles applied. The key to these is good effective hand hygiene which you have practised (see above). The most effective form of isolation is a single room with a self-contained toilet and bathing facilities (basin or shower). However, in an outbreak of an infection where there are a number of patients with the same organism (type, onset and location) and there are too few single room facilities, then a further option is 'cohort nursing'. This procedure entails all the patients being cared for as a group (cohort) within a bay of a ward or a separate ward. If bays are used, then these must have a means to physically separate them from other patients, i.e. doors. Additional isolation precautions are only required when there is a specific risk from specific infections (tropical infections) and all hospitals and care areas will have their own policies and infection control teams to be responsible and follow advice with the best evidence-based care.

In the cases of any type of vomiting or diarrhoeal illness, patients must remain isolated/barrier nursed until they are asymptomatic for a minimum period of 48 hours clear of their last symptomatic episode.

In a community or residential setting the same principles apply, however, the specifics may be different. For a patient in their own home, isolation would mean staying within their home or residence and maintaining their own 'patient zone', ideally with their own dedicated toilet and sleeping or living areas. This can be difficult with a family present. However, maintenance of good personal hygiene is critical particularly hand hygiene at key moments such as after using the toilet or before eating. Outbreaks in residential environments require isolation as outlined above and precautions as much as possible in Box 15.2. Unnecessary movements to other locations (day centres, public venues) are to be avoided until the infection is ended. For outbreaks such as gastro-enteritis, this may mean up to 48 hours after the last symptom has ceased since the patient may still be infectious for a period after the symptoms subside. This is important especially when dealing with vulnerable people in the community such as young children, elderly people or those who are confused, anxious or disorientated (Box 15.3).

Waste disposal

The effective and safe disposal of waste starts with the healthcare worker who may be the nurse (RCN, 2007). Most healthcare waste is similar to domestic waste (cardboard, paper, etc.), however, a small proportion is infectious or hazardous (body fluids) and poses a risk to human health and the environment. Healthcare staff have a responsibility to consider waste and particularly assess the risk, take precautions in handling waste, and have systems in place to ensure no harm arises from the waste to service users, other staff and the environment (Control of Substances Hazardous to Health, 2002) (DoH, 2008; HSE, 2009).

The revised classification of waste highlights what is hazardous and what is non-hazardous. Furthermore, each of these categories is divided into clinical and non-clinical fields. The waste does need sorting in order for it to be disposed of appropriately. This has led to anxieties and confusion and the revised classification is simpler.

Clinical waste

This is divided into two categories: waste that poses a risk of infection; and waste that is medicinal waste. Risk of infection waste includes those with a known infection or waste which contains body fluids. Medicinal waste is expired, used, or contaminated medicine products, including vaccines and sera. It also includes equipment and devices used in the handling of contaminated waste, such as bottles, vials, sharps and packaging. Only cytotoxic (cytostatic) medicines are classified as hazardous and need to be separated for disposal. The new national coding scheme is recommended for disposal of waste and is now standardised across the UK (RCN, 2007; DoH, 2011). This can be seen in Table 15.3.

These bags are recommended to be positioned in places where the origin of the waste is generated, not filled more than three-quarters full, tied securely and appropriately labelled if needed by the local policy. Any liquid or solidified waste should be put into a solid or leakproof container and there should be arrangements in place at the ward or community setting to regularly transport the waste to a storage or disposal site. Recyclable uncontaminated and non-sharps waste items should be routinely segregated to be disposed of in appropriate recycling receptacles which are routinely found in clinical areas.

In the community there are additional challenges including the removal and transportation of waste. The Department of Health (2011) recommends that most bagged community nursing waste enters the orange stream (orange bags) and nurses carry yellow rigid boxes for any waste requiring incineration or, if cytotoxic, yellow boxes with purple lids. For patients with rare and highly infectious or dangerous infections should be contacted the Health Protection Agency should be contacted for advice not only on care but also on the waste disposal procedures of wound or other bodily fluids.

Box 15.2 Practical considerations for isolation procedures

Preparation

- Explain the need for isolation and gain consent
- Decontaminate hands before and after any contact with the patient and their belongings
- Single room or group area
- Physical separation maintained (closed doors, no unnecessary opening or going into and out of isolated area)
- An appropriate colour-coded isolation precaution sign (according to the suspected or confirmed infection) must be displayed outside the room on the door
- Wear appropriate PPE, i.e. gloves and aprons which should be available in the room and used to provide care to the patient
- Provide specifically designated equipment, e.g. sphygmomanometers, thermometers, commodes
- Maintain confidentiality of a patient's diagnosis while ensuring that healthcare workers and visitors are aware of the appropriate precautions for prevention and control of infection.

During the infection period

- Limit the number of staff entering the isolation room
- Consider the psychological needs of the patient during isolation
- Use single-use plastic apron for close patient contact (e.g. bed bathing, moving patient), when in close contact with potentially infected material (e.g. bed making), and any other situation when contamination of clothing may occur
- Remove apron, then gloves and discard promptly into yellow clinical waste bag
- Wash and dry hands thoroughly after having removed protective clothing and before leaving the isolation room. Use the alcohol hand rub/gel outside the room
- Protection of eyes, nose and mouth may be necessary if blood/body fluid sprays or splashes are possible – depends on infection, interventions and be guided by local Infection Control advisors
- Dispose of all excreta promptly, preferably by discarding it directly into the bedpan washer/macerator or the patient's own toilet. It should be considered hazardous waste for disposal
- All linen within the isolation room must be placed into water-soluble alginate bags
- Deal with any blood/body fluid spillage immediately, wearing appropriate protective clothing and disinfecting the spillage with locally recommended chemicals
- All crockery/cutlery should be decontaminated in a dishwasher with a final rinse temperature of 80°C
- The Infection Control Team/advisors advise on the frequency of cleaning the isolation rooms and solutions to be used
- Patients requiring therapy in their rooms should be seen last where possible and the equipment cleaned in-between patient use
- Minimal movement between departments/clinics is advised
- Equipment which is NOT single use should be cleaned between patients in accordance with local policy and manufacturer's instructions
- All staff and visitors to adhere to PPE and hand hygiene on entering an isolation room/area
- Documents and charts ought be kept outside the patient's room.

Following (end of isolation)

- The vacated bed, mattress and bed area on the ward must be thoroughly cleaned
- Enhanced cleaning of isolated area. Curtains and walls need only be washed if visibly soiled
- Enhanced cleaning of equipment according to local policy.

Box 15.3 Considerations in caring for an older patient with *Clostridium difficile* diarrhoea

- Source of organism: *faeces*
- Spread: *direct/indirect contact; airborne*
- Additional risk factors: *vomiting, incontinence; antibiotics*
- Mental/physical condition of patient: *potential confusion; immobility; unrecognised underlying diseases*
- Others at risk: *other older patients; those in same bay/nearby/sharing toilet facilities*
- Staffing/facilities: *availability of side rooms.*

What could be contaminated? Hands (of patient, carers); clothing; linen; refuse; toilet facilities; any areas contaminated with faeces or spores.

Table 15.3 Revised colour codes of waste segregation bags for safe disposal of waste

Colour	Type of waste (example)	Disposal description
Waste bags		
Purple/yellow (rigid containers or waste bags)	Infectious consisting of or contaminated by cytotoxic products	Incineration
Yellow bags	Infectious and other waste, e.g. anatomical, diagnostic specimens or chemicals	Incineration
Orange bags	Same as above	Requires rendering safe prior to disposal – in licensed or permitted facility Incinerated
Black bags (may be clear bags)	Non-infectious, non sharps, non-medicinal domestic waste e.g. packaging, flowers, etc.	Landfill
Yellow with back stripe	Offensive hygiene waste, e.g. sanitary wear, nappies	Landfill
Sharps boxes		
Yellow with orange lid	Sharps contaminated not with medicinal products (including cytotoxics) only bodily fluids	Requires rendering safe prior to disposal – in licensed or permitted facility Incinerated
Yellow with yellow lid	Undischarged or partially discharged sharps	Incineration
Yellow with purple lid	Sharps contaminated with cytotoxic material	Incineration

Sharps disposal

Sharps may include hypodermic, suture or biopsy needles, razor or scalpel blades, broken glass or other sharp objects. Many opportunities for injury can occur, e.g. inoculation, needle-stick injury, puncture wounds, cuts, grazes or scratches. Sharp tissues, e.g. spicules of bones or teeth, may also pose a risk of injury. These objects then need to be carefully discarded without causing any risks to those disposing of them. The highest risk of transmission of bloodborne infection via a sharp is through a hollow-bore needle-stick injury, either during use or after use but before disposal. Re-sheathing needles carries a high risk of injury and is not recommended. To aid safe practice, the following guidelines are proposed:

■ Never re-sheath needles. If re-sheathing is absolutely necessary, e.g. insulin syringes, use 'one-handed scoop' technique (WHO, 2001) (Figure 15.11)
■ Sharps should not be used in patients' rest areas or day rooms
■ Practise a safe handling technique, do not pass sharps from hand to hand – use a neutral zone (i.e. tray).

Scoop Technique – not to be used routinely only if ABSOLUTELY necessary (e.g with insulin syringes)

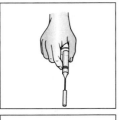

• Only re-sheath if a device is available that allows this to be done using one hand only.

• If no device available the single handed scoop method may be used.

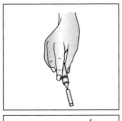

• Hold the barrel of the syringe with one hand and scoop the needle cap from a hard flat surface on to the end of the needle (whilst in a rigid container, i.e. injection tray/kidney bowl).

• Only when the needle tip is covered should re-sheathing be completed with the other hand.

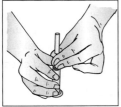

• When the cap covers the needle completely, use the other hand to secure the cap on the needle hub. Be careful to handle the cap at the bottom only (near the hub).

Figure 15.11 **One-handed scoop technique for re-sheathing needles**

The person using the sharps must dispose of them in a sharps box immediately after use and never leave them for someone else to clear away. If sharps are dropped, they should be left to fall with no attempt to catch them otherwise this would increase the risk of injury. In specialist areas such as operating theatres, it is recommended that used suture needles and scalpel blades be kept for safety on the appropriate sterile adhesive pad (e.g. Discard-a-pad) during the surgical procedure, prior to counting before disposal into the recommended sharps container. Syringes and needles should be discarded as a single unit wherever possible into a sharps container. In many clinical areas now safety syringes are being introduced which automatically retract the needle. Used needles and syringes, intravenous lines and cannulae must be placed in the sharps box immediately after use. Needles ought never be broken or bent or lines cut into pieces as this increases risk of injury. This is the same advice for patients using needles when injecting at home. For people with drug problems or using illegal drugs, many areas in the United Kingdom have needle and syringe programmes that provide free supplies of clean needles and advice on disposing of used needles safely in sharps boxes. These patients are also strongly advised not to reuse needles or share them due to the risk of transmitting blood-borne diseases such as Hepatitis B or C.

Safe practice with sharps also includes care with sharps boxes. Sharps containers should be correctly assembled prior to use, to prevent spillage of the contents, only filled to three-quarters of its capacity in order to reduce the risk of external contamination of the box, to prevent overfilling and to accept cannulae, wound drainage bottles, etc. before being sealed prior to its disposal without risk of injury to user. Boxes should be located in positions in wards/departments convenient to users of sharps to encourage immediate disposal after use. Wherever possible, take a sharps box to the bedside when undertaking procedures using sharps, e.g. giving injections. Injection trays with sharps boxes are generally available on wards and departments to aid safe practice. It is important that sharps boxes are not stored on the floor where they are a trip hazard and also should be away from the public reach and particular vulnerable people (children, the elderly, those with learning difficulties). In the main, boxes are to remain in ward/department in a safe area prior to collection. Sealed sharps boxes should be handled with care, do not throw, drop or invert them, carry them only by the handle. Disposal must always be by incineration.

Exposure-prone procedures (EPPs)

These are invasive procedures where there is a risk that injury to the worker from exposure of the patient's open tissues to the blood of the worker. These procedures include those where the worker's gloved hands may be in contact with sharp instruments, needle tips or sharp tissues (spicules of bone or teeth) inside a patient's open body cavity, wound or confined anatomical space where the hands or fingertips may not be completely visible at all times (Public Health England and DoH, 2014). Staff with blood borne infections are restricted from EPPs.

Accidents and incidents

The Safe Management of Health Care: Waste document by the Department of Health (2011) advises clinical areas to have written policies for waste disposal, and also for accidents or incidents. These should include: first aid measures, reporting routes to a designated responsible person, recording procedures, retention or investigation of the event and any remedial action.

Spillages of blood and potentially infected body fluids onto a floor, equipment or other surfaces must be cleaned as soon as they occur in order to prevent unnecessary exposure. To do this, staff must protect themselves with suitable protective clothing: gloves, aprons. Spillage kits are often available in healthcare settings especially for spillages of products such as mercury or other products, as a requirement by law if the product is to be used (COSHH, 2002). If no spillage kits are provided for bodily fluid spills, the preferred method for cleaning up spillages is use of disinfection products (as identified in the local policy), then wiped up with disposable cloths and disposed of in a clinical waste (yellow or orange) bag. If unusual or concerning infections are suspected, then advice from the appropriately qualified personnel, i.e. the Infection Control Team should be sought.

Cleaning and decontamination

Some equipment or instruments which may be used in patient care are reusable. All equipment will require cleaning. Some equipment will also require disinfecting or sterilising. Manufacturers of medical instruments (e.g. commodes, sphygmomanometers) are required to provide decontamination guidance for reusable products. The choice of method also depends on the purpose of the equipment and other risk factors such as whether it will be in close contact with the skin or mucous membranes (may need to be sterilised), is single use (sterilised), or may require disinfection or for low-risk cleaning.

- *Sterilisation*: this means an instrument or object is free from all micro-organisms. In hospitals this is done through heat or steam at high temperatures (autoclave). Ideally this is carried out in specialised sterilisation and disinfection units. The nurse needs to ensure the equipment is kept sterile until use and needs to check that the packaging is intact and does not exceed the expiry date
- *Disinfection*: this procedure ensures removal of harmful bacteria but not spores and is recommended for all instruments or equipment which has been in contact with body fluids, tissues or used on patients with known or suspected infection or on patients who are severely immune-compromised (poor immune systems and defences). Disinfection is necessary to prevent cross-infection transmission. It is required for most articles that may be contaminated with pathogenic micro-organisms, e.g. bedpans or that come into contact with mucous membranes, e.g. oral thermometers, endoscopes. The preferred method of disinfection is by heat
- *Cleaning*: ordinary cleaning with a neutral detergent and water is adequate where there is no decontamination with blood or body fluid and no contact with patients having known or suspected infections. Cleaning should ideally take place away from patient care areas with clean disposable cloths, and the equipment or patient area (bed, locker) should be rinsed and dried. Electrical equipment must not be immersed in water and must be disconnected from mains supply. Cleaning may be carried out using a detergent wipe or, alternatively, an alcohol wipe if there is no visible soiling.

Watch out

Research indicates that some equipment and belongings of patients are difficult to clean but local policies should be in place to advise. Fleming and Randle (2006) identified that toys harbour micro-organisms and are a significant risk in paediatric intensive care.

Summary

Micro-organisms are in the environment (air, inanimate objects, and people) and awareness of this is an important part of controlling their transmission. A fully functioning immune system and vaccination or protection are important but there are times when patients and vulnerable groups are unable to resist infections. The nurse has a key role to play using simple measures to control transmission of micro-organisms (hand washing, single-use devices), however, this still remains a problem. Constant vigilance and attention to sources of micro-organisms, routes of transmission and how to minimise these are important. Box 15.4 summarises good practice guidance for schools and childcare facilities (HPA, 2010).

Activity 15.7

Label the following **YES** if you think non-sterile gloves are necessary and **NO** if you think they are not.

- Administering naso-gastric feeding
- Taking a blood pressure post operatively
- Changing a catheter bag
- Making a bed
- Giving a patient a suppository
- Bed bathing an uninfected patient
- Giving a patient a drink
- Cleaning a bed following patient discharge from hospital.

Look back at Case study 15.1 in what instances would you wear gloves?

Box 15.4 Good practice guidance for schools and childcare facilities (HPA, 2010)

Good hygiene practice: A guide for schools and childcare facilities

- Handwashing is important: after using the toilet, before eating or handling food/animals. All cuts and abrasions must be covered with waterproof dressings
- 'Coughs and sneezes spread diseases' so wash hands after using disposing of tissues. Discourage spitting or clearing of noses without a tissue
- Disposable gloves and disposable plastic aprons must be worn where there is a risk of splashing or contamination with blood/body fluids (e.g., nappy or pad changing)
- Cleaning of the environment is necessary, including toys and equipment. This should be frequent, thorough and follow national guidance. For example, use colour-coded equipment, COSHH and correct decontamination of cleaning equipment
- All spillages of blood, faeces, saliva, vomit, nasal and eye discharges should be cleaned up immediately (always wear PPE). When spillages occur, clean using a product that combines both a detergent and a disinfectant. Use disposable paper towels and discard clinical waste as in the local policy. A spillage kit should be available for blood spills
- Soiled linen should be washed separately at the hottest wash the fabric will tolerate. Wear PPE when handling soiled linen
- Separate domestic and clinical waste. Used nappies/pads, gloves, aprons and soiled dressings should be stored in correct clinical waste bags in foot-operated bins.
- Animals in school (permanent or visiting) ought be kept separate to children's eating and sleeping areas. Waste should be disposed of regularly, and litter boxes should not be accessible to children.

References

DoH (Department of Health) (2008) *Clean Safe Care: Reducing Infections, Saving Lives.* London: HMSO.

DoH (Department of Health) (2010) Reducing Healthcare Associated Infections. Available at: http://hcai.dh.gov.uk/reducinghcais/ (accessed 20 January 2016).

DoH (Department of Health) (2011) Safe management of healthcare waste, v1.0. Available at: http://webarchive.nationalarchives.gov.uk/+/www.dh.gov.uk/prod_consum_dh/groups/dh_digitalassets/documents/digitalasset/dh_126348.pdf (accessed 20 January 2016).

DoH (Department of Health) (2013) Prevention and control of infection in care homes: an information resource. Available at: www.gov.uk/government/uploads/system/uploads/attachment_data/file/214929/Care-home-resource-18-February-2013.pdf (accessed 20 January 2016).

ECDPC (European Centre for Disease Prevention and Control) (2008) *Annual Epidemiological Report on Communicable Diseases in Europe.* Stockholm: European Centre for Disease Prevention and Control.

Efstathiou, G., Papastavrou, E., Raftopoulos, V. and Merkouris, A. (2011) Factors influencing nurses' compliance with Standard Precautions in order to avoid occupational exposure to microorganisms: a focus group study. *BMC Nursing* Available at: www.biomedcentral. com/1472-6955/10/1 (accessed 20 January 2016).

Fleming, K. and Randle, J. (2006) Toys – friend or foe? A study of infection risk in a paediatric intensive care unit. *Paediatric Nursing* 18(4): 14–18.

Gould, D., Chudleigh, J., Drey, N.S. and Moralejo, D. (2007) Measuring handwashing performance in health service audits and research studies. *Journal of Hospital Infection*, 66: 109–115.

HPA (Health Protection Agency) (2010) *Guidance on Infection Control in Schools and Other Child Care Settings.* Available at: www.hpa.org.uk/webc/HPAwebFile/ HPAweb_C/1194947358374 (accessed 10 November 2015).

HPA (Health Protection Agency) (2011) *Hand Hygiene for Health Care and Social Care Staff.* Available at: www.hpa.org.uk/webc/HPAwebFile/HPAweb_C/1194947403810 (accessed 6 February 2012).

HSE (Health and Safety Executive (2009) *Control of Substances Hazardous to Health Regulations (COSHH) 2002.* Available at: www.hse.gov.uk/coshh/ (accessed 20 December 2015).

COSHH (Control of Substances Hazardous to Health Regulations) (2002) 2677 regulation 7.

Huang, C., Wenjun, M. and Stack, S. (2012) The hygienic efficacy of different hand-drying methods: a review of the evidence. *Mayo Clinic Proceedings*, 87(8): 791–798.

Loveday, H.P., Wilson, J.A., Pratt, R.J. et al. (2014) epic3: National Evidence-Based Guidelines for Preventing Healthcare-Associated Infections in NHS Hospitals in England. *Journal of Hospital Infection*, 86S1 (2014): S1–S70.

MHRA (Medicines and Healthcare Regulatory Authority) (2011) Single-use devices. Available at: www.mhra.gov.uk/home/groups/dts-iac/documents/publication/con2025015. pdf (accessed 20 January 2016).

NAO (National Audit Office) (2009) Reducing Healthcare Associated Infections in Hospitals in England. London. The Stationery Office.

NICE (National Institute for Clinical Excellence) (2014) Infection prevention and control NICE quality standard [QS61]. Available at: www.nice.org.uk/guidance/qs61/chapter/ introduction (accessed 10 January 2016).

NMC (Nursing and Midwifery Council) (2010) *Standards for Pre-Registration Nursing Education.* London: NMC.

NNRU (National Nursing Research Unit) (2007) Does 'cohort nursing' help control healthcare acquired infection? Policy Plus Evidence 4. 1–2, Available at: www.kcl.ac.uk/ content/1/c6/03/09/92/PolicyIssue4.pdf (accessed 6 February 2015).

Public Health England and DoH (Department of Health) (2014) *The Management of HIV Infected Healthcare Workers who Perform Exposure Prone Procedures: Updated Guidance, January 2014.* London: Crown Publications.

Public Health England and DoH (Department of Health) (2015) The complete immunisation schedule. Available at: www.gov.uk/government/uploads/system/uploads/attachment_ data/file/500214/9406_PHE_2016_Complete_Immunisation_Schedule_A4_02.pdf (accessed 20 January 2016).

Royal College of Nursing (2007) *Safe Management of Healthcare Waste: RCN Guidance.* London: Royal College of Nursing.

WHO (World Health Organisation) (2001) *Injection Safety Toolbox.* Available at: www. who.int/injection_safety/toolbox/en/LeafletBestPracticesPrinter.pdf (accessed 6 February 2015).

WHO (World Health Organisation) (2009a) Clean care is safer care. Available at: www.who.int/gpsc/5may/tools/en/index.html (accessed 6 February 2015).

WHO (World Health Organisation) (2009b) *WHO Guidelines on Hand Hygiene in Health Care*. Available at: http://whqlibdoc.who.int/publications/2009/9789241597906_eng.pdf (accessed 6 February 2015).

WHO (World Health Organisation) (2011) *WHO Hand Hygiene Self-Assessment Framework*. Available at: www.who.int/gpsc/5may/hhsa_framework/en/ (accessed 28 February 2015).

Chapter 16

Safe and accurate administration of medicines

Sheila Cunningham

The administration of a medicine is a common but important clinical procedure and an important aspect of professional practice. The Nursing and Midwifery Council recognizes that it is not a mechanical task to be performed in strict compliance with the instructions of the prescriber but requires thought and the exercise of professional judgement.

(NMC, 2015)

Key concepts

Drug actions in the body
Medication routes and medication
    formulations
Administering medications
    safely

Legal aspects of medication
    administration
Considerations of medications for
    vulnerable groups
Drug calculations

Learning outcomes

By the end of this chapter you will be able to

- Discuss the actions of medications in the human body and their desirable and non-desirable effects
- Explain the legal implications of medication administration
- Describe the 'Rights' of safe medication administration
- Describe the routes of medication administration and explain safe practice in administering medicines via these routes
- Be familiar with drug calculations (oral and parenteral), including weight and volume conversions

■ Discuss individual differences and specific issues of safe medication administration for elderly, young and other vulnerable client groups

■ Self-evaluate your own practice in infection control knowledge and skills and develop an appropriate self-development plan.

Introduction

This chapter introduces the key theoretical and practical skills of medication action and administration to enable you as a nurse to practise safely and responsibly. The rights of the patients and the responsibilities of the people involved in the administration of medication are described. This chapter cannot address all aspects of drug action so you may wish to refer to a good quality pharmacology book after seeing some of the drug examples that will be used in this chapter and subsequent chapters, as pharmacological explanations are not provided. The examples in this chapter are used to illustrate the main points (names, labels, forms).

Activity 16.1

Before commencing reading this chapter, try to answer the following questions. What are your strengths and are there areas you need to develop?

1 What is a drug prescription? _____

2 Who are the main people involved in the prescription process? _____
_____

3 How many 'Rights' of drug administration are there? _____

4 Can medications be given up to 30 minutes before or after the time stated in the prescription chart? _____

5 Identify three reasons why patients/clients may not comply with taking medication and the nurses' responsibility to these patients. _____
_____

6 What does the 'generic' name of a drug mean? _____

The manner in which a medicine is administered will determine to some extent whether or not the patient gains any clinical benefit, and whether they suffer any adverse effect from their medicines. There have been incredible scientific advances in the past fifty years and these have enabled medicines to make a positive contribution to human morbidity and mortality. People are living longer, and with the use of powerful and effective drugs, at times complex drug regimens combined with technological advances mean that healthcare and nursing professionals have an increasing responsibility to have up-to-date knowledge and practice to ensure medication safety as well as keeping abreast of the relevant advances.

Alongside this are other potential problems. Drug reactions or non-adherence to medicines will have an effect on the medicine. Between one-third and half of prescribed medication for long-term conditions are not used as recommended (DoH, 2012); and as many as 50 per cent of older people may not be taking their medicines as prescribed (NICE, 2015). One of the most common types of adverse events is medication error, which is the most frequent cause of morbidity and preventable death in hospitals (Adams and Koch, 2010). NICE (2015) report that up to that 38 per cent of medication errors are serious or fatal, and 42 per cent of those are preventable. However, the incidence of medication errors in the NHS is unknown, so vigilance and preparation are still key to safe medication administration. Medication errors can take many forms, and may occur at different parts of the medication administration process (from prescription, dispensing or administration) and thus may involve a range of healthcare professionals (prescribers, pharmacists and nurses). Examples of factors contributing to these errors are:

- Poor medication labelling
- Poor communication about patients moving through care settings
- Lack of medicine verification on prescription and on administration (checking and double checking)
- An incomplete prescription
- Inadequate staffing levels
- Poor monitoring of patient response to medication or patient understanding of medication (Smith, 2004)
- Mistakes in dosage knowledge and calculation.

This has a potentially huge impact on the patient's health, and on the costs to the NHS and society as a whole. Nurses are responsible for administering medications and so are associated with approximately 26–38 per cent of medication errors in hospitalised patients (Bates, 2007). The nurse is the last person who can check the medication is correctly prescribed and dispensed before it is administered (Davey *et al.*, 2008).

Medications and the human body

The definition of a medicine used in the Medicines Act 1968 is: 'A medicine is any substance used for treating, preventing or diagnosing disease, for contraception, for inducing anesthesia or modifying a normal physiological function.'

The purpose of administering medications is to achieve a certain predicted effect in the body (Barber and Robertson, 2015) by being in a sufficient amount called the therapeutic level. Too little medication is ineffective and too much is potentially hazardous or fatal. Pharmacology is the science of medicines' action on and interaction with live organisms; in this chapter, this refers to humans. The four main divisions of pharmacology are:

- *Pharmacodynamics* – the study of what the medicine does to the body
- *Pharmacokinetics* – the study of what the body does to the medicine
- *Pharmaco-economics* – the study of the cost and benefit ratio compared with other treatments
- *Pharmaco-vigilance* – the study of medicine safety in the longer term.

Only the first two will be addressed briefly in relation to safe medicine administration.

Pharmacodynamics refers to the action of the drug at the cell level in the body. All body actions are controlled by components such as enzymes, receptors on cell surfaces, carrier molecules and cell integral proteins. Most drugs act by interfering with these control systems to bring about a change in function. This is then the drugs' effect. Most drugs produce their effects by binding to protein molecules (targets) such as enzymes, transport proteins, ion channels and cell receptors (Rang et al., 2012). Medications acting on cell receptors either inside or on the surface of cells bind with the receptor like a 'key with a lock', due to complementary binding sites, to instigate a response. The response can be to activate or to block a reaction in the cell known as an agonist or antagonist respectively. The medication therefore mimics the binding and actions of molecules naturally occurring within the body. An example would be morphine, which binds to cell opioid receptors in the nervous system. This then ultimately has the action of altering pain signals being transmitted to the brain and causing pain relief (analgesia). For more information, consult a good pharmacology text.

Pharmacokinetics refers to the effect of the body on the medicine or movement of the medicine through the body. You may recall from your clinical experiences when one medication worked better than another for a particular problem (e.g. blood pressure medications). This relates to individuals' responses to medicines from a genetic or other individual reason. There are four elements to pharmacokinetics relating to the entry of the medicine until the exit from the body: absorption, distribution, metabolism and excretion (ADME).

- *Absorption*: this is the process by which the medicine enters the bloodstream either orally (absorbed through the gastro-intestinal tract), via injection or via various other routes. Oral medications after absorption pass through the liver (first pass effect) where they may start being broken down by detoxification though some medicines use this process to be activated (e.g. atenolol, a beta blocker for hypertension)
- *Distribution*: this is the process by which the medicine passes from the bloodstream to the body tissues and cells
- *Metabolism*: this process is a series of enzyme reactions generally where the medicine is prepared for excretion
- *Excretion:* this process is the removal of the metabolised medicine from the body generally via the kidneys but also sometimes via the liver or the skin and lungs.

Medicines in blood levels and their actions are dependent on understanding the processes above. Thus, the frequency of giving a medication ensures a therapeutic level of medicine in the blood and the desired action, though this usually refers to adults with fully formed and functioning bodies. Achievement of therapeutic levels varies with the very young, the elderly and other vulnerable groups, as well as their differing body responses.

The World Health Organisation (1975) defines an adverse drug reaction (ADR) as an unintended harmful reaction to medicines. They state that no medicine is risk-free and as such effects and unintended (or side) effects are to be monitored (Table 16.1). Furthermore, the MHRA (2012) adds that an unwanted or harmful effect may also arise from combinations of medicines which may be those that the patients buy and self-administer or from herbal or nutritional supplements taken alongside prescribed

Case study 16.1

Nanna Griffiths is looking after her pregnant grand-daughter Nicole and Nicole's 5-year-old son Josh. As Josh is a lively child with learning difficulties Nicole needs some help as she is exhausted from her pregnancy. Nanna usually lives alone and is very independent, even with her high blood pressure. This is well controlled on beta blockers, statins and diuretics which she sets out in her 'dosette' box every Sunday evening for the week. Nanna really loves having Nicole and Josh stay but is amazed at how tiring it is.

Factors that influence the effect of drugs

- Nanna has been so busy over the last few weeks, she is forgetting to eat and today she forgot to take her lunchtime blood pressure medicine and takes both doses (lunchtime and evening one) together. What are the implications for Nanna? Why?
- Nicole has a headache and decides to take two tablets of paracetamol. What advice would you give her?
- Josh also says he has a headache and wants the same medicine as his mum. Is this OK?

Are there any other vulnerable groups or patient conditions you can identify (clue: nutrition, age, ethnicity, emotional and mental factors)?

Table 16.1 Examples of drug reactions

Medicine	Reactions
Erythromycin estolate (antibacterial)	Hepatitis (liver disorder)
Oral contraceptives	Thromboembolism (blood clots)

Source: WHO (2012).

medicines. One example cited was liver toxicity by Kava or Block Coshosh or the use of heavy metals which are toxic in some herbal preparations (MHRA, 2012). The concern is more with unregulated herbal products but the patients' use of such treatments does need to be identified. This emphasises the importance of communicating with patients and evaluating their understanding of medicines and medication actions and interactions.

Legal aspects of medications

The control of medicines in the United Kingdom is primarily through two key pieces of legislation: the Medicines Act (1968) and the Misuse of Drugs Act (1971), plus associated British and European Union legislation. Legislation on medicines applies to all healthcare workers and not just nurses and so is very broad. The Medicines Act (1968) is very comprehensive and addresses administration systems, packaging, licensing, sale and supply of medicines, to the public. This Act classifies medicines into three categories which designate how they can be obtained: (1) general sales list (GSL); (2) pharmacy only (P); and (3) prescription only medicines (PoMs). Since 2002, all new medicines are PoM for their first five years on the market (Crouch and Chapelhow, 2008). The key implications for nurses concern storage and possession of medicine container keys. It is also notable that only pharmacists (or dentists) can change the labels on medicinal products.

The Misuse of Drugs Act (1971) is the one most people have heard of from the media or current events. This has been subject to amendments and updates (called Regulations) to amend aspects of the Act. This Act and subsequent Regulations control medicines with the potential for abuse and regulate the import, export, supply and use of drugs, classifying them according to their potential for abuse. This is the Act the police and criminal authorities use to control the movement of drugs and impose penalties for improper supply or use. This Act classifies drugs into classes (A, B or C) with Class A being the most dangerous. The implications for nurses are in understanding the danger of certain drugs, in particular, those used therapeutically, and they need to be aware of the storage, reporting and chain of evidence issues around these medicines. With regard to lawful possession (for healthcare professionals) and supply, a different set of categories apply which are set out in the Misuse of Drugs Regulations 2001. This sets out five schedules, each with its own restrictions. Schedule 1 contains substances which allegedly have no medicinal value such as hallucinogens, and their use is limited primarily to research, whereas schedules 2–5 contain the other regulated drugs also termed 'controlled drugs', which has implications for storage (in a locked cupboard within a cupboard) and for documentation. This means that although drugs may fall into the category of Class A, B, or C, they may also fall into one of the schedules for legitimate medicinal use. For example, morphine is a Class A drug under the Misuse of Drugs Act 1971, but, when lawfully supplied, falls under the category of a Schedule 2 controlled drug.

Clinical significance

Following recent amendments to legislation, previously trained community nurses who might have been able to prescribe and administer a limited number of controlled drugs to patients in their homes (morphine for pain) were not allowed legally to collect a prescription or carry them to the patient but this has been amended and now they are. You may see this in practice.

The drug administration process

Drug administration is a process involving a chain of healthcare professionals. The prescriber writes the drug prescription, the pharmacist dispenses the prescription, and the nurse or other healthcare professional administers the drug to the patient; each is responsible for the accuracy of the prescription. The legal responsibility for the prescription lies with the person who signs the prescription (DoH, 2008). Nurses are expected to administer medicines safely and in a timely manner (NMC, 2010); this also includes assisting patients with self-administration in a variety of settings. This section addresses this.

Who administers drugs?

A range of healthcare professionals can prescribe drugs, from general practitioners, hospital doctors, pharmacist independent prescribers, dentists and more. Although prescribers may administer drugs to patients, other professionals, namely, registered nurses, midwives, and specialist community nurses, are usually responsible for administering drugs according to the Standards for Medicines Management (NMC, 2007). In some situations, designated non-professional personnel administer drugs or medications to clients (residential homes) and this is generally following training and preparation for competence while also following local policies and maintaining strict records of administration (CPE, 2012) and assessment of risk. It is also important to attend to local policies and procedures including the documentation and reporting of medicine administration or alterations to it.

The 'Rights' of medication administration

In order to prepare and administer drugs, it is important that you understand and follow professional guidance (NMC, 2007) and focus on the 'Rights' or 'correct actions' of medication administration. In practice, there is no set number of 'Rights' to follow though the key is safe medicine administration. Historically nurses were reminded of five 'Rights' or 'correct' checks. These were:

1. Right Patient
2. Right Medicine
3. Right Dose
4. Right Route
5. Right Time, with an additional Right Documentation.

Elliott and Liu (2010) propose three additional elements: Right action, Right form and Right response (Figure 16.1).

Some institutions or clinical areas recognise additional rights, such as the patients *right to know*, or the *right to refuse*. Patients need to be informed and educated about their medications as they are a partner in their care and treatment, and if a patient refuses a medication, the reason must be documented and reported immediately. These 'rights' should be checked before administering any medications. Failure to achieve any of these rights constitutes a medication error.

The Right patient

Before administering any medication, it is essential to determine the identity of the recipient. This is self-evident since the medication is prescribed for a patient for a specific purpose. The NMC clearly states in Standard 8 of the Standards for Medicines Management (2007) that 'you must be *certain* of the identity of the patient to whom the medication is to be administered'. To be certain, you must check:

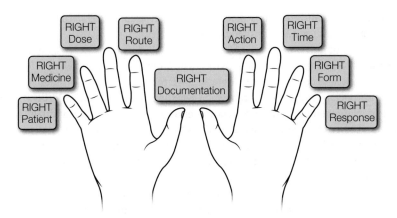

Figure 16.1 **The rights of medication administration**

■ Verbally – ask the patient their full name, date of birth, if an in-patient also the hospital number, if known. Asking 'Are you Mrs Jones?' may increase the risk of error since there may be more than one Mrs Jones, hence you should ask for more than one indicator of their identity

■ Visually – check the patient's name and (if an in-patient) against the name on the prescription chart

■ *Never use the patient's bed number or room number as identity*. Always verify the patient's identity as indicated above. The patient's details must match the prescription chart, i.e. patient's name, age and hospital number or address

■ Do note that not all patients or clients in healthcare settings wear identification bands, particularly mental health patients, learning disability clients or elderly persons in nursing homes. In these situations, extra vigilance is needed, as some patients may be confused or unable to identify themselves. The NMC (2007) suggests: 'Where there are difficulties in clarifying an individual's identity, e.g., in some areas of learning disabilities, patients with dementia or confused state, an up-to-date photograph should be attached to the prescription chart(s)'

■ In summary, nurses should know the local policy in place to ensure a firm system of identification.

The Right medicine

A medicine is a chemical substance that acts on the physiological processes in the human body. If nurses are unsure of the medicine and its action or purpose, they should check and, if necessary, confirm with the prescriber. Errors can occur if medicines have similar-sounding names, are referred to by their trade or proprietary names instead of their generic names or because the patient is allergic to them. For example, a patient who has type I diabetes mellitus would be given insulin since they cannot produce this themselves. Some drugs have more than one action. Aspirin, for example, is an antipyretic (fever-reducing), analgesic (pain-relieving), and anti-inflammatory medicine that also has anticoagulant properties (keeps the blood from clotting). A medicine may be taken for one, some, or all of its therapeutic properties.

The generic or non-proprietary name is the official accepted name of a drug, as listed in the British National Formulary (BNF) (Joint Formulary Committee, 2015). A drug has only one non-proprietary name, but can have many proprietary or trade names. By law, the European Union (EU) Directive on labelling of medicines 92/27/EEC requires the use of recommended international non-proprietary names (rINN) for drugs. In many instances, the British Approved Name (BAN) and the rINN were identical but where they were not, the BAN was modified to comply for consistency and safety. Many companies may manufacture the same drug using different proprietary (trade, patented, or brand) names (Table 16.2).

Activity 16.2

Look at the medicine trolley or cupboard on your clinical area. Make a list of five medicines in there. Identify the trade (proprietary name) and the generic name of these medicines.

Next look them up in a pharmacology textbook or formulary (such as the BNF). How many proprietary types could you find for each generic brand you identified in the cupboard?

Clinical significance

Patients may become confused with drug packaging changes, it is important the nurse understands the concepts of proprietary and non-proprietary forms of drugs and can advise, explain and support patients self-administering drugs to minimise anxiety and potential errors. There is a move to make designed drug packaging and labels clearer but patients still require support (NPSA, 2007). To minimise errors, medicines must be prescribed using only the non-proprietary names. There are also economic implications. Proprietary brands and sophisticated or colourful packaging may cost more than simpler, plain, non-proprietary brands of drugs. This may require extra vigilance by the nurse or whoever is administering the drug or even the patient who may be self-administering.

Watch out

Do note that some drugs have names that sound alike, or have names or packaging that look similar, thus a working knowledge of the names is essential. If in doubt, always consult a pharmacological text such as the British National Formulary (BNF) or the Electronic Medicines Compendium (EMC) or ask the local pharmacist. Table 16.2 includes a sample list of drugs whose names may be confused.

Table 16.2 Look-alike/sound-alike drugs

Drug name	Look-alike/sound-alike drug name
ceftazidime	cefotaxime
ephedrine	epinephrine
fluconazole	fluorouracil
folic acid	folinic acid
Losec	Lasix
vinblastine	vincristine

The right medication should also be one the patient is not allergic to. When administering a medication, the patient must be asked if they have any known allergies, and these *must* be documented in the appropriate place. Ask the patient about the allergic reactions they have experienced, as some may confuse a side-effect with an allergic reaction. Side-effects such as nausea, diarrhoea and sedation are frequently reported as allergies, when they are not. Do note allergies to components like protein are also important since medicine products contain constituents to fill them or provide colour or taste which may also cause an allergic reaction.

Don't forget!

The person who administers the drug has the last opportunity to identify an error before a patient might be injured or harmed. Rigorous checking should not be ignored even if it has already been done!

Top tip

Giving the wrong drug is a common medication error

In order to avoid errors, carefully read drug labels at the following times, even if the dose is pre-packaged, labelled, and ready to be administered:

- When reaching for the container
- Immediately before preparing the dose
- When replacing or discarding the container.

These are three additional check points to ensure safe administration.

Make sure the drug is not expired, and never give a drug from a container that is unlabelled or has an unreadable label.

The Right dose

As nurses are responsible for ensuring patient safety, they must also ensure that the prescribed dose is within the known dose range. Alongside this nurses should be vigilant when reading a patient's prescription. Errors could result from lack of clarity in written prescriptions (a decimal point in the wrong place could result in either a tenth or ten times the correct dose being administered), incorrect calculations or incorrect units of measurement (using symbols not words in full, e.g. μg interpreted as mg). The prescriber may write unclearly but the nurse administering the medication is also responsible.

Responses to drug actions differ according to the gender, race, genetics, nutritional and health status, age, and weight of the patient (especially children and the elderly), as well as the route and time of administration. *Body surface area* (BSA) is an estimate of the total skin area of a person measured in metres squared (m²). Body surface area is determined by formulas based on height and weight or by the use of a BSA nomogram. Many drug doses administered to children or used for cancer therapy are calculated based on BSA.

Procedure for administering drugs to patients

1   Carefully read the drug label to determine the *dosage strength*.
2   Perform and *check calculations* and pay special attention to decimal points.
3   Be sure to check for the recommended *safe dosage range* based on the patient's age, BSA or weight.
4   After you have calculated the dose, be certain to administer using appropriate standard *measuring devices* such as calibrated medicine droppers or syringes.

Table 16.3 sets out the steps in the procedure for medication administration regardless of route.

Clinical significance

The calibrated dropper supplied with a medication should be used ONLY for that medication. Be careful if using syringes for oral medicines – do not mix them up – oral syringes must not be used for injections.

The Right route

Medications must be administered through the route specified on the prescription. Medications are manufactured in a variety of forms: tablets, capsules, liquids, suppositories, creams, patches, or injectable medications (which are supplied in solution or in a powdered form to be reconstituted). The route indicates the site of entry into the body and method of drug delivery. Some forms of medication can be confused. There have been incident reports of death and harm in the UK and worldwide following wrong route errors when oral medicines dispensed in oral syringes have been administered intravenously in error (NPSA, 2007).

Table 16.3 **Principles of medication administration regardless of route**

Step	Procedure	Rationale
1	*Check:* *Patient notes and prescription chart:* for any known allergies *Prescribed dose:* ensure the dose is within the correct range for the patient *Prescribed date and time:* confirm this information *Prescription:* that it is clear and valid *Administration:* ensure the medicine has not already been given	Anticipatory checks PRIOR to administration to ensure safe administration of medication
2	Wash hands Prepare necessary equipment Inform patient of the medication, routes and reasons and gain consent to administer medication	Minimise infection transmission Gain patient cooperation
3	*Right patient* – check identity: *In hospital:* check the patient's name-band, hospital number and date of birth with details on the prescription chart (full) *In the community:* verbal confirmation of the patient's name from either the patient or the patient's carer; also a photo identification with the patient's name on it	To ensure appropriate treatment
4	Prepare *right medication* and check *right form* for *right route* and medicine not expired	To ensure safety
5	*Right time:* Also check that there are no other special requirements in relation to the administration of this medicine, e.g., after food, depending on blood pressure	To ensure optimal absorption of medicine
6	*Right dose:* Administer the medicine as prescribed. Do not leave the medicine unattended at any time	To ensure therapeutic levels of medicine through appropriate timing of doses
7	*Right action.* Observe the patient for any adverse reactions or signs of discomfort. If the patient experiences any adverse reactions to the medicine, this must be recorded and reported thereafter to medical staff	To monitor for desirable and undesirable effects reporting as necessary
8	*Right documentation.* Record that the medicine has been given or if not include the reason for not administering. Report as appropriate. Signatures must be legible and include both the date and time of administration	To comply with legal responsibility and be accountable for practice
9	Safely dispose of any soiled equipment. Refer to local policy guidelines for disposal of waste and infection control	Reduce infection or equipment hazards
10	Wash hands	

Source: Lister (2015).

Oral medications

Oral medications are administered *by mouth* (*per ora* or PO). Oral drugs are supplied in both solid and liquid form.

- The most common solid forms are *tablets* (tab), *capsules* (cap), and *caplets*
- *Scored* tablets have a groove down the centre so that the tablet can easily be broken in half. To avoid an incorrect dose, unscored tablets should never be broken for administration (Lister, 2015)
- *Enteric-coated* tablets are meant to dissolve in the intestine rather than in the stomach. Therefore, they should neither be chewed nor crushed
- A *capsule* contains a powder, liquid or granules in a gelatine case. *Sustained-release* (SR) or *extended-release* (XL) tablets or capsules slowly release a controlled amount of medication into the body over a period of time. Therefore, these drugs should not be opened, chewed, or crushed
- Tablets or *wafers* for *buccal* administration (absorbed by the mucosa of the mouth) and tablets for *sublingual* (SL) administration (absorbed under the tongue) should never be swallowed
- Oral drugs also come in liquid forms: *elixir*, *syrup* and *suspension*. An elixir is an alcohol solution, a syrup is a medication dissolved in a sugar and water solution, and a suspension consists of an insoluble drug in a liquid base.

Don't forget!

DO NOT substitute a different route for the prescribed route because a serious overdose or under-dosing may occur. Drug forms are made specifically for particular routes so tablets or capsules cannot be used for parenteral or injectable routes.

Parenteral medications

Parenteral medications are those that are injected (via needle) into the body by various routes. Drug forms for parenteral use are sterile and must be administered using aseptic (sterile) technique. The most common parenteral sites are the following:

- Intramuscular (IM): into the muscle
- Subcutaneous (SC): into the subcutaneous tissue
- Intravenous (IV): into the vein
- Intradermal (ID): beneath the skin.

Topical medications

Topical medications are those that are administered through the skin or mucous membrane. Routes include the following:

- ▢ *Cutaneous*: administered on the skin surface
- ▢ *Transdermal*: contained in a patch or disc and applied to the skin
- ▢ *Inhalation*: breathed into the respiratory tract through the nose or mouth
- ▢ *Solutions and ointments*: applied to the mucosa of the eyes (optic), nose (nasal), ears (otic), and mouth
- ▢ *Suppositories or pessaries*: are semi-solid and shaped for insertion into a body cavity (rectum or vagina) and dissolve at body temperature.

Sometimes a prescription may give a number of options of a route for the medication. The nurse must understand the differences between these routes such as the rate of absorption or onset of action. The form of the medication must be correct for the route of administration and fit with the timing as prescribed.

The Right time

The prescriber will indicate when and how often a medication should be administered. Medications must be administered at the correct time to ensure therapeutic serum levels. So how close to the prescribed time a medication should be administered? The guiding principle is that medications should be administered as closely to the prescribed time as possible. Bullock, et al (2007) state that if a medication is ordered to be given at particular time intervals, the nurse should never deviate from this time by more than half an hour. If administration occurs outside this 30-minute window period, the bioavailability of the medication and its therapeutic value may be affected. For some medications this could be disastrous, e.g., giving insulin too early with a time delay until a meal may result in a patient having a low blood sugar episode (hypoglycaemia) which could be dangerous. In addition, be aware of professional responsibilities: it is imperative that the patient is observed taking the drug, if it is left to take 'later', this constitutes negligence – once the administration process is commenced, the steps should be followed *all* the way through.

Administering medications at the right time also involves preparing the medication at the appropriate time. Medications should not be prepared many hours (or even one hour) before they are administered, unless the manufacturer recommends this. The right time of administration also involves administering the medication at the right rate as this may affect comfort. Be alert to allergic reactions or to other complications.

Oral medications can be given either before or after meals, depending on the action of the drug. Medications can be prescribed *once a day* (daily/od), *twice a day* (b.i.d./bd), *three times a day* (t.i.d./tds), and *four times a day* (q.i.d./qds). Drugs can also be prescribed to be administered as needed (*pro re nata* or prn). Table 16.4 shows the common abbreviations used. Most health or clinical institutions indicate specific times for these administrations and this is often clearly marked in the prescription chart. Community or other settings may not have charts but the nurse should check with the local policy and documentation to practice safely.

The Right documentation

The nurse must sign the medication chart immediately after administering the medication. This is a record of administration and a clear signal to other nurses taking over the

Table 16.4 Common abbreviations used for medication administration

Abbreviation	Meaning	Abbreviation	Meaning
Route:			
ID	intradermal	p. r. n.	pro re nata (when required)
IM	intramuscular	PO	by mouth
IV	intravenous	PR	by rectum
NG	nasogastric tube	SL	sublingual
PEG	percutaneous endoscopic gastrostomy	Supp	suppository
		Stat	immediately
PV	vaginal	top	topical
Frequency:		**General:**	
a.c.	ante cibum (before food)	g	gram
p. c.	post cibum (after food)	kg	kilogram
o. d.	omni die (every day)	L	litre
b. d.	bis die (twice daily)	mg	milligram
t. d. s.	ter die sumendum (to be taken three times daily)	mL	millilitre
t.i.d.	ter in die (three times daily)	NKA	no known allergies
q. d. s.	quater die sumendum (to be taken four times daily)	NBM	nil by mouth
o. m. or mane	omni mane (every morning)	SR	sustained release
o. n. or nocte	omni nocte (every night)		

Don't forget!

The term b.i.d.(twice daily) is not necessarily the same as 12 hourly. B.i.d. may mean administer at 10 a.m. and 6 p.m., whereas 12 hourly may mean administer at 10 a.m. and 10 p.m. (depending on the particular local institutional policy).

patient's care of the medication given as part of the nursing care. It is important to document any relevant information. For example, document patient allergies to medications, specific measurement, e.g. heart rate (when giving digoxin) or blood pressure (when giving antihypertensive drugs). All documentation must be legible. Remember the old saying, 'If it's not signed for, it's not done' and this may lead to confusion and potentially further unnecessary doses of medication being administered if assumed not given.

When administering medications 'as needed' (prn), the nurse should make a note of it in the patient's medical record as well as signing the chart. Documentation should include the medication's generic name, dose, time, route, reason for administration and the effect achieved. Nurses should be aware that accuracy of documentation is an important legal responsibility (Woodrow *et al.*, 2010).

Once a medication is administered, the nurse should monitor the patient to evaluate if the medication has the desired effect or response. This may be monitoring blood pressure or blood sugar depending on the type of medication. This observation is important also in evaluating any side-effects or undesirable effects. For example, codeine relieves pain, but its side-effects include constipation, nausea, drowsiness, and itching. These also need to be documented and reported to the prescriber.

The Right action

When administering a medication to a patient, the nurse must ensure that the medication is prescribed for the appropriate reason. For example, administering a sedating medication to a patient who appears very sedated or drowsy may be dangerous and should be questioned and checked with the prescriber. Similarly if a medication is for a purpose such as to lower blood pressure and the patient's blood pressure is very low, then this also should be brought to the attention of the prescriber. When a nurse is administering a medication, they should state to the patient the action of the medication and the reason for which it is prescribed, e.g., 'Here is your antibiotic for your chest infection'. This ensures the patient consents to receiving the medication but also is fully informed of the medication and will be a partner in their care and treatments. This could also be termed an additional 'right' or duty which is to inform and support patients to know their care and medication so they comply in their treatment regimen as informed partners.

Drug prescriptions

Before anyone can administer any medication, there must be a legal prescription for the medication. A *drug prescription* is a directive for a drug to be given to a patient and is based on patient consent to the treatment, recently more commonly known as a *Patient Specific Directive*. In order for a patient to receive a drug which is paid for by the NHS, a particular prescription must be completed (FP10). Some medicines are normally only available on prescription and not surprisingly these are referred to as prescription only medicines (or POMs), In addition, patients receive products on prescription that are not licensed medicinal products, e.g., appliances or dressings. Other medicines can be bought in pharmacies or from general retail outlets and this is a consideration for nurses when administering medications to patients to avoid situations of administering medications and patients self-administering their own purchased medication at the same time. Patients who are in-patients in a hospital will have medications prescribed on hospital prescription charts for use during the in-patient period only.

When checking prescriptions the following is advised by the Joint Formulary Committee (2015):

- Avoid unnecessary use of decimal points, e.g. 5 mg, not 5.0 mg
- Quantities less than 1 gram should be written in milligrams, e.g. 500 mg, not 0.5 g
- Quantities less than 1 mg should be written in micrograms, e.g. 100 micrograms, not 0.1 mg
- When decimals are unavoidable, a zero should be written in front of the decimal point where there is no other figure, e.g. 0.5 mL, not .5 mL

■ Micrograms and nanograms should *not* be abbreviated. Similarly units should *not* be abbreviated. For the purpose of this chapter abbreviations will be used.

Directions to the patient for use may be included but this will be clearly identified by the pharmacist dispensing the drug or medication following NPSA (2007) guidance.

Watch out

If persons administering drugs or medications have difficulty understanding, reading or interpreting the prescription, they must clarify with the prescriber. Consider the effect of administering Daonil (hypoglycaemic drug) instead of Amoxil (antibiotic) because the prescriber's handwriting was illegible.

Medication Administration Records (MARs)

Medicine Administration Records are often used in homes and residential care institutions, which should also be referred to in association with the patients' prescription and care plan. A Medication Administration Record (MAR) is a form that some healthcare institutions and other areas such as care homes and residential institutions increasingly use to document all the drugs administered to a patient. It is important to note that nurses or anyone else routinely administering medication should be prepared and informed of the responsibilities of drug and medicine administration. Invariably non-professional colleagues will administer oral or topical medications as injectable or other routes require specific training.

The national minimum standard for all care homes set by the Care Home Regulations (2001, cited in CSCI, 2008) is that the records detail for each person:

■ What is received
■ What is currently prescribed (including those self-administering medicines)
■ What is given by care workers
■ What is disposed of.

Homely remedy protocols are not prescriptions but protocols to enable administration of general sales list (GSL) and pharmacy only (P) listed medicines in settings, e.g., care homes, children's homes and some educational institutions. Although they have no legal standing, they are required for liability purposes. Any registrant using a homely remedy protocol must ensure there is a written instruction that has been drawn up and agreed in consultation with other relevant qualified professionals. (Where possible, this should be a medical practitioner or pharmacist.) The protocol should clarify which medicinal product may be administered and for which indication it may be administered, the dose, frequency and time limitation before referral to a GP. An example of a homely remedy could be paracetamol for a headache. All registrants using the protocol should be named and they should sign to confirm they are competent to administer the medicinal product, acknowledging they will be accountable for their actions (NMC Standards, 2007: guidance 22).

Clinical significance

Always read the expiry date! This is important because after the expiry date, the drug may lose its potency or act differently in a patient's body. Expired drugs should be discarded either in the clinical area or given to the pharmacy for disposal. Never give expired drugs to patients and patients should be advised not to keep drugs for a long time 'just in case' as they will not be as effective.

Administering medications safely

One of the first steps in administering medicines is to ensure the patient receives the right amount of medicine. You need to be confident and competent in calculating these amounts as well as understanding the units of measurement – this is too broad to address here but you are given a reminder of the key points for calculating oral tablet, oral liquid and parenteral injection medicines.

Oral medicines (tablets)

Oral medicines are given as tablets, capsules or liquids. These are generally presented in weight (tablets) or volume units of measurement. Weights are microgram (µgm), milligram (mg) or gram (g). Liquids are measured in millilitres (mL) or occasionally in litres (L). These are all metric units of measurement and are factors of 10 and there is a relationship between them. Perhaps the most common measurement is length, which is measured in millimetres (mm), centimetres (cm), metres (m) and kilometres (km). You need to understand the concept of units, tens, hundreds, thousands. and can see the connection between the units. The conversion between them is logical if you remember what the key prefixes mean, so kilo means a thousand (1000), centi means a hundred, etc. (Table 16.5).

Table 16.5 Converting one metric unit to another

	Kilo-	Fundamental Unit	Milli-	Micro-
Weight	**kilo**gram (kg)	gram (g)	**milli**gram (mg)	**micro**gram (mcg or µg)
Volume		litre (L)	**milli**litre (mL)	**micro**litre (mcL or µL)
Length	**kilo**metre (km)	metre (m)	**milli**metre (mm)	**micro**metre (mcm or µm)

To convert between grams and milligrams it is a factor of a 1000 because 1 g equals 1000 mg (Table 16.6). If you want to know what a millilitre is in litres, this is also a factor of a 1000 but this time is means 100 times smaller (or 1/1000th of a litre) so you need a decimal point because the number is less than 1. Thus, 1 mL = 0.001 L. One easy way to remember this is to move the decimal point (Box 16.1).

Table 16.6 Equivalences for measurement

1	Gram/litre
10	Decigram/litres (not generally used in practice)
100	Centigrams/litres
1000	Milligrams/litres
10 000	Micrograms/litres

Box 16.1 Converting metric values

To convert a large number to an equivalent smaller number (e.g. mL to L), move the decimal place three places to the <u>LEFT</u>:

1,750 mL = 1750.0 L = 1 7 5 0 . 0 L = 1.750 L = **1.75 L**

Use this to convert mcg to mg, mg to g (smaller value to larger)

To convert a small number to an equivalent larger number (e.g.. g to mg), move the decimal place three places to the <u>RIGHT</u>:

0.5 g = 0.500 mg = 0 . 5 0 0 mg = 0500.0 mg = **500 mg**

Use this to convert mL to mcL, mL to L (larger value to smaller)

Practice

1   What is 750 mg in g?
2   What is 600 mcg as mg?
3   What is 300 mg as g?
4   What is 2,500 mL as L?
5   What is 0.085 m as cm?
6   What is 50 mL as litres?
7   What is 0.07 g as mg?
8   What is 0.89 L as mL?
9   What is 0.00625 mg as mcg?
10 What is 15 g as mcg?

Calculations review

The key information you need is the dose required and the amount available. Thus, if a patient needs 1 gram of paracetamol and the bottle in the medicines cupboard states:

Paracetamol tablets 500 mg.

How much do you give? You need to know the relationship between grams and milligrams (mg). There are 1000 mg in 1 g. So 500 mg is half a gram. If you follow this thought through you will realise that 500 plus 500 equals 1000.

So, 500 mg × 2 = 1000mg or 1 gram. So you give 2 tablets.

This is an example of a logical relationship and working out medicines as you work out other numerical parts of your life (dividing bills in restaurants, adding VAT to purchases or calculating the cost of travel). There is an easy formula to remember this but do use your own logical sense too. Remember always to double check calculations with another nurse before giving medicines.

The formula is:

What you WANT divided by what you HAVE AVAILABLE multiplied by the AMOUNT (W/A × V)

Box 16.2 shows examples.

Box 16.2 Patient dosages

Patient 1

A patient needs Tolbutamide 0.5 g. The available tablets are Tolbutamide 500 mg. How much do you give?

1　What is the relationship between mg and gram? 1 g = 1000mg.
2　Work out that 0.5 g is the same as 500 mg.

The available medicine is Tolbutamide 500 mg, so you give 1 tablet.

Patient 2

Another patient needs Methotrexate tablets 7.5 mg. The available medicine is Methotrexate 2.5 mg tablets. How much do you give?

1　Work out the relationship between mg and mg – they are the same – so that is OK.
2　You want 7.5 mg. It is available as 2.5 mg per tablet. So use the equation:
　　7.5 mg/2.5 mg × 1 = 3

So you give 3 tablets. Double check: 2.5 × 3 = 7.5 mg, so this is correct.

Watch out

You need to ensure you are working with the same units of measurement. Do not confuse grams and milligrams – convert medicines to the same unit before completing calculations for accuracy!

In Case study 16.1, Josh becomes unwell. He now needs some oral antibiotics and is prescribed Amoxicillin syrup 125 mg every four hours by mouth. The medicine bottle Nicole has states:

Amoxicillin syrup: 250 mg/5mL

She is unsure how much to give and has an oral syringe – help her work this out:

1 What is the relationship between mg and volume? 250 mg in a volume of 5 mL
2 Now identify how much you want – since you need 125 mg, this is less than 5 mL but how much?

Use the formula:

Want	Available	Volume	Answer
125 mg	250 mg	5 mL	?
125 mg/250 mg × 5 mL = 2.5 mL			

The answer is 2.5 mL.

Activity 16.3

Practise these calculations:

1 A child is prescribed oral chloral hydrate 250 mg. The drug is available as an elixir containing 200 mg in 5 mL. How much do you prepare?
2 Prescription is oral phenobarbital (phenobarbitone) 45 mg. It is available as 15 mg in 5 mL. How much do you prepare?
3 Oral paracetamol 80 mg is prescribed. It is available as a syrup with 120 mg in 5 mL. How much do you prepare?
4 The prescription reads co-trimoxazole 480 mg. The medicine is available as syrup containing 240 mg in 5 mL. How much do you prepare?
5 A patient is to have 125 mcg digoxin orally. The medicine is available as tablets and the label states each is 0.0625 mg. How much do you prepare?

Injections (parenteral)

This formula works for injection preparation too. Mr Cleary needs an injection of 75 mg pethidine for pain. You have ampoules of prepared pethidine containing 100 mg in 2 mLs. How much do you draw up?

Think logically to estimate – is it more or less than 2 mLs? It is less. Then use the calculation formula:

Want	Available	Volume	Answer
75 mg	100 mg	2 mL	?
75 mg/100 mg × 2 mL = 1.5 mL			

There are other more complex calculations involving patient's body weight, flow of infusions over time. Do seek a good calculation book to practise these.

Box 16.3 shows how to read a prescription.

Practical administration skills

Oral medications

Before administering, follow steps 1 and 2 in general principles, as shown in Table 16.3.

Procedure for administering oral medication

1   Ensure the correct form of the medication is available and prepare equipment: medicine pots, tissues, cups and water/milk to swallow medicines.
2   Re-check the prescription.
3   Calculate the required number of tablets/capsules or liquids to achieve the prescribed dose.
4   Place the correct dose into a medicine pot – avoid handling the medicines (use the non-touch technique with lids of medicine pot) (Figure 16.2).
5   When all medicines are ready, re-check the patient's identity according to local policy.
6   Hand medicines to the patient together with an appropriate drink to swallow the medicines. Ensure the patient has swallowed the medicines.
7   Do not interfere with time-release capsule or enteric-coated tables. Do not crush or open. Do not hide medicines in food (covert administration) this is deceitful and unethical (NMC, 2007). Ask patients to swallow these whole and not to chew them.
8   Sublingual tablets must be placed under the tongue. Buccal tablets must be placed between the gum and the cheek and not chewed but allowed to dissolve.
9   When administering liquid medicines to very young, to very old persons, emaciated or vulnerable persons, these can only accurately be measured with an oral syringe. This is preferred to a spoon. If using a syringe, the correct procedure is to place the tip of the syringe into the mouth towards the side and let the contents slowly

Box 16.3 Reading a prescription

Prescriber:	Dr D O Good
Prescriber address:	100 High Road, New Town
Prescriber phone number:	0111 222 333
Date prescription written:	02/07/2016
Patient's full name:	Mr Patrick Patient
Patient address:	Flat 1, Tower Block, Newtown, TE22 1ST
Patient date of birth:	02/04/1992
Drug name:	Amoxycillin
Dosage:	25 mg/5 mLs
Route:	PO
Frequency:	Three times a day
Amount to be dispensed:	105 mLs
Directions to the patient:	Take 125 mg three times a day for 7 days ensure the course is completed
Refill instructions:	No more refills on this prescription

Example

Read the prescription and complete the following information.

Date prescription is written: _____

Who is the doctor prescribing the medicine?_____

Patient address: _____

Patient date of birth: _____

Generic drug name: _____

What form is the medicine? _____

What route must this be taken? _____

Frequency:_____

Amount to be dispensed: _____

Directions to the patient: _____

discharge towards the inside of the cheek. Pause to let the medicine be swallowed. If these groups are uncooperative, it may help to place the barrel of the syringe between the teeth but care needs to be taken not to harm the patient. The process needs to be documented in the care plan and on the medicine record.

10   Afterwards, observe patient for any reactions, ask them how they feel.

11   Dispose of any packaging (e.g. blister packs) according to local policy.

Injections

An *ampoule* is a glass container that holds a single dose of medication. It has a narrowed neck that is designed to snap open. The medication is aspirated into a syringe by gently

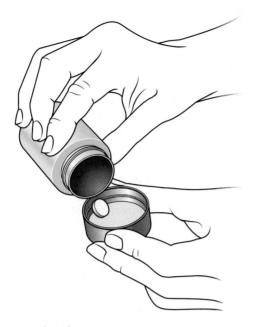

Figure 16.2 **The non-touch technique**

pulling back on the plunger, which creates a negative pressure and allows the liquid to be pulled into the syringe (Figure 16.3).

A *vial* is a glass or plastic container that has a rubber stopper on the top. This stopper is covered with a lid that maintains the sterility of the stopper until the vial is used for the first time. Multidose vials contain more than one dose of a medication. Single-dose vials contain a single dose of medication, and many drugs are now prepared in this format to reduce the chance of error. The medication in a vial may be in liquid or powdered form and may need to be 'reconstituted' with a liquid called a *diluent*. Commonly sterile water and 0.9% sodium chloride 'normal saline' are used to then become the medicine to be administered. Drugs and medications in this form need to be given as soon as they are reconstituted due to their limited stability (NPSA, 2007).

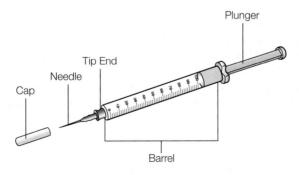

Figure 16.3 **A syringe**

Procedure for preparing a syringe

1   Open the syringe packaging at the plunger end and remove the syringe.
2   Do not touch the tip end of the syringe, hold this in one hand while carefully opening the needle packaging.
3   Attach the needle to the tip of the syringe, ensuring you do not touch the sterile ends.
4   Do not remove the needle cap yet but ensure the syringe plunger is functional. Place in tray while preparing the medicine.

Procedure for preparing the injectable medicines

This should be in an area which is as clean, uncluttered and free from interruption and distraction as possible. Ideally, preparation should take place as an area dedicated to this process.

Ampoule (solution)

1   If drawing up from a glass ampoule/vial, tap the ampoule to ensure all the medicine is at the bottom of the vial. Check solution for cloudiness or visible particles, do not use if this is present and report the medicine to pharmacy.
2   Snap off the top, ensuring you cover the neck of the ampoule with a sterile swab or the syringe packaging to protect your fingers. Some medicines may be provided with small files to enable snapping off of the top. If using a plastic ampoule/vial, then break off the top ensuring you do not touch the open part. Inspect the ampoule contents for glass or plastic fragments. If present, these must be discarded and reported.
3   Use a 'non-touch' technique, i.e. avoid touching areas where bacterial contamination may be introduced, e.g. syringe-tips, needles, vial tops. Never put down a syringe attached to an unsheathed needle. Wash hands and wear gloves.
4   Place the syringe firmly in your dominant hand and the medicine in the other. Let the needle cover slide off the needle into the tray, insert the needle into the ampoule/vial and into the solution.
5   Draw up the medicine by pulling back with the plunger – you may need to rest your index finger on the flange of the syringe to do this using your other fingers to manipulate the plunger.
6   Replace sheath on needle carefully (NB: this is a sterile needle and this is NOT *resheathing*). Tap to dislodge any air bubbles. Check you have the correct amount of medicine in the syringe
7   Attach a new needle and discard used needle into the sharps box.

Ampoule (powder requiring reconstitution)

1   Ensure you have correct diluents (type and amount).
2   Follow steps 1–4 above for powder and diluent ampoules. Add the drawn-up diluents to the powder in the ampoule. Gently mix the diluents and powder without

removing the needle. Check the solution and when clear, draw up the prescribed amount

3   Replace needle sheath and attach new needle (as above).

Multidose vial (powder)

1   Use a 'non-touch' technique, i.e. avoid touching areas where bacterial contamination may be introduced, e.g. syringe tips, needles, vial tops. Never put down a syringe attached to an unsheathed needle. Wash hands and wear gloves.

2   Remove the tamperproof cover of the multidose vial and clean the rubber seal according to local policy and let this dry for at least 30 seconds.

3   To minimise environmental exposure of the drug when drawing up (Doughty and Lister, 2015, p. 228), and to prepare the solution, insert a 21G needle into the vial to allow air to escape when adding the diluent for injection. Then add the diluents to the vial, remove needle and syringe and cover the remaining first needle with a sterile swab. The carefully shake the vial to mix the powder and diluent. Draw up the reconstituted medication solution.

4   Check the vial for cloudiness or particles. The medicine should be clear.

5   Reinsert the syringe and needle, invert the vial and draw up the correct amount of medicine required. The second needle should be above the fluid, then withdraw the medication solution to the desired amount as indicated in the marks of the syringe. It is important to remove air from the syringe by injecting back into the vial and not spraying it into the atmosphere. Inspect the syringe to ensure no pieces of rubber have been detached and drawn up, a process known as 'coring' by the bevel of the needle. This can be minimised by inserting the needle at an angle of 45–60 degrees.

6   Attach a new needle for administering to the patient.

7   Should there be other forms of vials and connections which are provided by the manufacturer (e.g. vials with transfer connectors), the nurse or whoever is preparing the medication should follow the manufacturer's instructions.

Multidose (solution/suspension)

1   Use a 'non-touch' technique, i.e. avoid touching areas where bacterial contamination may be introduced, e.g. syringe tips, needles, vial tops. Never put down a syringe attached to an unsheathed needle (NPSA, 2007). Wash hands and wear gloves.

2   Remove the tamperproof cover of the multidose vial and clean rubber seal according to local policy and let this dry for at least 30 seconds.

3   With the needle sheathed, draw into the syringe a volume of air equivalent to the required volume of solution to be drawn up.

4   Remove the needle cover and insert the needle into the vial through the rubber septum.

5   Invert the vial. Keep the needle in the solution and slowly press the plunger to push air into the vial. This 'equilibrium method' helps to minimise the build-up of pressure in the vial.

6   Release the plunger so that the solution flows back into the syringe.

7   The vial(s) and any unused medicine should be kept until administration to the patient is complete.

Subcutaneous injections

Procedure for administering subcutaneous injections

1   Follow steps 1 and 2 in the general principles in Table 16.3. Qualified nurses are only to administer injections, students may be able to do this under direct supervision depending on local policy

2   Ensure the correct form of the medication is available and prepare the equipment: prescribed medicine, clean tray/receiver, syringe of appropriate size (0.5–2 mL), appropriate needle (25 g), clinical wipe/alcohol swabs, sharps bin.

3   Check to ensure equipment is not out of date and the packaging is intact. If the medicine is pre-prepared (e.g. heparin), the medicine will be in the syringe so there is no need to draw this up, so omit the drawing up section below.

4   Re-check the prescription (steps 4–6, general principles in Table 16.3).

5   Wash hands, put on gloves.

6   Calculate the amount of medicine to be given and draw this up.

7   Select the site on the patient for administration of the medicine (Figure 16.4b). If frequent injections, the sites may be rotated for comfort and to avoid over-use or fat deposits on one site. Assess selected site for inflammation or lesions and report as necessary.

8   Ensure the patient is in the correct position and maintain patient's dignity.

9   Clean the injection site with an alcohol swab – local policy may indicate the skin is not cleaned if it is hygienically clean and healthy.

10   Gently pinch skin into a fold.

11   Insert needles into the skin at a 45 degree angle (or 90 degree for insulin) (Figure 16.4a). You do not need to withdraw as the needle is unlikely to penetrate a blood vessel. Release pinched skin and inject slowly.

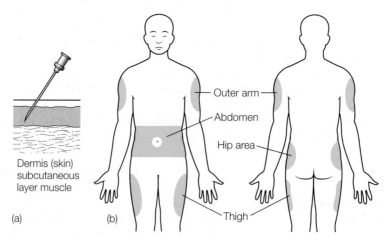

Figure 16.4 **Positions for subcutaneous injections**

12 Withdraw needle. Do not apply pressure on the injection site but if the site bleeds slightly, use a sterile swab to stop the bleeding.

13 Dispose of syringe and needle in sharps box immediately. Do not resheath the needle. Observe patient for response and ensure they are comfortable. Document administration. Wash hands.

Intramuscular injections

Procedure for administering intramuscular injections

1 Follow steps 1 and 2 in general principles in Table 16.3. Qualified nurses are only to administer injections, students may be able to do this under direct supervision depending on local policy.

2 Ensure the correct form of the medication is available and prepare equipment: prescribed medicine, clean tray/receiver, syringe of appropriate size (2–5 mL), appropriate needle (21 g for adults), clinical wipe/alcohol swabs, sharps bin.

3 Check to ensure equipment is not out of date and packaging is intact.

4 Re-check the prescription (steps 4–6, general principles in Table 16.3).

5 Wash hands, put on gloves.

6 Select the site on the patient for administration of the medicine. Sites may include: mid deltoid, dorso gluteal, vastus lateralis or ventrogluteal (see Figures 16.5–8).

7 Ensure patient is in the correct position and maintain patient's dignity.

8 Assess selected site for inflammation or lesions and report as necessary.

9 Clean the injection site with an alcohol swab, allow to dry for at least 30 seconds or according to local policy which may indicate the skin is not cleaned if it is hygienically clean and healthy.

10 Stretch the skin around the injection site with the non-dominant hand.

11 Insert needle swiftly and directly into the injection site at an angle of 90 degrees (right angle) leaving approximately 1 cm of the needle showing.

12 Aspirate by pulling back the plunger to ascertain if the needle has entered a blood vessel. If blood appears, remove the needle, replace needle and attempt injection again. Do explain to the patient the reason for this. If no blood appears, inject the medicine at a rate of approximately 1 mL every 10 seconds. NB some injections, e.g. depot injections are thicker.

13 When the medicine is injected, wait 10 seconds and then withdraw the needle rapidly. Using a clean swab, press on the injection site to stop the bleeding.

An alternative method is the Z track technique which is reported to cause less discomfort and cause less leakage of medicines at the injection site.

Procedure using the Z track technique

1 Follow steps 6–8 above.

2 Using the non-dominant hand, pull the patient's skin 2–3 cm sideways or downwards from the injection site (causing skin and subcutaneous fat to slide over the muscle).

3 Using the dominant hand, inject the needle at a 90 degree angle into the muscle as above.

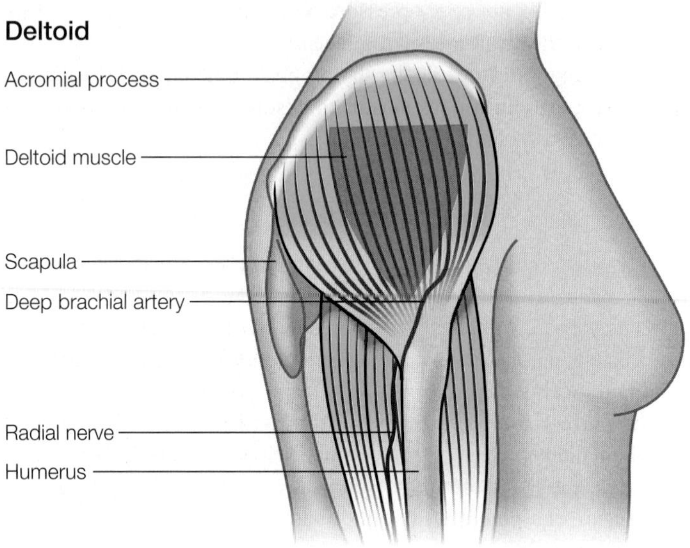

Deltoid

Acromial process ————

Deltoid muscle ————

Scapula ————

Deep brachial artery ————

Radial nerve ————

Humerus ————

Figure 16.5 **Deltoid muscle**

4   Aspirate for blood (as above). Slowly inject the medicine as above, hold needle in place for 10 seconds. Withdraw needle quickly and release tension on the skin, causing the tissues to return to their normal position which seals the injection site preventing leakage of medicine.

5   Dispose of syringe and needle in sharps box immediately. Do not resheath the needle.

6   Observe patient for response and ensure they are comfortable. Document administration. Wash hands.

Possible injection sites

Deltoid (upper arm)

Easily accessible but not a huge muscle and thus can only accept small volumes (e.g. 1 mL). It is like a triangle shape on the upper arm. Injection sites are usually found approximately 5 cm below the acromial process.

Dorsogluteal (buttock)

This area is used for deep IM and Z track injections (like depot). A large muscle so can accommodate 4 mL volume (Figure 16.6).

Home to the gluteal artery and sciatic nerve. To avoid these in IM injections the term 'upper outer quadrant' has been used. Consider the buttock as a grid of four quadrants, then split the top outer part into four more quadrants – the injection site is then in the upper outermost quadrant.

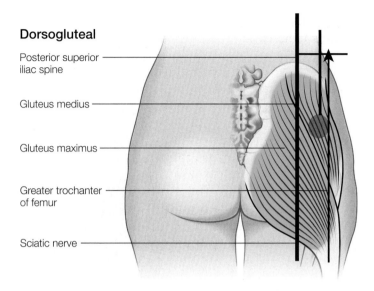

Dorsogluteal

Posterior superior iliac spine

Gluteus medius

Gluteus maximus

Greater trochanter of femur

Sciatic nerve

Figure 16.6 **Dorsogluteal**

Vastus lateralis and rectus femoris (outer and upper thigh)

These areas are used for deep and Z track injections. They can accommodate up to 5 mL though in infants this is much reduced (1–3 mL). The rectus is found halfway between the superior iliac crest (hip bone) and the patella (knee) (Figure 16.7). The vastus is on the outer part of the thigh and is found by measuring a hand's breadth from the greater trochanter (hip joint) (middle third of quadriceps).

Ventrogluteal

These areas are used for deep and Z track injections. This site is found by placing the palm of the hand on the patient's opposite trochanter (i.e. right palm on left hip). The index finger then points to the anterior iliac spine making a V shape with the middle finger (as seen in the dark shaded section in Figure 16.8). This identifies the largest part of the muscle and the optimal injection site.

Medications via nasogastric or gastrostomy routes

Where medications must be given through an enteral feeding tube, the nurse needs to know if the distal tip of the tube is situated in the stomach or small intestine. Some medications are absorbed in the stomach and others in the small intestine; it is vital to recognise the site of absorption of any drug given this way. For example, the medicine digoxin is absorbed in the stomach so there is little point giving it via a jejunal feeding tube. Absorption of medication through an enteral feeding tube can be adversely affected by the type of feed or feeding regimen. To minimise disruption of the feeding regime, the

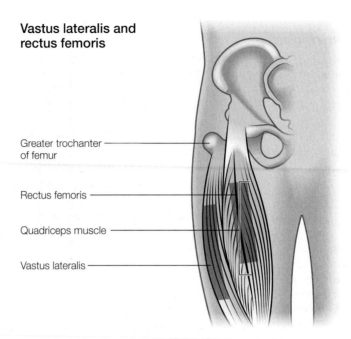

Vastus lateralis and rectus femoris

Greater trochanter of femur

Rectus femoris

Quadriceps muscle

Vastus lateralis

Figure 16.7 **Vastus lateralis and rectus femoris**

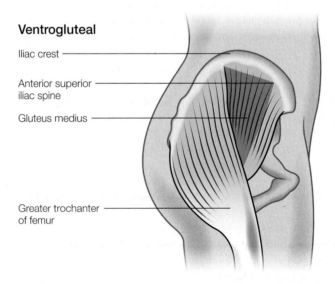

Ventrogluteal

Iliac crest

Anterior superior iliac spine

Gluteus medius

Greater trochanter of femur

Figure 16.8 **Ventrogluteal**

timing of certain medications will need to be considered carefully. As a rule, medication should not be given while the enteral feed is in progress because the combination of feed and medication within the tube not only increases the risk of coagulation and tube blockage but may also reduce the level of drug absorbed. In cases when a patient receiving feed needs to be given medication, the feed should be stopped and the enteral feeding tube flushed with at least 30 ml of water (BAPEN, 2007).

Procedure for administering enteral medicines

1   Follow steps 1 and 2 in general principles in Table 16.3. Qualified nurses are only to administer enteral medicines, students may be able to do this under direct supervision depending on local policy.
2   Check if patients are able to take their medication orally. It may be necessary to ask the prescriber to review this and consider the form of the medication to enable oral administration.
3   Seek further advice for fluid-restricted or paediatric patients as flushing volumes may need to be reduced.
4   Check if medicines can be given with feed or after a break in the feeding regimen.
5   Ensure the correct form of the medication is available and prepare equipment: prescribed medicine, clean tray/receiver, oral or enteral syringe of appropriate size (50 mL oral, enteral or catheter-tipped syringe). Prepare each medicine separately.
6   Calculate the amount of medicines needed.
7   Never mix drugs unless instructed by a pharmacist. Do make note of problem medicines which may react or block the tube and seek advice.
8   Check to ensure equipment is not out of date and the packaging is intact. Only use labelled oral/enteral syringes that cannot be connected to intravenous catheters or ports to measure and administer oral liquid medicines.
9   Re-check the prescription (steps 4–6, general principles in Table 16.3).
10   Wash hands.
11   Stop the feed and flush the tube with at least 30 mL water (check local policy for type).
12   Re-check the prescription (steps 4–6, general principles in Table 16.3).
13   Wash hands, put on gloves.

Differing medicine forms will be described:

1   Soluble/dispersible tablets: dissolve in 10–15 mL water and administer through tube. Rinse syringe with 10 mL water and administer through tube to ensure full dose of medicine is given.
2   Liquid/syrups: dilute with equal quantities of water and administer down the tube. Rinse syringe with 10 mL water and administer through tube to ensure full dose of medicine is given.
3   Tablets: AS A LAST RESORT (following advice) do the following. Crush uncoated and sugar-coated tablets using a pestle and mortar or suitable device. *Do NOT crush enteric-coated (EC) medicines, modified release (MR, SR, LA, XL) medicines, hormone preparations*, or *cytotoxics*. Seek advice from pharmacist and prescriber.

4   Mix with 10–15 mL water and administer down the tube. Rinse syringe with 10 mL water and administer through tube to ensure full dose of medicine is given.

5   Capsules: open capsule and place powder into a syringe, mix with 10 mL water and administer down the tube. Rinse syringe with 10 mL water and administer through tube to ensure full dose of medicine is given.

6   If more than one medicine is to be administered – flush between drugs with at least 10 mL of water to ensure that the drug is cleared from the tube.

7   Check if the patient needs to have a break before continuing with the feed.

8   Observe patient for response and ensure they are comfortable. Restart feed when advised. Document administration. Wash hands.

Topical (skin/patches)

Procedure for applying a topical medicine

1   Follow steps 1 and 2 in general principles in Table 16.3.

2   Ensure the correct form of the medication is available and prepare equipment: medicine, applicators, clean non-sterile gloves, sterile topical swabs.

3   Re-check the prescription (steps 4–6 in general principles in Table 16.3).

4   Wash hands and put on non-sterile gloves.

5   Ensure the patient is in the required position with the area receiving the medicine exposed. Maintain patient dignity by ensuring the room door or curtains are closed.

6   Use aseptic technique if the skin is broken.

7   Dispense the required amount of topical medicine and apply to the affected area checking with the process (i.e. rubbing or thin layer using an applicator, etc.).

8   If the medication causes skin or clothing staining, do inform the patient of this.

9   If patches are the form of medication, do ensure they are used. Patches are a source of medicine such as nicotine, hormone replacement or analgesia that is continuously delivered through the skin over a period of time.

10   General instructions include: ensure the skin is clean and not too cool or hot, i.e. just after a bath (this will affect the rate of absorption). Do not apply moisturiser or powders to the area of the patch will be as this will reduce the adhesiveness.

11   Pull off the plastic backing to expose the adhesive. Do not touch the sticky surface of the patch. Apply the patch firmly with the sticky side down to a clean, dry, non-hairy area of skin, on the area of the body specified in the instructions supplied with the patches. DO NOT place on broken or inflamed skin areas as this may cause further irritation.

12   Observe patient for response and ensure they are comfortable. Document administration. Discard gloves or old patches safely and wash hands.

Other: opthalmic medicine

Procedure for applying opthalmic medicine

1   Follow steps 1 and 2 in general principles in Table 16.3. Explain to the patient that their vision may be blurred for a period of time following instillation of the eye medicine.

2   Re-check the prescription (steps 4–6 in general principles in Table 16.3).

3   Wash hands. Wear an apron, use gloves only if the patient has infected eyes.

4   Ensure the correct form of the medication is available and prepare equipment: eye drops/ointment, gauze or cotton wool. Determine if the medicine is to be given in one or both eyes. This is a clean procedure. Where both eyes may require treatment, each eye must be treated separately. If infection is present, there should be two bottles of medication, one for each eye (labelled) to prevent cross-contamination. If only one container, the least affected eye should be treated first to minimise the likelihood of transfer of infection from one eye to the other. If more than one medication is being inserted into the eye, care must be taken to give time for the first medication to be absorbed, before applying further medication.

5   Re-check the prescription (steps 4–6 in general principles in Table 16.3).

6   Wash hands and put on non-sterile apron.

7   Ensure the patient is in the required position with the head tilted back and supported.

8   Using a clean gauze swab, gently pull down on the lower lid margin to form a small pocket for the eye drops or ointment.

9   Ask the patient to look upwards before instilling the drops/ointment.

10   Hold the dispenser between the forefinger and thumb approximately 2 cm from the patient's eye.

11   Eye drops: squeeze the required amount of drops into the affected eye. Do this one drop at a time, asking the patient to blink between drops. Do not touch the eye with the dropper.

12   Eye ointment: squeeze the tube gently until a small amount (1 or 2 cm) forms a ribbon and place this into and along the lower lid. Ask patient to blink gently. Do not touch the eye with the ointment tip.

13   Wipe away any excess medication which runs down the face with a clean swab.

14   Replace the cap of the medicine container and store safely.

15   Observe patient for response and ensure they are comfortable. Document administration. Discard gloves aprons safely and wash hands.

Otic (ear) medicine

Procedure for applying ear medicine

1   Follow steps 1 and 2 in general principles in Table 16.3.

2   Re-check the prescription (steps 4–6, general principles in Table 16.3).

3   Wash hands.

4   Ensure the correct form of the medication is available and prepare equipment: medicine, gauze or cotton wool. Determine if the medicine is to be given in one or both ears. Warm the ear drops to body temperature if possible.

5   Ask the patient to lie on their side with the affected ear accessible.

6   Remove cap from eardrops dispenser – do not touch the tip of the dispenser.

7   Gently pull the pinna of the ear upwards and backwards.

8   Squeeze the bottle or dispenser to administer the prescribed number of drops into the ear.

9   Allow the drops to fall into the ear canal.

10 Request the patient remain in this position for two minutes to allow the medication to reach the eardrum. Gently wipe away any excess fluid seeping from ears.

11 If this is to be repeated on the other ear – there may be another bottle of eardrops. Follow the same procedure on the alternate side. Ask patient to also remain in position for two minutes at the end of the instillation.

12 Replace the cap of the eardrops and put medicine securely in storage.

13 Observe patient for response and ensure they are comfortable. Document administration.

14 Wash hands.

Rectal: enema administration or suppositories

Enemas are administered rectally and can be given to soothe and treat bowel mucosa in chronic inflammatory bowel disease such as ulcerative colitis and Crohn's disease (Figure 16.9). This section will not address details of evacuant enemas only for medicine administration. A suppository is a medication which is formulated as a solid material to melt at body temperature following insertion into the rectum. Suppositories are also used to clear the bowels but are also a means of administering medication into the system and are especially useful if the patient cannot tolerate oral medicines (due to nausea or vomiting) or if they are in a situations where other access is impossible i.e. epileptic fit.

Procedure to insert an enema

1 Follow steps 1 and 2 in general principles in Table 16.3.

2 Re-check the prescription (steps 4–6, general principles in Table 16.3).

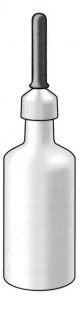

Figure 16.9 Enema

3   Explain the procedure and any potential risks to the patient and obtain consent again.

4   Wash hands.

5   Ensure the correct form of the medication is available and prepare equipment: disposable incontinence pad, disposable plastic gloves, topical swabs, lubricating jelly, enema solution or medicine. Warm the enema to body temperature for comfort.

6   Encourage the patient to empty their bladder as fluid entering the rectum may cause discomfort to an already full bladder.

7   Ensure the patient has privacy and maintain dignity as much as possible (doors or curtains closed, speak in low voice).

8   Make sure that a commode or toilet is nearby because inserting an enema often gives the patient urgency to defecate.

9   Remove any clothing below the waist and ensure that the patient is covered with a blanket.

10 Assist the patient to lie, if possible, in the left lateral position with knees flexed and their buttocks near the edge of the bed (Figures 16.10 (a) and (b)). If this position is not possible, then either the prone position or the other side will suffice.

11 Place an incontinence pad beneath the patient's hips and buttocks.

12 Wash hands and wear an apron and non-sterile gloves.

13 Remove cap from enema and lubricate the end of the nozzle of the enema or the suppository.

14 Ask the patient to relax and take some deep breaths.

   a   For an enema, part the buttocks with one hand. With the other hand, hold the nozzle of the enema and gently insert into the anal canal to a depth of the administration tube (10 cm).

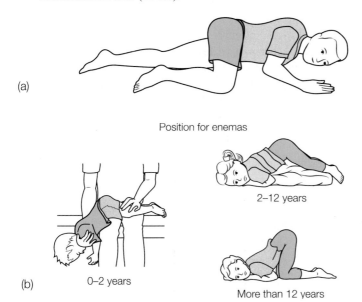

(a)

Position for enemas

2–12 years

0–2 years

More than 12 years

(b)

Figure 16.10 (a) Adult position for a suppository/enema; (b) child positions for a suppository/enema

      b   Squeeze the enema bag until all the contents have been deposited and gently withdraw the nozzle.

      c   For a suppository, part the buttocks with one hand and insert the suppository blunt end first. advancing it for 2–4 cm. Repeat this procedure if a second suppository is to be used.

      d   Wipe away the lubricant, ensure the patient is comfortable, dry and covered. Ask them to remain on their side for 15–30 minutes to allow retention and absorption of the fluid or suppository.

      e   Do not insert a suppository into a faecal mass.

15   Ensure the patient has access to the nurse call bell, is near a bedpan, commode or toilet. A suppository will take approximately 20 minutes to dissolve.

17   Remove and dispose of equipment appropriately. Observe patient for response and ensure they are comfortable.

17   Wash hands and discard apron and gloves.

18   Document administration and effects.

Watch out

Phosphate enemas must be avoided in certain patients – do be aware of which are vulnerable, e.g. those with colitis, proctitis, or inflammatory bowel conditions.

Summary

Many patients will need medicines given through a variety of routes. Nurses must practise to ensure safe administration, including checks at every step of the administration process. Procedures discussed include the 'rights' and checks of medication administration; how to interpret prescriptions, calculate medicines and how to skilfully administer them to a variety of routes. The legal implications are addressed briefly here and emphasise the seriousness of knowing about medicines and storage and careful documentation.

- The 'Rights' of medication administration serve as a guide for *safe* administration of medications to patients. Failure to achieve any of the 'Rights' constitutes a medication error
- Carefully read the label to determine dosage strength and check calculations, paying special attention to decimal points
- Medications must be administered in the form and via the route specified in the prescription
- Storage of medicines relies on knowledge of the key legislation.

References

Adams, M. and Koch, R. (2010) *Pharmacology Connections to Nursing Practice*, 3rd edn. Englewood Cliffs, NJ: Prentice Hall Pearson.

BAPEN (British Association for Parenteral and Enteral Nutrition and The British Pharmaceutical Nutrition Group) (2007) *Administering Drugs via Enteral Feeding Tubes: A Practical Guide*. Available at: www.bapen.org.uk/pdfs/d_and_e/de_pract_guide.pdf (accessed 6 February 2015).

Barber, P. and Robertson, D. (2015) *Essentials of Pharmacology for Nurses*. Oxford: Open University Press.

Bates, D. (2007) Preventing medication errors: a summary. *American Journal of Health-System Pharmacy*, 64(14) (Suppl. 9): S3–S9.

Bullock, S., Manias, E. and Galbraith, A. (2007) *Fundamentals of Pharmacology*. London. Pearson.

CPE (Centre for Policy on Ageing) (2012*) Report: Working Together to Develop Practical Solutions: An Integrated Approach to Medication in Care Homes*. Available at: www.cpa. org.uk/information/reviews/Managing_and_Administering_Medication_in_Care_Homes. pdf

Crouch, S. and Chapelhow, C. (2008) *Medicines Management: A Nursing Perspective*. Oxford: Pearsons Education Limited.

CSCI (Commission for Social Care inspection) (2008) *Professional Advice: Medicine Administration Records (MAR) in Care Homes and Domiciliary Care*. QPM document 124/08. London: CSCI.

Davey, A., Britland, A. and Naylor, R. (2008) Decreasing paediatric prescribing errors in a district general hospital. *Quality and Safety in Health Care*, 17(2): 146–149.

DoH (Department of Health) (2008) Supplementary prescribing. Available at: www. dh.gov.uk/en/Healthcare/Medicinespharmacyandindustry/Prescriptions/TheNon-MedicalPrescribingProgramme/Supplementaryprescribing/index.htm (accessed 28 October 2015).

DoH (Department of Health) (2012) *Long Term Conditions Compendium of Information*, 3rd edn. London: HMSO.

Doughty, L. and Lister, S. (2015) *The Royal Marsden Manual of Clinical Nursing Procedures: Professional Edition,* 9th edn. Oxford: Wiley-Blackwell.

Elliott, M. and Liu, Y. (2010) The nine rights of medication administration. *British Journal of Nursing*, 19(5): 300–305.

Joint Formulary Committee (2015) *British National Formulary*, edition 71. London: BMJ Group and Pharmaceutical Press.

Lister, S. (2015) Drug administration general principles. In L. Doughty and S. Lister (eds) *The Royal Marsden Hospital Manual of Clinical Nursing Procedures*, 9th edn. Oxford: Wiley-Blackwell.

NICE (National Institute for Health and Clinical Excellence) (2009) *Medicines Adherence: Involving Patients in Decisions about Prescribed Medicines and Supporting Adherence*. London: NICE.

NICE (National Institute for Health and Clinical Excellence) (2015) *Medicines Optimisation: The Safe and Effective Use of Medicines to Enable the Best Possible Outcomes*. London: NICE.

Medicines and Healthcare Regulatory Authority (MHRA) (2011) Single use devices. [online] http://www.mhra.gov.uk/home/groups/dts-iac/documents/publication/con2025015.pdf (accessed 20 January 2016).

NMC (Nursing and Midwifery Council) (2007) *Standards for Medicines Management.*

London: Nursing and Midwifery Council. Available at: www.nmc-uk.org/aDisplayDocument.aspx?DocumentID=3251 (accessed 1 July 2014).

NMC (Nursing and Midwifery Council) (2010) *Standards for Medicine Management*. London: NMC.

NMC (Nursing and Midwifery Council) (2015) *The Code: Professional Standards of Practice and Behaviour for Nurses and Midwives*. London: NMC.

NPC (National Prescribing Centre) (2004) Patient group directions: a practical guide and framework of competencies for all professionals using patient group directions. Available at: www.npc.co.uk/publications/pgd/pgd.pdf (accessed 6 February 2015).

NPSA (National Patient Safety Agency) (2007) Promoting safer measurement and administration of liquid medicines via oral and other enteral routes. Available at: www.nrls.npsa.nhs.uk/resources/?entryid45=59808 (accessed 6 February 2015).

NPSA (National Patient Safety Agency) (2008) *Clean Hands Save Lives: Patient Safety Alert*. London: NPSA.

Rang, H., Dale, M., Ritter, J. and Flower, R. (2012) *Rang & Dale's Pharmacology*, 8th edn. London: Elsevier.

Royal Pharmaceutical Society of Great Britain (2003) *The Administration and Control of Medicines in Care Homes and Children's Services*. London. RPSGB.

WHO (World Health Organisation) (1975) *Requirements for Adverse Reaction Reporting*. Geneva: World Health Organisation.

Woodrow, R., Colbert, B. and Smith, D. (2010) *Essentials of Pharmacology for Health Occupations*, 6th edn. New York. Delmar Cengage Learning.

Part V

Nutrition and fluid balance

Chapter 17

Nutrition

Susan Kaur Lawrence

Every careful observer of the sick will agree in this that thousands of patients are annually starved in the midst of plenty, from want of attention to the ways which alone make it possible for them to take food.

(Florence Nightingale, 1860)

Florence Nightingale's reflections in 1860 provide insight that the challenges of nursing patients' nutritional needs have not changed much in the passing years. Sadly, her comment is just as valid now as it was during her time of practice.

Key concepts

Role of the nurse
Nutritional requirements
Nutritional assessments

Mainutrition
Nutritional support

Learning outcomes

By the end of the chapter you will be able to:

- Demonstrate knowledge and understanding of the components of a healthy diet, including nutritional requirements
- Undertake a comprehensive assessment of the patient's nutritional needs
- Analyse the role of the nurse in promoting healthy eating
- Recognise the characteristics of malnutrition and the contributing factors
- Understand the need for alternative methods of nutritional intake for patients who cannot achieve this in the conventional way.

Introduction

Recently, nutrition has become a high profile topic for the UK population, with initiatives being focused to address problem areas in schools and hospitals. The previous Labour government in 2000, introduced the 'Change for Life' campaign (DoH, 2009) in a bid to address the nation's changing lifestyle needs, with diet being a central focus. This has been coupled with high profile stories in the press, of patients starving while being in-patients and entrusted into the care of hospital staff (Age UK, 2006; Francis Report, 2013).

In 2011, the Care Quality Commission (CQC) performed 100 unannounced visits to hospitals and 17 of the 100 hospitals inspected failed to meet acceptable standards. While this figure is too high, it must be highlighted that there are a number of great initiatives and interventions (locally and nationally), directly addressing the nutritional needs of patients. Practitioners, whatever their discipline, have a statutory obligation to 'make every contact count' when meeting their clients/patients, while ensuring that the mental and physical health and well-being of their patients are maintained or improved (DoH, 2012).

This chapter will discuss the important role of nutrition, together with suggestions on how to address patients' nutritional needs.

Healthy eating

There are many tools to assist with nutritional guidance. The Eatwell Plate (DoH, 2011a) is one that is widely used in practice settings to enable practitioners to support individuals with healthy choices (Figure 17.1). As well as the visual tool, the Department for Health (Food Standards Agency, 2016) has created simple-to-follow advice through their eight helpful tips on making healthier choices:

1   Base meals on starchy foods
2   Eat lots of fruit and vegetables
3   Eat more fish – including a portion of oily fish each week
4   Cut down on saturated fat and sugar
5   Try to eat less salt – no more than 6 g a day
6   Get active and try to be a healthy weight
7   Drink plenty of water
8   Don't skip breakfast.

Daily requirements

The Eatwell Plate (DoH, 2011a) clearly demonstrates that an individual requires some proportion of each of the five main categories of foods in order to maintain a healthy, well-balanced diet and a healthy lifestyle without nutritional or potential nutritional problems (e.g. following bowel surgery). Within the healthcare setting, the dietitian normally takes the lead in addressing patients' nutritional needs. However, nurses must reinforce the information, assess and monitor patients' dietary needs.

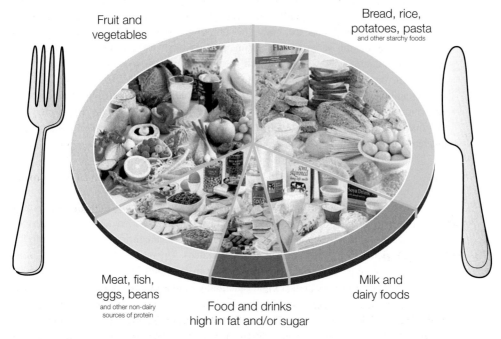

The eatwell plate

Use the eatwell plate to help you get the balance right. It shows how much of what you eat should come from each group

Fruit and vegetables

Bread, rice, potatoes, pasta
and other starchy foods

Meat, fish, eggs, beans
and other non-dairy sources of protein

Food and drinks
high in fat and/or sugar

Milk and dairy foods

Figure 17.1 **The Department of Health's Eatwell Plate (2011a)**

Carbohydrates

A third of an individual's daily food intake can be derived from this food group (DoH, 2009), it is a form of energy for the body but also it is a source of glucose. When consumed in a disproportionate amount, it can be detrimental to the body's functioning and can accelerate weight gain.

This group is made up of foods that are simple sugars or complex carbohydrates and depending on which category the food falls into determines how it will be broken down and absorbed within the body. Carbohydrates are essentially sugars and a long-term over-consumption of carbohydrates can lead to elevated blood sugars. This could subsequently predispose an individual to an increased risk of type 2 diabetes.

Sugars are the simplest form of carbohydrate and are produced by plants and animals. Sugars fall into two sub categories:

1a Monosaccharide (single molecule), e.g. fructose, galactose, and glucose.
1b Disaccharides (pairs of monosaccharides), e.g. sucrose, lactose and maltose.
2 Polysaccharides (comprised of long chains of units), e.g. amylase and amylopectin.

Starch is the most common form of carbohydrates. Large amounts of starch are found in grains, unripe fruit and certain vegetables.

Fibre

Fibre is also a source of complex carbohydrates that are plant-based which humans cannot digest. Fibre assists the body by supplying 'roughage' that helps satisfy the appetite, while at the same time enabling the digestive tract to function fully in its role of eliminating waste. Fibre can be found in the skin, seeds and pulp of fruits, vegetables, bran and grains. Consuming carbohydrates that are derived from natural sources enhances the individual's ability to absorb essential vitamins such as calcium and vitamin D. When individuals eat fresh produce, they are getting a lot more from their diet than if they were to consume processed food which is usually much less likely to be nutrient-rich, and is definitely more calorific.

Fats/Lipids

Often dietary advice advocates the consumption of 'good' fats while limiting the intake of 'bad fats'. There are four categories of fats: (1) monounsaturated; (2) polyunsaturated; (3) saturated; and (4) hydrogenated. Understanding these categories can be confusing for individuals when trying to make healthy food choices. The ratio of fats in foods can vary according to the type of food, e.g. meat is higher in saturated fat rather than polyunsaturated fat. And oily fish contains a higher amount of monosaturated fat.

- *Monounsaturated and polyunsaturated* fats are classified as 'good' fats: these fats do not impact on your blood cholesterol levels. Examples of monounsaturated fats are found in foods such as avocados, olive oil and almonds. Polyunsaturated fats are seen in corn oil, margarine, oily fish, like mackerel, salmon, herring.
- *Saturated and hydrogenated* fats are referred to as 'bad fats' and are found in meat products and animal-derived foods such as butter, cream, full dairy produce, cakes and biscuits. If an individual consumes a large amount of saturated fat, it increases the amount of blood cholesterol that contributes to heart disease.

Activity 17.1

- Think of examples in your diet of 'good' and 'bad' fats
- Write down how much fat you consume in your average week's diet. Look at the fat content on food packaging for this information.

Nutritionist advice on the consumption of these various fats states 30 per cent of our total daily calories should be from fats and only 10 per cent should come from saturated fats. Some 10–15 per cent of our total daily intake should be from monounsaturated fats. It is recommended that polyunsaturated fats should contribute to less than 10 per cent of total daily calorie intake.

Cholesterol

Cholesterol is a fatty substance that occurs naturally in the body. It plays an important part in maintaining the structure and permeability of cell membranes. Cholesterol assists in creating bile acids as well as synthesising steroid hormones. Bile acids aid the body's ability to digest foods, by emulsifying fats and breaking them into tiny particles. A large amount of the body's cholesterol is produced in the liver, however, it is also absorbed from an individual's diet.

There are two main types of cholesterol: low density lipoprotein (LDL) and high density lipoprotein (HDL). As a fat it needs a transporter – low density lipoprotein transports the cholesterol from the liver to the body's tissues, an excessive amount can contribute to a build-up on the inside walls of blood vessels, causing them to narrow and restrict circulation. This mechanism is why LDL and cholesterol is often known as the 'bad' cholesterol.

To counterbalance the effects of LDL, HDL enables the body to remove excess cholesterol from the body's tissues and return it to the liver from where it can be eradicated. This type of cholesterol is what the body needs to maintain a healthy balance.

The current guidance on cholesterol states that individuals should aim to keep their total cholesterol level below 5 mmol/L, specifically keeping the LDL level below 3 mmol/L. Elevated levels of cholesterol can increase an individual's risk of heart disease and associated problems.

Proteins

Protein is an important factor in the body's functioning as every cell within the body requires protein as part of its basic structure. Proteins are broken down during digestion and provide the body with amino acids. Proteins consist of amino acids (the chemical subunits of proteins). There are 20 types of amino acids, of which eight cannot be reproduced by the body, meaning that their presence is entirely dependent on dietary intake. These eight are also known as 'essential amino acids'. Non-essential amino acids can be produced in the body from the amino acids ingested through diet.

Proteins can also be separated into two further categories: complete or incomplete. Complete proteins (e.g. from meat, fish, dairy products, and eggs) contain all the essential amino acids as well as some non-essential amino acids. Incomplete proteins can be found in vegetables and contain one or more of the essential amino acids, making it important that these are included in an individual's diet. Some patients require high protein diets containing meat, fish, dairy produce, beans, peas and peanut butter to assist recovery following intensive treatments, such as chemotherapy, where the protein is required to help the body repair itself.

When caring for a patient who requires a high protein diet, it is important that they are offered foods that contain complete proteins. If the patient is unable to eat much food, they can be given nutritional supplements to increase protein intake.

Vitamins

Vitamins are organic substances that are derived from either plants or animals. They are required to help speed up chemical reactions within the body's metabolic processes. An individual's diet must include a certain amount of each essential vitamin, as the body cannot produce these and is therefore dependent on the individual's consumption. A lack of essential vitamins can cause certain metabolic disturbances that result in physical disorders, one such example is the lack of vitamin C that results in a condition known as scurvy.

Another complexity is that the body is unable to store certain vitamins, meaning that it needs a daily supply from your diet (Box 17.1). This is due to the body's ability to store a certain amount of fat-soluble substances, which are those that dissolve in fat, but it is unable to replicate the same action with water-soluble substances such as vitamin C and B complex. These need to dissolve in water before the body is able to absorb them. Vitamins come in both forms. Any of the water-soluble vitamins that remain unused by the body, get filtered by the kidney. Fat-soluble vitamins are stored in the liver and fatty tissues. An over-consumption of these fat-soluble vitamins can be harmful. Table 17.1 shows the source of both water-soluble and fat-soluble vitamins.

Table 17.1 Sources of both fat-soluble and water-soluble vitamins

Vitamins	Sources
A	Liver, kidney, egg yolk, oily fish, dairy products (full fat), as well as any fruit/vegetables that are orange, red, yellow or green
D	Egg yolk, butter, oily fish, and the action of the skin absorbing the sunlight
E	Available in many foods the best sources are nuts, seeds, vegetable oil as well as some cereals with almonds delivering the highest amount of vitamin E than any other nut
K	Available in many cereals and vegetables
Thiamin (B1)	Liver, eggs, vegetables, fruit, wholegrain cereals, milk and liver
Riboflavin (B2)	Milk and milk products
Niacin (B3)	Fish, pulses, meat and some fortified cereals
Cobalamins (B12)	Meat, eggs, fish, dairy products, and other animal products. (note: for strict vegans they may require supplements)
Folic Acid/ Folates (B group)	Green vegetables, liver oranges, fortified breakfast cereals and yeast extract
Ascorbic Acid (vitamin c)	Citrus fruit, tomatoes, green leafy vegetables, strawberries and blackcurrants.

Notes:
■ Water-soluble vitamin ▪ Fat-soluble vitamins

Box 17.1 Vitamins

In order to optimise vitamin consumption, fresh foods are better eaten soon after they are harvested (storage and processing can affect the vitamin content of these foods). It is essential for nurses to pay attention to a patient's intake of vitamins while they are in hospital as often long periods in hospital can lead to vitamin deficiencies.

Watch out

Rickets is a condition that affects bones. Although vitamin D is mainly produced through exposure to natural sunlight, it can also be absorbed from foods such as oily fish and eggs. This is a fat-soluble vitamin that assists the body in absorbing calcium.

Minerals

These substances are inorganic, meaning they originate from the soil or water and they are absorbed by plants or ingested by animals. Minerals are required for cellular and bodily functions. They are necessary for building bones, teeth, assisting the body in controlling intra-cellular and extra-cellular fluid composition, as well as converting the food into useable energy. Once ingested, minerals exist in the body as free ions, meaning they carry an electrical charge which is used to assist with cellular communication and transmitting of impulses.

There are two categories of minerals: macrominerals (calcium, sodium, potassium, magnesium, chloride, sulphur, and phosphorus) and microminerals (iron, zinc, iodine, fluoride, copper, cobalt, manganese, chromium, and selenium), also known as trace minerals.

Water

Water is an invaluable part of an individual's diet, especially as the body's composition is 60 per cent water (Chapter 18). Its importance as a factor of a healthy diet is well recognised. It is essential for normal bodily functions, such as ingestion and digestion, as well as being a vehicle for carrying other important nutrients. The recommended daily intake of water is 2 litres for an adult, for an infant 680–1000 mls per day; toddler (1–2) 1100–1200 mL/day, older child – 9–13. 2100–1900 mL per day (The European Food Safety Authority, 2010).

Daily nutritional requirements

Daily nutritional requirements are dependent on many variables, one of which is age. In infancy and adolescence, an individual's nutritional requirements are far greater than in old age, due to an increased metabolic rate and growth 'spurts', increasing the amount of energy expended in one day.

Gender also plays a role in nutritional requirements as men require more calories than women, due to hormones and body structure. Men need larger amounts of lean protein whereas women have a greater need for calcium and iron.

Health needs such as diabetes, high cholesterol, and high blood pressure also determine what should be considered. The body requires energy for physical activity, this energy is measured in calories and is either obtained from the body's fat stores or the food that is eaten.

There has been a change in dietary habits, with the influx of pre-packed and processed meals, balanced against the cost of eating healthily and having five portions of fruit/vegetables a day.

Obesity is also a growing concern. It is estimated that in the UK 23 per cent of adults are obese and 37 per cent are overweight (DoH, 2011b). Obesity is not unique to any one particular age group and its prevalence is increasingly being highlighted as of 'epidemic' proportions (Hall and Elliman, 2006). It is recognised that there are many drivers that contribute to the increase in obesity, although a major one is the increased sedentary lifestyle of the population, particularly among the younger generation.

Increasing numbers of patients who are classified as obese are being cared for by healthcare professionals who require support. When nurses are thinking of discussing dietary advice with patients, caution should be placed on advising them to restrict major food groups, they should also take into account an individual's personal preferences and enable the individual to take a flexible approach to reducing their calorie intake (NICE, 2015). It is considered good practice to involve a dietitian in any cases where you have concerns, to help advise and guide both you and the patient. NICE Clinical guidelines focuses on managing obesity in adults and children (NICE, 2015). It outlines best practice with comprehensive advice and guidance (NICE, 2016) for professionals.

The importance of nutrition

The term nutrition includes the concepts of the supply of nutrients to the body, their absorption and the overall effects on health, as well as covering a broad range of related topics (Dudek, 2010). It is well documented that nutrition plays a vital role in the healing and recovery process from disease and ill health, as well as supporting daily functioning. Nutritional status forms a large component of the nurse's assessment and it takes both practice and time to develop this important skill.

All ages have specific dietary requirements that help to facilitate growth, reproduction and preservation. Nutrition can be described as the food an individual consumes and how this nourishes their body. It is a culmination of processes that interpret the intake of nutrients from the environment in order to aid vital functioning. A healthy diet contributes not only to the physical, but also the psychological well-being of individuals. A balanced diet is essential for the maintenance of good health. Eating appropriate portions of foods from the five major food groups is essential for good health. These include fruit, vegetables, complex carbohydrates (starchy food), proteins (dairy produce, pulses, meat, fish and eggs), fats, sugars and water (Table 17.2). Water is important as it assists the body's metabolic status, as well as playing a vital role in digestion and

Table 17.2 **Dietary recommendations as set out by the Committee on Medical Aspects of Food and Nutrition Policy (COMA) and Scientific Advisory Committee on Nutrition (2008)**

Recommendation		Population group	Reason for recommendation
Fruit and vegetables	At least 5 × 80 g portions/ day (400 g) (portion sizes are smaller for children under age 5)	Adults	Reduces risk of some cancers, cardiovascular disease and many other chronic conditions
Oily fish	At least 1 portion/week (140 g)	Adults	Reduce the risk of cardiovascular disease
Red and processed meat	Individual consumption should not rise and high consumers should consider a reduction	All red meat consumers	To reduce cancer risk
Non-milk extrinsic sugars (NMES)	No more than 11% food energy (maximum)	All	NMES contribute to the development of dental caries
Fat	Population average 35% food energy (maximum)	All	To reduce the risk of cardiovascular disease and reduce energy density of diets
Saturated fat	Population average 11% food energy (maximum)	All	As above
Non-starch poly-saccharides	An average intake of 18 g/day	Adults	To improve gastrointestinal health

absorption of food and nutrients. Within a hospital setting, an individual's consumption of water is even more vital as dehydration can exacerbate a patient's condition, creating complications and even extending their hospital stay as a result.

Infants' nutritional needs

It is recognised that, primarily, breast milk is the most valuable feed to promote the growth, development and overall health of babies. The Pan American Health Organization (2013), endorsed by the World Health Organisation, recommends colostrum, which is the first milk produced by a mother (usually produced in the first three days) as the perfect feed for a newborn and states ideally breastfeeding should be commenced within an hour post birth. They also go as far as recommending that mothers should breastfeed exclusively until their child is aged 6 months.

Breast milk contains all the nutrients that a growing infant needs as well as being rich in antibodies to help boost their immunity and protect them from various common childhood infections. WHO (2009) suggests that those babies who are breastfed are not just healthy babies but they go on to become healthy adults; they often have lower levels of cholesterol, lower blood pressure and also have a reduced incidence of type 2 diabetes. Despite the initiative of the WHO in promoting breast milk as the only option for infants, some infants are unable to intake or tolerate it. This means that they have to go onto infant formula milk. It is advised that infants below 12 months should not be given cow's milk, as it does not contain adequate nutrients, and it also is not easy to digest for children of that age.

Feeding children solely with breast milk up until the age of 6 months is recommended by the WHO (2009), and their advice on introducing solids is that the process of 'weaning' should be commenced at the age of 6 months. The infant's digestive system is not mature enough to aid digestion until the age of 6 months, therefore introduction to solids should start with mashed/pureed fruit and vegetables. Once this is tolerated by the infant, meat and fish should be introduced.

Toddlers' nutritional needs

As part of a healthy diet, toddlers require a higher amount of fat and a lower amount of fibre, in contrast to children over the age of 5 and adults. Ideally their diet should consist of three meals and two or three nutritious snacks in a day.

The Infant Toddler Forum also have web-based specific information on nutritional advice for toddlers and children, at: www.infantandtoddlerforum.org.

Dietary habits

Our individual eating habits and patterns are influenced in early childhood. By the age of 1, an infant's diet should include all the basic food groups (Berk, 2009). Children will tend to imitate the food preferences of their role models, i.e. parents, siblings, significant family members. For example, preschool children in Mexico who are used to seeing their parents enjoying peppery food also consume chilli peppers without any issue.

The dietary habits of an adolescent can affect an individual's future eating habits and preferences. This corroborates the evidence presented by developmental theorists, that successful progression through developmental milestones can have an impact on future adult life choices.

Freud is one such theorist who states that every child goes through the oral stage between birth–1 year where the child's focus is on oral satisfaction. Generally it is the pre-school age 1–5 years when children are being weaned and are starting school, that food habits are formed. There can be many contributing factors that lead an individual to make their personal food choices which need to be taken into consideration when assessing nutritional status. These drivers are often subconscious thoughts that are as a result of learned behaviour through childhood (Figure 17.2).

Activity 17.2

- Think of any other factors that would influence a person's eating habits
- How could ill health affect an individual's food intake? Reflect on some of the patients that you have cared for while on placement.

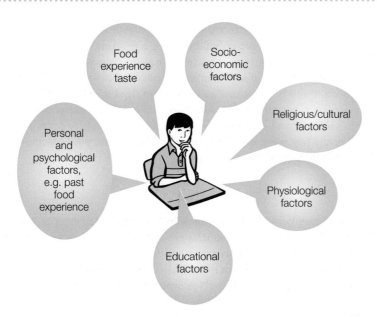

Figure 17.2 **Factors influencing a person's eating habits**

Case study 17.1

Peter, a 15-year-old, used to be very active as a child. Since his teenage years he is very reluctant to go out and stays at home playing on his electronic game console. He hates anything to do with a 'healthy diet' and his favourite foods consist of sugary drinks, egg and chips. Peter has been admitted to the ward with low mood – he weighs 101 kgs and is very conscious of his body image. He believes that people are making fun of his weight. He wants to lose weight and has asked for your help.

- What advice would you give him?
- How would you educate him to 'live healthily'?

Psychological effects of diet

The brain has a vast need for energy and the amount of nutrients ingested determine the brain's chemistry. The level of nutrients available to the brain affects the levels of chemicals (neurotransmitters), that can help relay messages and signals from one nerve to another. The availability of the number of neurotransmitters can influence sleep patterns, thought and mood. An imbalance in the vitamins and minerals available to the brain can cause nerve damage in the brain, which in turn can cause changes to memory and problem-solving abilities.

The link between mental illness and poor food choices is clear, with patients often replacing healthy foods for more unhealthy foods, e.g. crisps, chocolate, ready meals, takeaways. This can lead to physical problems such as heart disease, stroke, and diabetes.

A link between low levels of serotonin and suicide has been reported. It is implicated that lower levels of this neurotransmitter can, in part, lead to an overall insensitivity to future consequences, triggering risky, impulsive and aggressive behaviours which may culminate in suicide, the ultimate act of inwardly directed impulsive aggression.

Depression and low mood often mean that individuals have poor appetites, skipping meals, and a dominant desire for sweet foods.

Malnutrition

All cells require nutrition of one form or another, in order for them to function and maintain their structure. These requirements are almost directly dependent on our nutritional intake. Nutrition is vital in promoting health and has an inherent role in recovery from ill health, trauma or surgery. An individual's daily requirement can double in some cases, as a result of ill health, and recovery is dependent on specific energy consumption.

Malnutrition can be a problem for some patients, and is the state in which there is a deficiency in energy, protein and other essential nutrients causing adverse effects on body tissue, function and composition. Preventative measures include an early assessment of the patient's nutritional needs using a validated assessment tool. It is estimated that malnutrition costs the NHS a staggering £7.3 billion each year (Age UK, 2006). BAPEN (2012) suggest that 25–34 per cent of all hospital admissions are at risk of malnutrition. In 2007, the estimation of deaths attributable to malnutrition was 239 (Age UK, 2010), however, it is important to highlight that as Age UK suggest, malnutrition in hospital settings can go unreported and this incidence could indeed be a great deal higher.

The main causes of malnutrition can be placed into four categories, as stated by NICE (2006):

- An impaired intake
- Impaired ingestion/absorption
- Altered metabolic nutrient requirements
- Excess nutrient losses.

Factors contributing to a deteriorating nutritional state are described in Box 17.2.
Signs and symptoms of malnutrition include:

- Unplanned weight loss, loss of appetite
- Fragile bones, osteoporosis and muscle loss and/or weakness
- Feeling tired all the time and lacking energy
- Increased vulnerability to infection
- Delayed wound healing
- Dizziness
- Irritability
- Brittle, nails, dry and flaky skin
- Depression

Box 17.2 Factors contributing to a deteriorating nutritional state

- A decreased oral intake due to nausea/vomiting/inability to swallow (from surgery, stroke, coma, obstruction or even an impaired mental state).
- Periods of hospitalisation resulting in anxiety from a change of environment, a variance in mealtimes, unusual foods and being kept nil by mouth.
- The body's altered requirements, i.e. where the individual has impaired digestion and absorption, or the increased requirement from burns, fever, and fractures.
- Drug therapy and its variety of side effects.
- Lack of availability of skilled staff to assist individuals with eating.

(Age Concern UK, 2006).

- Swollen and/or bleeding gums
- Soft, flaccid muscles
- Indigestion, diarrhoea, constipation
- Inability to regulate salt and fluid retention (BAPEN, 2012).

Age Concern (2006) has also identified seven steps to reducing malnutrition in hospitals (Box 17.3). The guidance explicitly identifies steps for implementation of this with older patients. However, there are elements of good practice within the guidance that can be implemented in other fields of practice. Especially the idea of nurses becoming more 'food aware' of what the situation with their patient/client is in terms of nutritional intake preceding their admission/contact with health services.

Most Trusts now operate a colour-coded approach to meal times. Special trays have been introduced to the wards at the hospital in an attempt to ensure that those who needed help at meal times were given it. Food for patients who need help eating is sent up from the kitchen on a red tray, mustard trays are used for those patients who need supplements and green trays are for normal meals.

Some Trusts also operate a no visiting policy during breakfast, lunch and dinner times. This may be counterproductive as many relatives have been viewed as essential at meal times as they are involved in helping to feed their loved ones. There are some patients who will only eat when given food by their family members.

The RCN has also issued guidance on malnourishment in children: www.rcn.org.uk/publications/pdf/malnutrition.pdf

There are also certain medical conditions that require a certain type of diet as part of the treatment. The following are examples of physiological conditions (the first three are conditions that come under the heading of inflammatory bowel disease (IBD)):

- *Colitis*: refers to the inflammation of the colon attributable to a variety of causes including infections, restricted blood flow, and auto-immune responses

Box 17.3 Seven steps to reducing malnutrition in hospitals

1   Hospital staff must listen to older people, their relatives and carers, and act on what they say.
2   All ward staff must become 'food aware', by knowing whether patients have been eating/not eating before admission, whether they need assistance to eat or if they require special diets.
3   Hospital staff must follow their own professional codes and guidance from other bodies.
4   Older people must be assessed for the signs of malnourishment on admission and again at regular intervals during the admission.
5   Introduce 'protected' mealtimes – mealtimes that are focused around the needs of the patient. Limit unnecessary interruptions and interventions.
6   Implement a 'red tray' system whereby it signifies a patient who requires assistance to eat their meal.
7   Use mealtime volunteers where possible.

(Age Concern, 2006).

Activity 17.3

■   Think about your chosen field of practice – what practices have you observed being implemented in trying to prevent malnutrition?
■   What do you think constitutes a healthy diet?

■   *Ulcerative colitis*: affects the colon, and specifically the internal mucosa of the bowel is affected, this is where ulcers develop, where there is inflammation often exposing underlying tissue. Generally patients are recommended to take in a healthy diet. Sometimes they are also advised to increase their fibre intake to help with symptoms of constipation
■   *Crohn's disease*: can affect any part of the digestive tract in which all layers of the bowel can become affected. The most common reported site for the first occurrence is the ileum. While an individual is experiencing an acute flare-up of symptoms, they are usually advised to follow an elemental diet. This is a liquid diet that contains the necessary nutrients including proteins. Once the acute symptoms settle, the individual is restarted back onto a 'normal' diet
■   *Diabetes*: depending on the type of diabetes, it will explain the action of insulin efficacy and production. In type 1 diabetes, an auto-immune response has destroyed the cells that produce insulin. Without insulin, the body is unable to utilise glucose as energy and therefore this can be dangerous. The individual will need to have

insulin injections to rectify this problem and allow the body's cells to utilise the glucose appropriately, as energy

- In type 2 diabetes, the body is producing insulin but either it is not enough or it does not have the desired effect. Individuals are advised to change their eating habits to incorporate a balanced diet. Those with type 1 are educated in how to count their carbohydrate intake as a method of gaining a better control over their blood glucose levels. These patients may also have to have insulin at some point
- *Coeliac disease*: is an auto-immune disease, where an individual is intolerant of gluten. Exposure to it causes damage to the lining of the small intestine and can produce a range of symptoms from diarrhoea to weight loss. Gluten can be found in wheat, barley and rye, meaning if an individual consumed foods containing these elements, they would experience symptoms.

The above list is not intended to be a prescriptive list, it is more of an example, to highlight the potential complexities of nursing patients for an acute medical condition, while maintaining/controlling their pre-existing condition, as often the two are not the same.

Activity 17.4

Now reflect on what you have read, consider the following questions:

- What foods would you advise a patient with hypertension to avoid?
- What foods should an individual on a gluten-free diet avoid?
- What advice would you give an individual with high cholesterol?
- What interventions could you use when advising an adult who was overweight? How would this differ when advising a parent about their child's weight?

Nutritional assessment

In order to appropriately provide nutritional care and support to patients it is imperative that a comprehensive nutritional assessment is performed. The purpose of the assessment should be to identify patients who are at risk or those who are undernourished and those who are obese. A nutritional assessment includes both a subjective assessment (information from the patient/carer) as well as an 'objective' clinical assessment that involves the interpretation of information derived from dietary, laboratory, clinical assessment and clinical studies.

A nutritional assessment is a mandatory requirement for all patients admitted to hospital (NICE, 2006) and involves vulnerable patients for whom an admission to hospital can be quite upsetting. This could be individuals with learning difficulties, impaired mental health status, children and older persons. Arguably, every individual has the potential to be vulnerable to both mental health and/or physical problems.

Nurses should note and record food histories from both patients and their carers (Age Concern, 2006), to get a view of what has been happening in regards to food intake. Questions should also be asked about personal preferences, religious influences, dislikes and eating routines. It should be realised that food and eating may be a contentious issue, hence, this should be approached sensitively. Often they have a great deal of information about eating routines, favourite foods and least favourite foods. This should be completed along with any other observations that they may have regarding the individual, that would enhance the plan of care to be delivered to the patient.

Today, there is a greater cultural awareness of particular dietary preferences for certain ethnic groups, such as the requirement of halal food for Muslim patients and kosher food for Jewish patients. It is good practice even with this knowledge to assess the patient's dietary habits, preferences/eating practice undertaking this before/during/after eating.

With the younger patients, it is appropriate to ask questions about when the child started weaning and what stage are they at now, as well as noting any difficulties with achieving developmental milestones, in relation to eating. At times of stress or ill health, children tend to regress and go back a stage in their development in response to these situations. This can be quite distressing for parents/carers, so providing clear explanations and support during this time is important.

As well as the food history, a physical assessment should also be undertaken. This should include:

- Physical appearance: whether they appear emaciated or they are wearing very loose clothing
- Weight
- Height
- BMI (body mass index)
- Observation of skin turgor
- Presence of skin breakdown or pressure sores, indicating a poor immune system as a result of vitamin deficiency and/or under-nourishment
- Mobility, which can be weakened/reduced due to a reduction in muscle mass
- Vital signs including blood pressure: this will provide a baseline for reassessment especially useful for the undernourished patient who requires initiation of nutritional support. These will aid in the detection of re-feeding syndrome.

When undertaking any kind of assessment of a patient, the procedure and purpose should be explained, so that the patient can make an informed decision about whether to consent. Only once consent is obtained should the assessment be undertaken, with an explanation of each step given to the patient.

A nutritional assessment tool is usually referred to when conducting an assessment in hospital as it provides a structured approach with aids a unified approach. There are many tools in use, and one such tool is the Malnutrition Universal Screening Tool (MUST) (Stratton et al., 2004). This tool has been designed to address universal screening of malnutrition in adults in response to standardising care. It examines BMI, weight loss and disease factors and in return denotes a classification of nutritional status (ibid.).

Body Mass Index (BMI)

Body Mass Index is a measurement used to classify patient's weight and analyse whether it is within healthy parameters.

BMI = weight (kg) ÷ height (m²)

Example: BMI for a young man who is 1.6 m tall and weighs 60 kgs

$$BMI = \frac{60}{1.6 \times 1.6} = \frac{60}{2.56} = 23.44 \text{ kgm}^2$$

A BMI of 18.5–24.9 is classified as normal weight:

less than 18.5 = underweight
25–29.9 = overweight,
BMI greater than 30 = obese

The Royal College of Paediatrics and Child Health (RCPCH) have issued specific advice as to the measuring and plotting of weight in children please read via the following link:
UK-WHO growth chart resources (rcpch.ac.uk).

Don't forget!

Sick children require their weight to be monitored more frequently than adults as they can lose weight a faster rate. It is recommended that children over 2 years should be weighed at least weekly. In addition, healthcare professionals should look at the previous weight and height of the child. Attention in the younger than the 5-year-old age group should be paid to their centile charts, in their 'red' books (personal child health record). As part of discharge planning from hospital, the professional responsible should document the child's weight.

Assistance with feeding

It is important to have the right tools to assist your patient to maintain their independence in eating and drinking. An assessment by an occupational therapist can be requested in order to ensure that the patient has the right level of support, particularly in relation to feeding equipment and aids.

For some patients the only support that they may need is for someone to sit and encourage them, others may need assistance in cutting their food. Patients will have individual needs when it comes to assistance. The goal should always be to involve the patient by promoting their independence. The physical task of feeding a patient should only be undertaken when a patient can not undertake this task independently.

There are various pieces of practical equipment that can aid patients who require assistance with feeding, as shown in Figures 17.3–17.7.

A conscious effort should be made by healthcare professionals to ensure that mealtimes are 'protected' and that all unnecessary interventions are stopped in order to enable time for staff and patients to focus on eating. There are various ways of ensuring that this is possible. They do require a team effort to implement and maintain. Every practice setting should identify individuals to regulate and champion mealtimes (this can be healthcare assistants, housekeepers). Eating should be encouraged as a social event. Tips on promoting eating are highlighted in Box 17.4.

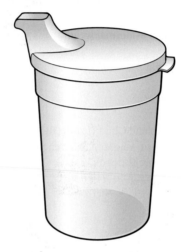

Figure 17.3 Beaker with a spout

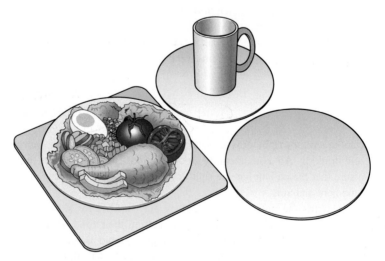

Figure 17.4 Non-slip mats to keep plates in place

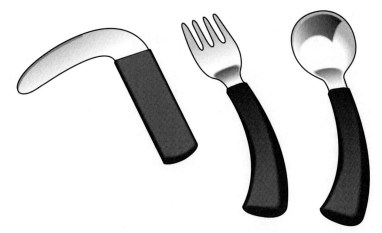

Figure 17.5 Specially moulded cutlery

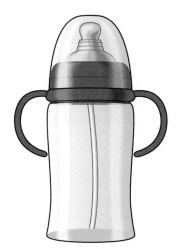

Figure 17.6 Bottle for children

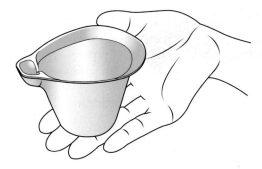

Figure 17.7 Cup used for premature babies

Box 17.4 Tips on promoting eating

- Involve patients in making food choices.
- Ensure where possible that patients can sit out away from their bed
- Clear beside tables in preparation for mealtimes
- Ensure that patients are ready to eat (e.g. that they have their dentures/mouth cleaned and, if a diabetic, they have had their insulin)
- Offer patients the facility and opportunity to wash their hands
- Ensure that the food is at the correct temperature
- Ensure that the food looks appealing and appetising to eat
- Provide the appropriate equipment (as mentioned earlier)
- Being available to support or assist as necessary
- Minimise disruptions (interventions and visitors)
- When the patient is finished, ensure that the plates and cutlery are cleared away
- If a patient misses mealtime, ensure that they still have access to food.

Individuals can require nutritional support at varying points in their treatment. This can be in the form of nutritional supplements being added to their diet to being fed totally via a feeding tube. This form of nutritional support is also known as enteral feeding, which also encompasses supplementary feeding orally as well as via a gastrostomy and a jejunostomy. A gastrostomy is a feeding tube, which is passed into the stomach and a jejunostomy is a feeding tube, passed into the middle section of the small bowel (Figures 17.8 and 17.9).

Enteral feeding

Nasogastric feeds can be given as a supplement to normal nutrition, where requirements are met through oral intake completely or partially. They are designed to provide short-term supplements for 2–4 weeks. This method is used in a variety of practice settings, e.g. paediatrics and adult surgical/medical care, adolescent eating disorders units, critical care units, to name a few. It can provide both short- and long-term solutions to nutritional problems. Nurses can insert the nasogastric tube but ONLY in patients who are assessed as having an adequate 'cough and gag' reflexes. If in doubt, patients can be referred to a speech and language therapist for assessment. For the patient without adequate cough or gag reflexes, e.g. someone who is unconscious, the nasogastric tube will need to be performed by a doctor or anaesthetist. This is to prevent aspiration of stomach contents into the lungs – if this happens – there can be fatal consequences for the patient.

Insertion of a nasogastric tube (without an introducer)

During this procedure, the nasogastric tube (NG) is passed through one of the patient's nostrils, and advanced down through the nasopharynx, oropharynx into the oesophagus and further down the alimentary canal until it reaches the stomach (Figure 17.10). The tube is confirmed as being in position through obtaining an aspirate and testing its

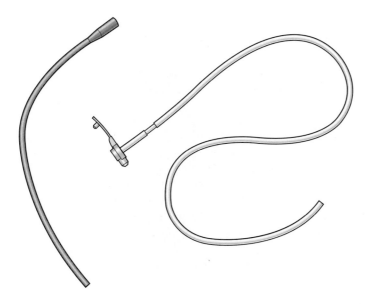

Figure 17.8 Jejunostomy tube

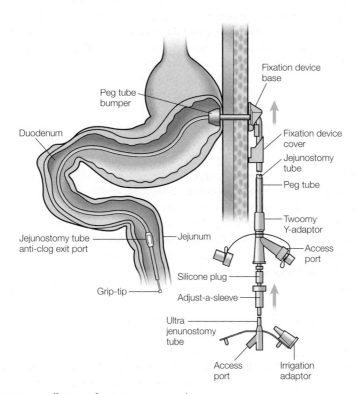

Figure 17.9 Installation of a jejunostomy tube

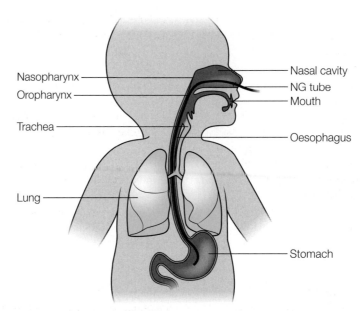

Nasopharynx

Oropharynx

Trachea

Lung

Nasal cavity

NG tube

Mouth

Oesophagus

Stomach

Figure 17.10 **Nasogastric tube in place**

pH value on a pH indicator strip, the required value should be less than 5.5 (NPSA, 2005). The placement does not need to be checked via x-ray making it a relatively safe procedure. Although the nasogastric route is relatively easy to access and it does not require surgical intervention, it does still have associated risks, such as misplacement, or migration of the tube into the lungs. Any professional involved with nasogastric tube insertion or position checks should have been assessed as competent through theoretical and practical learning (NSPA, 2012).

Equipment needed at the bedside

- Disposable plastic gloves
- Appropriate-sized finebore nasogastric tube (child/adult)
- Introducer (for tube if required)
- Receiver
- 20 mL (for child) or 50 mL for adult (enteral syringe)
- Sterile water
- pH testing paper and reference chart
- Hypo-allergenic tape to secure the tube in place
- Glass of clean water.

Pre-procedure for passing a NG tube

1   Before a decision is made to insert a nasogastric tube, an initial assessment on the suitability of this method of feeding should be made, with clear documentation in the patient's notes.

2   Placement of the tube should be delayed if there is not sufficient experienced support available to accurately confirm nasogastric tube placement, unless clinically urgent. The rationale for these decisions should be recorded in the patient's notes.

3   Nasogastric feeding tubes are radio-opaque throughout their length with externally visible markings.

4   Nasogastric tubes are not flushed, nor should any liquid/feed be introduced through the tube following its initial placement until the tube position is confirmed as being in the stomach by either pH testing or x-ray.

5   pH testing should be the first line method of testing tube position, with the pH of between 1–5.5 being a safe range. Each test and its result should be documented in the patient's bedside notes.

6   X-rays should only be a second line method when no aspirate can be obtained or the pH indicator strip has failed to confirm the position of the tube.

Procedure

1   Explain the procedure to the patient to ensure they are ready for the procedure. Gain consent. For the child, this can be very distressing, so use of play, and cooperation from parents is essential.

2   Identify a method by which the patient can indicate that they want you to stop (e.g. raising a hand).

3   Wash and dry hands before and after the procedure.

4   Ensure that patient is sitting comfortably and as upright as possible with the head supported with pillows.

5   Put on gloves, all aspects of the insertion procedure should follow the aseptic non-touch technique (ANTT). ANTT is a nationally recognised method for undertaking clinical tasks while reducing the risk of infection.

6   Measure the distance that the tube is to be passed down to. This is done by measuring from the patient's earlobe to the bridge of the nose, then an additional measurement from the bridge of the nose to the bottom of the xiphisternum. Both points of measurement together are the required distance (see Figure 17.11).

7   Pass the tube through the chosen nostril and advance past the nasopharynx and oropharynx and further down the oesophagus. This nostril should be clean and free from any sores. If possible ask the patient to cooperate by sipping some water (if they are able to) as you pass the tube as this will make the passage easier.

8   If the patient is a small child, you may need to swaddle the infant to ensure their safety. Always ensure that parents/carers are totally involved in the procedure by explaining all steps of the process to them.

9   If you encounter any undue resistance when attempting to pass the tube, DO NOT use force as this may cause damage to the internal structures of the patient. Instead you should withdraw the tube and try again.

10 Once the tube has been passed to the required length, test the tube by attaching the 20 mL syringe to the tube and pull back to obtain some stomach content/ aspirate.

11 Test the aspirate on the pH testing indicator, and read it against the recommended

reference chart. If the reading is less than 5.5, the tube is in the correct position. The NPSA (2005) alert clearly states that pH testing is the primary test for nasogastric tube positioning and x-rays are the second choice.

12   Secure the tube to the patient's face using an appropriate tape/dressing.

13   Remove gloves and wash hands.

14   Document the insertion of the tube in the patient's notes (NMC, 2015), ensuring it is documented which nostril used, the size of tube and to what length it was passed. Include a clear record of what the pH test result was.

15   If using an introducer, ensure that manufacturer's instructions are read and understood before insertion. You should also ensure that the introducer is able to move within the tube (to make removal post insertion easier). Once the tube is inserted, remove the introducer with gentle traction (if there is difficulty in extracting the introducer, then remove the tube as well), informing the nurse in charge or doctor. Once the introducer is removed, keep it somewhere safe, in case the tube requires re-inserting due to dislodgement.

16   Monitor the patient's condition for any problems, e.g. respiratory, non-compliance with the tube (pulling it out), pain.

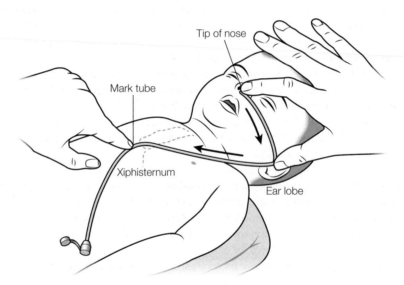

Figure 17.11 Measuring the NG tube for insertion

Top tip

Take precautions to use hypo-allergenic tape as well as a dressing in between the tube and the patient's skin so as to minimise friction and trauma to the epidermis.

Post procedure

The National Patient Safety Agency (NPSA, 2005) issued guidance on reducing harm caused by misplaced nasogastric feeding tubes in adults, children and infants. The guidance highlighted the risk factors associated with feeding via this route, through learning from national events related to nasogastric feeding. The alert provided clear guidance on checking and confirming tube positioning, as previously there had not been a clear national consensus. Since then, the NPSA (2011; 2012) has issued an update to the previous alert, as its findings reflect that the original advice is not always followed. The guidance can also be accessed via this link: www.nrls.npsa.nhs.uk.

The advice for healthcare professionals is:

1   The x-ray request form should clearly state the purpose of the x-ray is to establish the position of the tube for feeding.
2   The radiographer should take responsibility to ensure that the nasogastric tube can be clearly seen on the x-ray to be used to confirm position.
3   Documentation of the tube placement checking process includes confirmation that the x-ray viewed is the most current for the correct patient, how placement was interpreted, with clear instructions as to any required actions (e.g. such as movement of the tube). Any tubes that are identified as being in the lung are removed immediately.
4   'Whoosh' tests' (putting air through the tube and listening to the stomach for sound), acid/alkaline tests using litmus paper, the interpretation of the appearance of aspirate, putting the end of the tube in water and observing for bubbling *are never used* to confirm positioning as they are unreliable.
5   A full multi-disciplinary risk assessment is made and documented prior to a patient with a nasogastric tube being discharged from acute hospital care into the community.

Patients/carers need to have access to information that they can access at any time to reinforce the information given by professionals. There are many web-based resources available. One such portal for paediatrics, is the Coventry and Warwickshire children and young people's teaching framework website: www.act.org.uk.

Gastrostomy/Percutaneous Endoscopically placed Gastrostomy (PEG) tube

The PEG tube is a longer-term feeding tube that is placed directly into the stomach through a surgical procedure, or by using a percutaneous endoscope where the gastrostomy is made from the inside out (Figure 17.12). This method of enteral feeding is safer, as the tube has a reduced risk of aspiration or dislodgement.

The gastrostomy is an opening (stoma) to the abdomen from the outside of the body. The stoma creates a passageway between the stomach and the abdominal wall. A gastro-scope is a flexible instrument with an inbuilt camera which is passed through the mouth, down the oesophagus and into the stomach. At this point, the stomach is filled with air and a needle is passed through the outer skin into the stomach. The tube is inserted by it being threaded down the oesophagus, into the stomach and out through the hole made

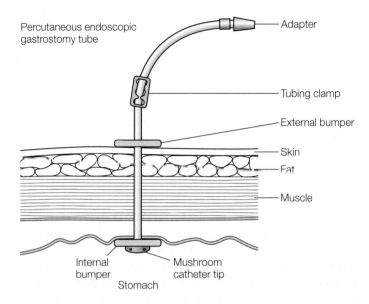

Percutaneous endoscopic gastrostomy tube

Adapter

Tubing clamp

External bumper

Skin

Fat

Muscle

Internal bumper

Mushroom catheter tip

Stomach

Figure 17.12 **PEG feeding tube**

by the needle. The internal retention disc, otherwise known as a flange, remains inside the stomach and then an external fixation plate is applied next to the skin, this holds the tubing in place. Connectors and clamps are attached to the external tubing before the patient is woken from the anaesthetic.

The added benefit is that patients/carers can be taught how to care for this tube independently and quite easily, as it is easier to manage than the nasogastric tube. However, if the tube is dislodged, there is an increased urgency to re-passing it (within 1–2 hours). Patients should always have a spare gastrostomy tube in case of tube dislodgement or rupture. Attention should also be paid to the patient's (adult/child) personal view of their body and whether they have any psychological issues as a result of a change to their body.

There are different types of PEG tubes, some have a balloon otherwise known as 'buttons' due to their appearance (popular with paediatric patients due to safety and discretion). The balloon is part of the tube that helps to maintain position once the balloon is inflated with sterile water to keep the tube sitting flush with the internal abdominal wall. There is also another type of PEG that has an extended external catheter and a disc that helps to maintain its position.

The gastrostomy site should be observed for any signs of infection. The site should be cleaned daily. Early signs that should be acted upon are:

- Redness
- Swelling
- Hot site
- Offensive smelling odour

■ Increased exudates (fluid that leaks out of blood vessels due to inflammation and is deposited into nearby tissue).

Caring for a PEG tube

Equipment

■ 1 x Dressing pack (should include gauze, gallipot, and clinical waste bag).
■ Cleaning solution: in hospital, 0.9% sodium chloride, at home, the patient is normally be advised to use either cooled boiled water or warm soapy water.

Procedure

1 Explain the procedure to the patient and where possible gain consent. For the child, play may need to be initiated.
2 Wash and dry hands before and after the procedure.
3 If the post-operative dressing is in place (for a newly placed gastrostomy), then remove it and write down your observations of the site. Note whether there is any odour, swelling, or discharge from the site. Discharge from the site is to be expected up to ten days after insertion.
4 Use aseptic non-touch technique (ANTT) to clean the site in a clockwise fashion, only using one piece of gauze in a sweeping fashion, then discard in the clinical waste bag (Chapter 12).
5 Rotate the gastrostomy tube 360 degrees in order to prevent the tube sticking to the sides of the stoma.
6 If the gastrostomy is new (under three months old), then the pH needs to be checked prior to every use.
7 The gastrostomy requires frequent flushing, to maintain the patency. Ideally you should flush the tube with 20 mLs of water (if the patient is under 1 year old, then it should be cooled boiled water).

This is a long-term solution that requires an increased amount of effort to manage, parents/carers have to be willing to take the care on as it requires constant vigilance. This method requires individuals to take a structured approach to ensuring an aseptic non-touch technique as the feeding tube is bypassing the stomach acids. The tube requires frequent flushing to maintain patency as it has an increased risk of blocking.

Total Parenteral Nutrition (TPN)

Total parenteral nutrition is a method of feeding directly into the bloodstream. This route is normally selected when the usual method of eating, digesting and absorbing is not possible. Listed below are some reasons as to why an individual could require TPN:

■ A non-functioning gut
■ Inaccessible gastro-intestinal tract
■ Intestinal failure

▪ Patients who have been 'nil by mouth' or have eaten minimally for more than five days
▪ Patients who are malnourished
▪ Oncology patients with complications of treatment (such as mucositis)
▪ Bowel obstruction.

The above situations highlight indications for short-term parenteral nutrition, however, there are those that may need this in the long term, e.g.

▪ Major trauma
▪ Severe malabsorption
▪ Severe disease or damage to the intestine (in Crohn's disease and short bowel syndrome).

The majority of patients can be managed via the oral/enteral route, it is only a few whose health needs result in them requiring intravenous assistance. As mentioned earlier, patients should be supported to achieve optimum independence rather than the ease of the task itself.

TPN is given via either a central or a peripheral line depending on the type of TPN to be administered as well as the duration. Prior to any decision about commencing this therapy being made, it is important that the patient is fully informed and has had the opportunity to discuss this openly with the medical/nursing team. It is also vital that the dietician and the Trust's nutrition team are involved.

All TPN must be prescribed on a drug chart by a doctor, and it is supplied by pharmacy and administered by a nurse. The nurse administering it or caring for a child with it should be deemed as intravenous competent, and also have had training specific to the administration of TPN. The nurse will use the ANTT method to prepare and administer the TPN bags and infuse them via an appropriate machine for a prescribed period of time.

Patient monitoring during the use of TPN

A baseline assessment should be undertaken before commencing a patient on TPN, this would include:

▪ Height and weight
▪ Biochemistry: urea and electrolytes (including calcium, magnesium and phosphate). liver function tests, and blood glucose monitoring
▪ Fluid balance
▪ Temperature.

This baseline assessment should be reassessed and there should also be ongoing monitoring of a patient's urinary functioning for secretion of sodium, potassium and nitrogen.

Staff caring for a patient receiving TPN should take considerable care in managing the line through which the nutrition is being infused, so as to minimise risk of infection and/or extravasation injury.

Top tip

All bags of TPN are sensitive to the light, therefore when a nurse has set the infusion up and it is running, the solution should be covered with an opaque plastic bag.

Once the infusion is running, it should not be disconnected for any reason; if after commencement the circuit is broken for any reason, then that TPN must be discarded for safety as it carries the risk of infection.

Nutrition and the role of the nurse

Nutrition is now, more than ever, an issue that is at the forefront of the nurse's professional responsibility when delivering person-centred nursing care. It was one of the Department of Health's (2001) Essence of Care benchmarks, for staff to ensure that best practice was achieved. In a bid to re-emphasise the relevance of nutrition to all the fields of nursing, the NMC has entrenched it within its guidance for pre-registration nursing and its 'essential skills clusters' (NMC, 2010) and the role of transferable skills within all fields of nursing. There are five clusters, of which nutrition and fluid management are one, and this clearly marks a move back to ensuring the basics of nursing care are addressed and delivered.

Nurses need to understand their role and responsibilities and abide by the code of professional conduct (NMC, 2015) in relation to caring for an individual with nutritional needs. This includes an understanding of when and how to make appropriate referrals to colleagues within the multi-disciplinary team, e.g., the dietician and speech and language therapist.

The nurse's role is not just limited to assisting patients with eating and the physical aspects of the activity. It is also one of health promotion and advice on dietary habits and healthy eating. It is in the nurse's interest to promote positive well-being, as a decreased nutritional state can prolong a patient's stay and increase the likelihood of potential complications.

It is also important to remember that although the activity of feeding is an everyday activity, feeding another individual with very specific needs is a totally different concept. It requires training and assessment of competence in the skill. Therefore, a nurse must ensure that they have the necessary training and are both confident and competent to undertake the task. If this is not the case, then they should seek advice and guidance from a senior member of staff. It is also the responsibility for the person delegating the task to you, the nurse, to check your level of understanding and competence. The NMC code of professional conduct (NMC, 2015) is explicit in its guidance on professional responsibility for delegation and undertaking particular tasks.

Summary

This chapter has discussed aspects that should be taken into consideration when providing care for patients with normal and changing nutritional needs. The importance that this basic daily task has in aiding the recovery and well-being of an individual is highlighted. Nutritional care is one of the cornerstones of good nursing practice that has been recognised since nursing began and its relevance and importance to practice have not changed. The only thing that has changed is the way nurses view it and the tools and expertise that are now available to provide truly individualised care to those who are most vulnerable. Early assessment and detection of a change in a patient's nutritional status are the key to positive outcomes and a quick return to optimal health, which is everyone's goal.

References

Age Concern (2006) *Hungry to Be Heard*. London: Age Concern.

Age UK (2006) *Malnutrition in Older People*. London: Age UK.

Age UK (2010) *Still Hungry to Be Heard*. London: Age UK.

BAPEN (British Association for Parenteral and Enteral Nutrition) (2012) *Malnutrition and Nutritional Care in the UK*. Available at: www.bapen.org.uk (accessed 1 March 2016).

Berk, L.E. (2009) *Child Development*, 8th edn. Harlow: Pearson.

Care Quality Commission (2011) *Dignity and Nutrition*. Available at: www.cqc.org.uk/content/dignity-and-nutrition-older-people-2011-inspection-programme (accessed 1 March 2016).

DoH (Department of Health) (2001) *Essence of Care*. London: The Stationery Office.

DoH (Department of Health) (2009) *Change for Life*. Available at: www.nhs.uk/change4life/Pages/change-for-life.aspx (accessed 1 March 2016).

DoH (Department of Health) (2011a) *Eatwell Plate*. Available at: www.nhs.uk/Livewell/Goodfood/Documents/Eatwellplate.pdf (accessed 6 March 2016).

DoH (Department of Health) (2011b) *Equality Analysis: A Call to Action on Obesity in England*. Available at: www.gov.uk/government/uploads/system/uploads/attachment_data/file/213721/dh_130511.pdf (accessed 1 March 2016).

DoH (Department of Health) (2012) NHS Future Forum calls on healthcare professionals to lead way on patient-centred care. Available at: http://tinyurl.com/86q78mn (accessed 1 March 2016).

Dudek, S.G. (2010) *Nutrition Essentials for Nursing Practice*, 6th edn. Philadelphia, PA: Wolters Kluwer Health Lippincott Williams and Wilkins.

EFSA (European Food Safety Authority) (2010) EFSA Panel on Dietetic Products, Nutrition, and Allergies (NDA); Scientific Opinion on Dietary reference values for water. *EFSA Journal*, 8(3):1459. doi:10.2903/j.efsa.2010.1459. Available at: www.efsa.europa.eu (accessed 1 March 2016).

Food Standards Agency (2016) *Eat well Guide: Helping you eat a healthy, balanced diet*. food.gov.uk

Francis, R. (2013) *Report of the Mid Staffordshire NHS Foundation Trust, Public Inquiry*, Volume 3 present and Future Annexes. London, The Stationary Office.

Hall, D. and Elliman, D. (2006) *Health for All Children*, revised 4th edn. New York: Oxford University Press.

Mental Health Foundation (2015) How to look after your mental health Available at: www.mentalhealth.org.uk/sites/default/files/How%20to%20look%20after%20your%20mental%20health.pdf

NICE (National Institute for Health and Care Excellence) (2006) *Nutrition Support in Adults: Oral Nutrition Support, Enteral Tube Feeding and Parenteral Nutrition*. Clinical guidance No. cg32. London: National Institute for Health and Care Excellence.

NICE (National Institute for Health and Care Excellence) (2015) *Clinical Knowledge Summaries: Available at:* http://cks.nice.org.uk/obesity (accessed 6 March 2016).

NICE (National Institute for Health and Care Excellence (2015) Obesity in children and young people: Prevention lifestyle weight management programme. https://www.nice.org.uk/guidance/lifestyle-and-wellbeing/diet--nutrition-and-obesity (accessed 6 March 2016).

NICE (National Institute for Health and Care Excellence (2016) Obesity in Adults: Prevention lifestyle weight management programme. https://www.nice.org.uk/guidance/lifestyle-and-wellbeing/diet--nutrition-and-obesity (accessed 6 March 2016).

Nightingale, F. (1860) *Nursing: Notes on What it is and What it is Not.* New York: Appleton and Company.

NMC (Nursing and Midwifery Council) (2010) *Standards for Pre-registration Nursing Education.* London: NMC.

NMC (Nursing and Midwifery Council) (2015) *The Code: Professional Standards of Practice and Behaviour for Nurses and Midwives.* London: NMC.

NPSA (National Patient Safety Agency) (2005) Reducing the harm caused by misplaced nasogastric feeding tubes: Patient safety alert 5. London: National Patient Safety Agency.

NPSA (National Patient Safety Agency) (2011) Reducing the harm caused by misplaced nasogastric feeding tubes in adults, children and infants. London: National Patient Safety Agency.

NPSA (National Patient Safety Agency) (2012) Harm from flushing of nasogastric tubes before confirmation of placement. Rapid response report (RRR001). London:-National Patient Ssafety Agency.

PAHO (2013) *Beyond Survival*, 2nd edn. Washington, DC: Pan American Health Organisation.

Public Health England (2014) *Your Guide to Eatwell Plate: Helping You Eat a Healthier Diet.* London: Department of Health.

Scientific Advisory Committee on Nutrition (2008) *The Nutritional Wellbeing of the British Population.* Edinburgh: The Stationery Office.

Stratton, R.J., Hackston, A., Longmore, D., *et al.* (2004) Malnutrition in hospital outpatients and inpatients: prevalence, concurrent validity and ease of use of the 'malnutrition universal screening tool' ('MUST') for adults. *British Journal of Nutrition*, 92(5): 799–808.

WHO (2009) *Infant and Young Child Feeding: Model Chapter for Textbooks for Medical Students and Allied Health Professionals.* Geneva: World Health Organisation.

Chapter 18

Hydration and fluid balance

Margaret Herlihy and Dee Anderson

The National Patient Safety Agency (NPSA), the National Institute for Health and Care Excellence (NICE), and the Royal College of Nursing (RCN) believe that hydration is a fundamental aspect of care and that everyone in healthcare environments has a role to play. According to NICE Quality Standard CG138 (NICE, 2012), patients ought to have a range of physical and psychological needs regularly assessed and addressed, this includes nutrition, hydration, pain relief, personal hygiene and anxiety.

Key concepts

Electrolytes

Homeostasis

Osmolality

Dehydration

Fluid balance

Fluid over-load

Blood transfusion

Transfusion reactions

Learning outcomes

By the end of this chapter you will be able to:

- Describe the physiological mechanisms required to maintain fluid and electrolyte balance in the adult and child
- Assess the patient's fluid and electrolyte status
- Identify clinical signs of dehydration or electrolyte imbalances in the adult and child
- Describe nursing interventions required to correct problems with fluid and electrolyte balance
- Outline the processes and complications associated with blood transfusion.

Introduction

Water is an essential requirement for humans and, unlike other deficiencies which may take a long period of time to develop, without water, life will only be sustained for a few days. This is closely linked to nutrition which ought to be considered alongside this and is addressed in Chapter 17. An adequate amount of water and electrolytes are needed to carry out all body functions at a cellular level. In a healthy person, fluid taken in is balanced with fluid loss and a fluid and electrolyte balance is necessary to maintain homeostasis. Dehydration occurs when insufficient water or other fluids are drunk, or excessive fluids are lost, even as little as 1 per cent of the body mass. This can lead to problems with the renal and cardiac systems, and in certain cases, subtle changes can lead to the death of a patient (RCN, 2007).

A moderately active adult needs to take in approximately 1.5–2.5 litres of fluid each day, and the ill adult may need far more. Fluid requirements in children vary depending on the age and weight of the child. There are numerous reasons for the ill person to lose fluids from the body, such as diarrhoea, vomiting, fever, haemorrhaging, burns, renal disease, drug therapies, and fasting. Attention to hydration during illness demands specific attention as at this time the body's need is greater to facilitate repair and recovery.

Hydration and the role of the nurse

Evidence suggests that many patients in hospital are not given sufficient fluids, with drinks being either put out of reach or not offered for long periods of time (Care Quality Commission, 2011). An adverse impact on the outcomes of some acutely ill hospitalised patients has been identified when nurses do not adequately manage a patient's fluid balance, or fail to keep accurate fluid balance records (NPSA, 2007). When hydration is overlooked, it can result in vulnerable individuals missing out on the support they need to help maintain a healthy level of hydration. The evidence for good hydration shows that it can assist in preventing or treating ailments such as: pressure ulcers, constipation, urinary infections and incontinence, kidney stones, heart disease, low blood pressure, cognitive impairment, dizziness and confusion leading to falls, poor oral health and skin conditions (RCN, 2007).

Activity 18.1

'TheThirst4Life hydration initiative' undertaken by Buckinghamshire NHS led to 45 per cent reduction in emergency admission in 2005 and in Surrey, in 2010, evaluation of the project showed marked improvements in elderly people's lives and those with dementia (RCN, 2007; NHS Surrey, 2010).

- Look up 'Thirst4life' and see what organisations in your area are doing in relation to this initiative
- How do you address water intake in your area of practice?
- Can you recognise patients or clients who would benefit from better water intake?

Water in the body

Water is the fluid in the body in which all life processes occur (Box 18.1). As the primary fluid in the body, water serves as a solvent for minerals, vitamins, amino acids, glucose and many other nutrients. Water is the medium for the safe elimination of toxins and waste products and whole-body thermoregulation.

Box 18.1 Functions of water

- Moistens tissues such as those in the eyes, mouth and nose
- Maintains and regulates body temperature
- Lubricates joints
- Protects body organs and tissues – insulator and shock absorber
- Helps prevent constipation
- Transports nutrients and oxygen to the cells
- Dissolves minerals and other nutrients to make them accessible to the body
- Flushes out waste products.

Body water is divided into a number of body compartments termed intracellular (ICF) and extracellular (ECF) spaces which comprise: blood, tissue fluid, lymph. They are kept there with dynamic processes (osmosis and diffusion). A good textbook will expand on this as it is core to homeostasis. A healthy young man is about 60–70 per cent water and a healthy young woman about 50 per cent (Figure 18.1). Thus, for a 75 kg man, this would equal a body water of 45L (Table 18.1). The proportion of body water decreases with ageing and in people over 60, it decreases to 50 per cent.

Table 18.1 Distribution of water in the body of a 75 kg man

75 kg man: Total Body Water: 60–70% (45–52L)		
Intracellular Fluid (ICF) 40–45% (30–33 L)	Extracellular Fluid (ECF) 20–25% (15–18 L)	
	Interstitial/Tissue Fluid 80% of ECF: 12–14 L	Plasma 20% of ECF: 3–3.6 L

Infants have the highest proportion of water, accounting for 70–80 per cent of their body weight and this can be higher in premature infants (Thibodeau and Patton, 2012). The percentage of water reduces with age from around 86 per cent at 26 weeks to 80 per cent at 32 weeks and to about 78 per cent at full term. This occurs as a result of the accumulation of body fat during development. In the newborn infant, body weight can be a good indicator of fluid loss and balance (Chow and Douglas, 2008).

Water balance of the adult body

Supply		Losses

Food:
1,100 mL

Drinks:
1,100 mL

Metabolism:
300 mL

Breathing:
400 mL

Sweat:
450 mL

Fecal matter:
150 mL

Urine:
1,500 mL

Total: 2,500 mL

Total: 2,500 mL

Figure 18.1 **Summary of water balance (intake and output) from the body**

Top tip

Children admitted to hospital suspected of dehydration or fluid overload should always be weighed on Class III clinical electronic scales.

Composition of body fluids

Body fluid is a composition of water and a variety of dissolved solutes, electrolytes and non-electrolytes. Non-electrolytes include glucose, lipids and urea. Nutrients and waste products constantly shift within the body's compartments of fluids and electrolytes between blood vessel or vascular space and body tissue. Electrolytes are the chemical substances such as salts, acids, and bases, which dissociate in water, forming electrically charged particles called ions. Alterations (excess or depletion) lead to problems. A summary of the electrolytes and their functions can be seen in Table 18.2.

Disorders of electrolyte balance

Electrolytes can be found inside and outside the cell, but only the levels in the bloodstream, outside the cell (ECF) are measured. Electrolytes are essential for the activity

Table 18.2 Electrolytes: broad function and dietary sources

	Source	Function
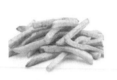	**Sodium** Found in many foods e.g. table salt, beef, pork, sardines, cheese, olives, bacon and ham. All processed and canned foods may have added salt, as well as crisps and snacks, nuts, butter, margarine, mayonnaise and sauces.	Main function is to control and regulate water balance also muscle and nerve function.
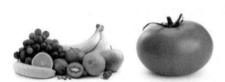	**Potassium** Found in range of fruits and vegetables especially leafy green vegetables such as spinach, kale, bananas, tomatoes, avocados, nuts, sweet potatoes and milk.	Helps maintain water balance. Aids skeletal, cardiac and smooth muscle activity and acid-base balance.
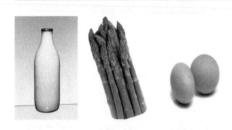	**Calcium** Commonly found in milk and milk products. It is also in meat, fish with bones such as sardines, eggs, fortified breakfast cereals, almonds, beans, certain fruits such as dried apricots, figs and asparagus.	Development of bones, regulating muscle contraction, relaxation and cardiac function.
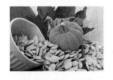 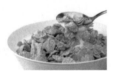	**Magnesium** Is in leafy green vegetables, nuts, cereals, beans, pumpkin and squash seeds, meat, chocolate and coffee. Also in 'hard water'.	Energy source (Adenosine Triphosphate or ATP) and in the stomach neutralises stomach acid.
	Phosphorus It is found in almost every food, and as such, deficiency is rare. Found in milk, meat, pumpkin, salmon, shellfish, brazil nuts, beans and lentils.	Cell functioning, growth, maintenance, and repair of cells and tissues, regulation of calcium, and for making ATP (energy).
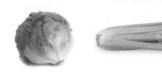	**Chloride** Chloride is found in salt or salt as sodium chloride. It is also found in many vegetables, e.g. seaweed, rye, tomatoes, lettuce, celery, and olives.	Major component of gastric acid. It is involved in regulating acid-base balance, fluid regulation and also blood pressure and volume.

of cells and their concentration in the blood is kept within a specific range (Table 18.3). Changes in levels or potential changes in these can be life-threatening. For example, a patient who has severe diarrhoea may have altered sodium or potassium and this will affect muscle contractions and cause cramping pains or cardiac problems. For children, alterations may occur more quickly and have profound effects. For patients with mental health problems, certain medicines can have severe effects for people, i.e. altering electrolytes for those taking lithium carbonate and sodium levels.

Rationale for fluid balance

The rationale for learning this skill is to monitor patients effectively and address problems is indicated as a key skill by the Nursing and Midwifery Council (NMC) (2010). Water intake normally balances with water loss. The normal daily turnover of water is approximately 4 per cent of total body weight in adults. This is equivalent to 2500–3000 mL day in a 70 kg adult. Most of our water needs are met by actually drinking water and other beverages and while most adults drink only approximately 1500 mL of fluid, another approximately 1000 mL is added by foods and oxidation of these foods during the metabolic processes. The water content of solid foods contributes approximately 750 mL per day. For example, the water content of fresh vegetables is approximately 90 per cent, of fresh fruits about 85 per cent, and of lean meats about 60 per cent. Water is also a by-product of food metabolism. This quantity is approximately 250 mL per day for the average adult.

Activity 18.2

Revise these terms for fluid and electrolyte homeostasis.

Diffusion	Passive movement of solutes from an area of high concentration to an area of lower concentration until equilibrium
Osmosis	Passive movement of water from where it is in high concentration to where it is in low concentration across a semi-permeable membrane until equilibrium is achieved
Hydrostatic pressure	The pressure created by blood flow and exerted on the walls of arteries.

Fluid requirements for adults and children

The reference values for total water intake include water from drinking water, beverages of all kinds, and from food moisture and only apply to conditions of moderate environmental temperature and moderate physical activity levels (European Food Safety Authority, 2010). Optimal intake is given in Table 18.4.

Fluid losses from the body counterbalance intake. Fluid loss occurs through:

■ Insensible means (through the skin as perspiration and via the lungs as water vapour in expired air)
■ Urine
■ Noticeable loss through the skin
■ Loss through the intestines in faeces.

Insensible losses occur through the skin and lungs and vary with perspiration and activity level. For example, with exercise or increased body temperature, this loss can increase.

Watch out

At birth, a baby's head makes up over 20 per cent of their total surface area, so exposing that skin leads to increased heat and moisture loss. Children younger than 36 months have a disproportionately large head in comparison to body size.

Factors that increase fluid loss add to fluid needs and include:

■ High temperature
■ Diarrhoea or vomiting
■ Low humidity
■ High altitude
■ High-fibre diet
■ High sodium intake
■ Caffeine and alcohol consumption
■ Exercise.

These all apply to the child but most common would be high temperature and diarrhoea and vomiting.

Watch out

People travelling in aeroplanes may well become dehydrated due to the recirculated air – they need on average to drink 250 ml extra an hour to compensate. This is especially important for children.

Table 18.3 Common electrolyte imbalances in adults

Electrolyte	Abnormality	Assessment findings	Causes
Sodium 133–146 mmol/L	Hypernatraemia	Non-specific – sticky or dry oral mucous membranes; thirst; restlessness, irritability, lethargy, convulsions; tachycardia, delirium, anxiety eventually coma – mostly due to decreased water in the brain	Excessive loss of water through intestines, (vomiting, diarrhoea) ; Inhalation of salt water in near drowning; Hypertonic tube feedings; Excessive infusion of saline solutions. Medications (e.g. loop diuretics)
	Hyponatraemia	Headache, lethargy, weakness, disorientation; Confusion, hostility; nausea & vomiting; absence of reflexes; muscle cramps, Delirium, convulsions, coma	Increased water intake with decreased sodium intake i.e., diuretics, excess intravenous fluids, gastric suction; medications such as some diuretics, drinking too much water or drugs (Ecstasy)
Potassium 3.5–5.3 mmol/L	Hyperkalaemia	Irritability and restlessness; cramps, weakness; paresthesias; ECG changes with cardiac irregularities; peaked T waves,, cardiac arrest	Renal failure; Excessive potassium replacement; Initial reaction to massive tissue damage (i.e., burns trauma, metabolic acidosis); potassium-sparing diuretics
	Hypokalaemia	Fatigue that progresses to paralysis; numbness (paresthesia); nausea, vomiting, anorexia, dizziness; confusion; cardiac arrest	Inadequate intake; Vomiting, diarrhoea, suctioning, wound drainage; Excessive diaphoresis; Metabolic alkalosis; Insulin treatment for Diabetic Ketoacidosis Diuretic therapy without adequate potassium replacement
Calcium 2.1–2.6 mmol/L	Hypercalcemia	Muscle weakness/atrophy; lethargy; coma; bone pain; polyuria; excessive thirst; anorexia, nausea vomiting, constipation; hypertension; ECG changes	Increased intestinal absorption; Excessive vitamin D; Increased bone resorption; Immobility; Decreased phosphorus, dehydration. Hyperparathyroidism; Multiple fractures. Hereditary factors. Secondary spread of cancer (metastases)
	Hypocalcaemia	Mild or life threatening. Paresthesias, tetany, seizures abdominal spasms, cramps, skeletal muscle cramps, laryngeal spasm, impaired memory, irritability, decreased cardiac output, bleeding	Renal failure; Protein malnutrition or malabsorption; Decreased intake; burns or infection; Hypoparathyroidism; Diarrhoea; Excessive antacid use; Multiple blood transfusions; Acute pancreatitis; Liver disease; Elevated phosphate
Magnesium (0.7–1.0 mmol/L)	Hypermagnesemia	Hypotension,, respiratory depression; lethargy, coma; bradycardia, cardiac arrest	Renal failure; Excessive intake from antacids and laxatives, severe dehydration with poor urine output
	Hypomagnesemia	Tremors, tetany, seizures, tachycardia, hypertension, cardiac arrhythmias, personality changes	Malnutrition; Alcoholism; Diuretics; Dehydration Diarrhoea
Chloride (95–108 mmol/L)	Hyperchloraemia	Dehydration, increased retention or intake, metabolic acidosis	No direct clinical symptoms. Symptoms generally associated with the underlying cause which is often related to pH abnormalities
	Hypochloraemia	Metabolic alkalosis due to vomiting or excessive ingestion of alkaline substances, aldosterone deficiency	

Note: the levels vary with age, gender, diet and any other illness. Ranges based on www.LabTestsOnline.org.uk but be aware ranges of normal levels may vary slightly with differing healthcare areas.

Table 18.4 **Optimal daily fluid intake**

Age	Amount
Infants 0–6 months of age	100–190 mL/kg per day
Infants 6–12 months of age	800–1000 mL/day
Second year of life	1100–1200 mL/day
Boys and girls 2–3 years of age	1300 mL/day
Boys and girls 4–8 years of age	1600 mL/day
9–13 years of age.	2100 mL/day for boys 1900 mL/day for girls
Adolescents of 14 years and older are considered as adults with respect to adequate water intake	
Adults	2.0 L/day for females 2.5 L/day for males
The same intake as for adults are defined for the elderly.	

Assessment of hydration status

The three elements required to assess fluid balance and hydration status are:

1 Clinical assessment
2 Body weight
3 Urine output.

Additionally information would also be obtained from:

1 Review of fluid balance charts
2 Review of blood chemistry.

Activity 18.3

■ How would you recognise that a change in patient's hydration status has occurred?
■ How to assess skin turgor in a child? In an elderly patient?
■ How to assess mucous membranes in a child? In an elderly patient?
■ What blood chemistry changes would you find in a patient who is over-hydrated? Under-hydrated?

The physical symptoms of mild dehydration include: impaired cognitive function; reduced physical performance; headaches, fatigue, sunken eyes and dry, less elastic skin. If dehydration persists, the circulating volume of blood can drop. This leads to: hypotension; tachycardia; a weak, thready pulse; cold hands and feet; and oliguria (reduced urine output). These are also the early signs of hypovolaemic shock and are very serious.

Procedure to assess hydration status

1   Approach the patient and inform them of what you are intending to do and obtain consent.
2   Ask the patient about any conditions, changes or lifestyle patterns which may affect their ability to drink. If any diarrhoea or vomiting or other points arise, note these and report immediately.
3   Ask the patient about their hydration preferences – type of drinks, frequency of drinking usually and its pattern during the day, to establish if they are usually well hydrated and to aid providing support if needed.
4   Observe the patient's skin, mucosa and conjunctiva: they ought to be moist and pink and the skin firm and relatively plump (not paper-like) which is termed skin turgor. The skin ought to return to its normal condition if pinched gently. This does depend on the age and general condition of the patient.
5   Record temperature, pulse, blood pressure, respiratory rate, breathing sounds. Alterations may be present to indicate dehydration or over-hydration.
6   Measure the patient's weight: generally stable but daily fluctuations may indicate increased or decreased fluid changes.
7   Measure their urine output, other fluid output and fluid intake noting the sources of these (see the fluid balance chart, Figure 18.2).
8   Evaluate the serum electrolyte levels in light of the clinical assessment to make a conclusion.

NHS

NHS Foundation trust

STANDARD FLUID BALANCE SHEET

FLUID RESTRICTION No

DATE 18 / 07 / 2016

Surname	Bloggs
First name	Simon
Hospital No.	123-123-1234
DOB	20 / 07 / 1964
Gender	Male

Volume in jug 2l

	INPUT						OUTPUT		
TIME	ORAL INTAKE	I.V. FLUIDS (including central)- BATCH % BAG NUMBER	VOL	OTHER (e.g. enetral)	VOL	running total	URINE	OTHER (e.g. drain, gastric contents)	running total
00.00									
01.00									
02.00									
03.00									
04.00									
05.00								Drain 200ml	200 ml
06.00							150 ml		350 ml
07.00		0.9% saline 123456	1l			1000 ml			
08.00									
09.00	150 ml					1150 ml			
10.00							500 ml		850 ml
11.00									
12.00									
Total	150 ml		1000 ml			1150ml			850 ml
13.00									
14.00	200 ml					1350 ml		Vomit 100ml	950 ml
15.00									
16.00							250 ml		1200 ml
17.00	100 ml					1450 ml			
18.00	100 ml					1550 ml			
19.00								Drain 100ml	1300 ml
20.00	150 ml					1700 ml			
21.00							300 ml		1600 ml
22.00									
23.00									
24hr total				TOTAL INTAKE:		1750 ml	TOTAL OUTPUT:		1600 ml
EVAPORATION = 800MLS					BALANCE -900 ml				

Figure 18.2 A fluid balance chart

Activity 18.4

How do nurses decide whether a patient requires a fluid balance chart?
Hint: think about vulnerable people or problems they may have.

Clinical significance

Water is good for health but drinking too much can cause problems. Over-hydration can be due to excessive intake of water and result in water accumulating in the brain and cause collapse. Psychogenic 'polydipsia' is an excessive water intake seen in some patients with mental illnesses such as schizophrenia, or developmental disabilities. It should be taken very seriously, as the amount of water ingested exceeds the amount that can be excreted by the kidneys.

Dehydration

Dehydration is not the same as hypovolemia, and refers to the loss of water alone, without a significant loss of electrolytes. As a result of this water loss, sodium is retained and there is an increase in serum sodium levels. However, water losses alone are unusual and more commonly sodium is lost in addition to water. Dehydration is defined as the loss of 1 per cent or more of bodyweight (BW) but a 1 or 2 per cent decrease is not harmful and should be corrected by being alert to the early signs of dehydration such as thirst and the replacement of the fluid loss by drinking. It is categorised by Thibodeau and Patten (2012) as:

- Mild: 4 per cent loss of BW
- Moderate: 5–8 per cent loss of BW
- Severe: 8–10 per cent loss of BW.

Dehydration results from decreased intake, increased output (renal, gastrointestinal or insensible losses), a shift of fluid (e.g. ascites, effusions), or capillary leak of fluid (e.g., burns and sepsis). Children are particularly susceptible to dehydration. The symptoms often begin with thirst and other symptoms of early dehydration. In extreme cases, symptoms include those indicating advanced dehydration and can progress to death. Table 18.5 shows risk factors in vulnerable groups.

Clinical assessment will determine over-hydration or dehydration and the next actions to take. The signs and symptoms of mild to moderate dehydration in adults are:

- Dry, sticky mouth
- Sleepiness or tiredness
- Agitation
- Thirst
- Decreased urine output

Table 18.5 Risk factors in vulnerable groups

Risk factors in older people	Risk factors in children
■ Reduced sense of thirst ■ Reduced renal function ■ Increased longevity ■ Female gender ■ Physical weakness and disabilities ■ Communication problems ■ Onset of dementia ■ Fear of incontinence linked to oral fluid intake ■ Multiple pre-existing medical conditions ■ Medications, in particular diuretics	■ Immature thirst mechanisms ■ Relatively high fluid loss (due to a large surface area to body mass ratio) and high activity levels ■ Less developed sweating and kidney function ■ Communication (relative to development)

Causes of dehydration:

■ Not drinking enough water – reasons include: tonsillitis, sore throat, mouth ulcers, difficulty swallowing, and/or a decreased thirst sensation (especially in older adults)
■ Gastroenteritis, nausea/vomiting, diarrhoea, fever pain
■ Indoor environment too hot
■ Inability to get water, e.g. mobility
■ Excessive urine output – uncontrolled diabetes, diuretic use
■ Medications – laxatives, sedatives/sleeping pills/anxiety medications
■ Decreased water intake due to a medical/health condition
■ Excessive exercise

■ Dark, concentrated urine with strong odour
■ Few or no tears when crying
■ Muscle weakness
■ Headache
■ Dizziness or light-headedness
■ Constipation
■ Loss of appetite.

In children, dehydration is very serious too. The principles of assessment remain the same and observation of the indicators in Table 18.6 will aid a nursing diagnosis.

Watch out

If a child appears unwell or is deteriorating, he/she has an altered responsiveness (irritable/lethargy), sunken eyes, rapid heart rate, rapid breathing rate and reduced skin turgor *they need immediate clinical intervention*.

Table 18.6 **Dehydration in children**

Mild to moderate dehydration in children	Severe dehydration in children
■ Loss of 1–5% body weight – mild ■ Loss of 6–10% body weight – mild–moderate ■ Restlessness/irritability ■ Sunken eyes ■ Very thirsty ■ Skin turgor – slow-skin fold is visible for less than 2 seconds ■ Dry mucous membranes (except mouth breather) ■ Reduced tears ■ Decreased urine output	■ Loss of 10% body weight severe In addition any two or more of the following raises alarms: ■ Increased lethargy/abnormal sleepiness ■ Sunken eyes ■ Drinking poorly or not at all ■ Skin turgor – very slow-skin fold visible for longer than 2 seconds ■ Weak rapid heart rate for age ■ Rapid breathing for age ■ Cool or blue extremities ■ Sunken anterior fontanelle

Case study 18.1 Adult

Betty is a 72-year-old who has recently been discharged home from hospital. The District Nurse makes a scheduled visit to Betty. Upon arrival she finds that Betty is not feeling well. She has been constipated for several days and today she notes that her vision is blurry. Betty also reports her mouth is very dry and she feels hotter than usual.

Upon further questioning, the District Nurse learns that Betty has been experiencing an increase in night-time urination so she has stopped drinking any fluids after dinner. She is now getting up just once a night but now her urine smells funny.

■ What are the signs and symptoms Betty is reporting that indicate she is dehydrated?

■ What caused Betty to stop drinking water?

■ What should the District Nurse suggest to help Betty increase the amount of fluid/water she is drinking?

■ What is the next step in Betty's care?

Management of dehydration in adults

The replacement of fluids is the main treatment in addition to managing the underlying condition. If possible, oral fluids are used but if not tolerated or if severely dehydrated, intravenous (IV) fluids are used (Figure 18.3). NICE (2013) have produced a useful algorithm (flow chart) with features and approaches to aiding rehydration: www.nice. org.uk/guidance/cg174/chapter/recommendations. Hypotonic solutions are used and the patient needs to be monitored for signs and symptoms of cerebral oedema which

Case study 18.2 Child

Zorina is the 3-year-old daughter of Ivan and Rehana. The family take advantage of the hot summer weather and spend a long weekend break away from home. While in the park Zorina walks over to her parents rubbing her tummy, saying that it hurts. But no sooner than Ivan had rubbed Zorina's tummy and cuddled her for a short while, then she springs up and pulls her daddy toward the slide to play. After half an hour Zorina slows down in her play activities and seems to be a little lethargic. Zorina says she wants to go home and sleep. Ivan and Rehana notice that Zorina's skin is clammy to touch and she looks hot and bothered. They offer her some diluted juice but she pushes it away from her face.

Rehana becomes concerned on return to their rented cottage, when Zorina has two episodes of watery diarrhoea and she notes that Zorina's urine is considerably darker than the clear straw colour it usually is.

Rehana discusses her concerns with her husband Ivan. Rehana has noticed that Zorina has not been drinking as much fluids as she normally would. They decide to take Zorina to the paediatric section of the local walk-in centre for assessment and management.

▪ What are the signs and symptoms that indicate Zorina is dehydrated?
▪ Why do you think Zorina pushed the juice away despite looking hot and bothered?
▪ What questions do you think staff should ask Zorina's parents to assess her fluid intake?
▪ How should Zorina's dehydration be managed?
▪ How should the staff in the walk-in centre help Zorina's parents to encourage her to drink?

Refer to NICE (2009) Diarrhoea and Vomiting in Children guidelines to help you.

include headache, irritability, lethargy, confusion, nausea, vomiting, decreased pulse rate, widening pulse pressure, and seizures. Patients with diabetes insipidus may be prescribed vasopressin (ADH). Fluid balance is assessed by monitoring blood sodium levels, urine osmolality and specific gravity, daily weights and an accurate record of fluid balance is maintained.

Management of dehydration in children

The treatment of mild to moderate dehydration in children does not require intravenous therapy as long as oral fluids are tolerated. An oral rehydration salt (ORS) solution should be used. If the child refuses to take sufficient quantities of the ORS solution and does not have warning signs or symptoms, they may have ORS solution supplemented with fluids such as milk feeds or water. Fruit juices and carbonated drinks should be avoided. In the case of babies, breast feeding should continue if possible (NICE, 2009).

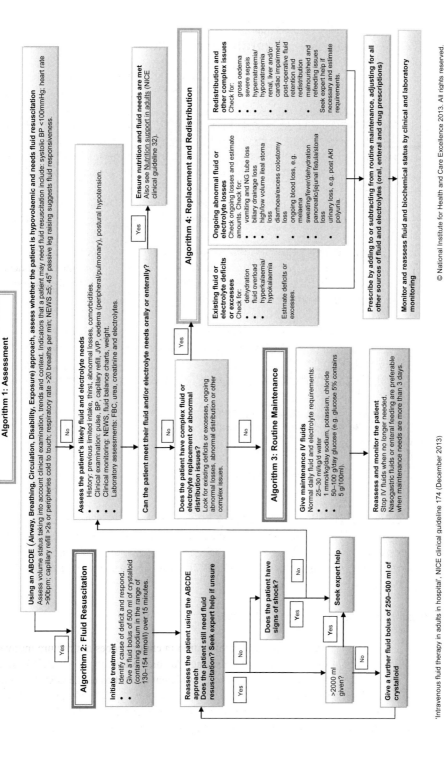

Figure 18.3 **Algorithms for IV fluid therapy in adults**

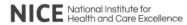

Algorithms for IV fluid therapy in adults

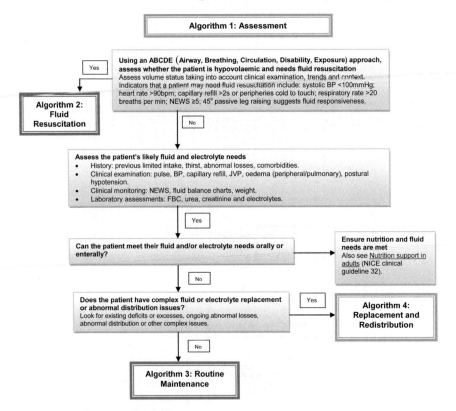

Figure 18.3 Algorithms for IV fluid therapy in adults (*continued*)

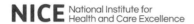 National Institute for Health and Care Excellence

Algorithms for IV fluid therapy in adults

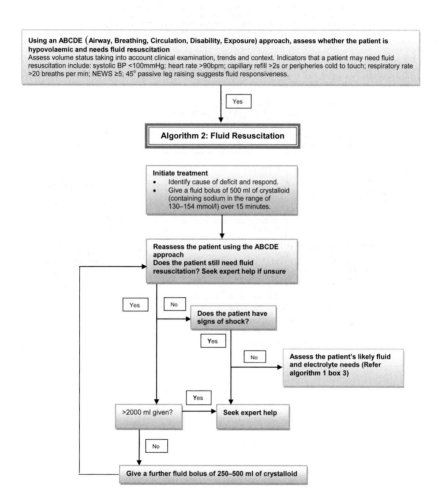

Figure 18.3 Algorithms for IV fluid therapy in adults *(continued)*

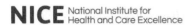

Algorithms for IV fluid therapy in adults

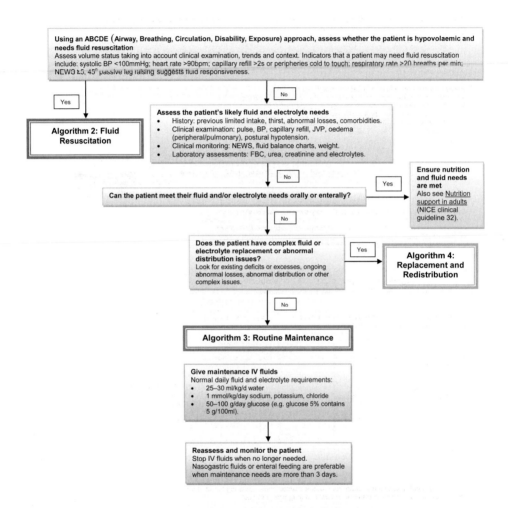

Figure 18.3 Algorithms for IV fluid therapy in adults (*continued*)

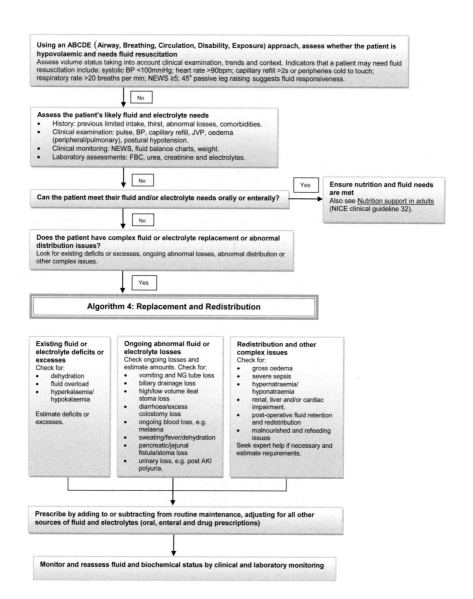

NICE National Institute for Health and Care Excellence

Algorithms for IV fluid therapy in adults

Using an ABCDE (Airway, Breathing, Circulation, Disability, Exposure) approach, assess whether the patient is **hypovolaemic and needs fluid resuscitation**
Assess volume status taking into account clinical examination, trends and context. Indicators that a patient may need fluid resuscitation include: systolic BP <100mmHg; heart rate >90bpm; capillary refill >2s or peripheries cold to touch; respiratory rate >20 breaths per min; NEWS ≥5; 45° passive leg raising suggests fluid responsiveness.

No

Assess the patient's likely fluid and electrolyte needs
- History: previous limited intake, thirst, abnormal losses, comorbidities.
- Clinical examination: pulse, BP, capillary refill, JVP, oedema (peripheral/pulmonary), postural hypotension.
- Clinical monitoring: NEWS, fluid balance charts, weight.
- Laboratory assessments: FBC, urea, creatinine and electrolytes.

No

Can the patient meet their fluid and/or electrolyte needs orally or enterally?   Yes → **Ensure nutrition and fluid needs are met**
Also see Nutrition support in adults (NICE clinical guideline 32).

No

Does the patient have complex fluid or electrolyte replacement or abnormal distribution issues?
Look for existing deficits or excesses, ongoing abnormal losses, abnormal distribution or other complex issues.

Yes

Algorithm 4: Replacement and Redistribution

Existing fluid or electrolyte deficits or excesses	**Ongoing abnormal fluid or electrolyte losses**	**Redistribution and other complex issues**
Check for:	Check ongoing losses and estimate amounts. Check for:	Check for:
• dehydration	• vomiting and NG tube loss	• gross oedema
• fluid overload	• biliary drainage loss	• severe sepsis
• hyperkalaemia/ hypokalaemia	• high/low volume ileal stoma loss	• hypernatraemia/ hyponatraemia
Estimate deficits or excesses.	• diarrhoea/excess colostomy loss	• renal, liver and/or cardiac impairment.
	• ongoing blood loss, e.g. melaena	• post-operative fluid retention and redistribution
	• sweating/fever/dehydration	• malnourished and refeeding issues
	• pancreatic/jejunal fistula/stoma loss	Seek expert help if necessary and estimate requirements.
	• urinary loss, e.g. post AKI polyuria.	

Prescribe by adding to or subtracting from routine maintenance, adjusting for all other sources of fluid and electrolytes (oral, enteral and drug prescriptions)

Monitor and reassess fluid and biochemical status by clinical and laboratory monitoring

'Intravenous fluid therapy in adults in hospital', NICE clinical guideline 174 (December 2013)

Figure 18.3 Algorithms for IV fluid therapy in adults (*continued*)

Fluid volume excess

Fluid volume excess or hypervolemia is an increase in sodium levels and retention of water. Hypervolemia can be due to a reduction of homeostatic mechanisms but it is most likely to occur due to the retention of sodium because of an underlying condition, such as renal failure, heart failure, and cirrhosis of the liver. Other causes are inappropriate administration of intravenous fluids containing sodium, fluid shifts, e.g. treatment of burns and prolonged corticosteroid therapy. Treatment is dependent on the cause and symptoms are treated by the administration of diuretics and fluids and sodium restriction (Table 18.7). The selection of diuretic is dependent on the severity of the hypervolemia, and the degree of renal function impairment.

Table 18.7 **Hypervolemia and diuretics for adults**

Signs and symptoms of hypervolemia in adults	Diuretics for adults
■ Distended jugular veins ■ Shortness of breath, crackles and cough ■ Acute weight gain ■ Peripheral oedema and ascites ■ Increased Central Venous Pressure (if in place) ■ Elevated BP, bounding pulse, increased respiratory rate ■ Increased urine output	■ Thiazides such as Bendrofluazide, Metolazone are prescribed for mild to moderate hypervolemia ■ Loop diuretics such as Furosemide, Bumetanide, and Torasemide are used for severe hypervolemia ■ Potassium sparing, e.g. Amiloride target cortical collecting ducts. Diuretics may cause electrolyte disturbances including hyponatremia and hypokalaemia and may require potassium supplements

Oedema

Oedema is swelling caused by excess interstitial fluid (Figure 18.4). There are different causative mechanisms: hydrostatic pressure builds in the vessels, forcing fluid into the tissues; decrease in colloid osmotic pressure due to low levels of protein in the plasma, e.g. malnutrition; tissue trauma, e.g. burns; inflammation which causes the capillaries to be more permeable and obstruction to the lymph flow.

In adults. oedema may be visible only in areas such as the sacrum and buttocks when the patient is lying down, or in the legs and feet when the patient is standing. Oedema in children tends to present as swelling in the feet, hands and face. With certain underlying conditions, overall swelling can be observed.

Pitting oedema is seen when, after pressure is applied to a small area, the indentation persists after the release of the pressure (Figure 18.4). It is evaluated on a scale of 1+ (minimal) to 4+ (severe). Weight gain occurs due to fluid retention (every 0.5 L of fluid gained equates to 0.5 kg weight gain). An increase in weight of 5–10 per cent indicates mild-to-moderate fluid gain; an increase of more than 10 per cent is severe fluid gain.

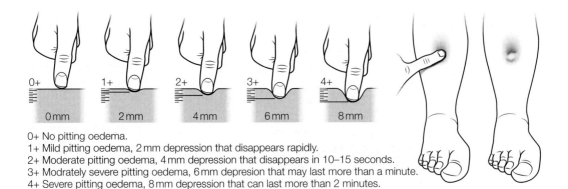

0+ No pitting oedema.
1+ Mild pitting oedema, 2 mm depression that disappears rapidly.
2+ Moderate pitting oedema, 4 mm depression that disappears in 10–15 seconds.
3+ Modrately severe pitting oedema, 6 mm depresion that may last more than a minute.
4+ Severe pitting oedema, 8 mm depression that can last more than 2 minutes.

Figure 18.4 Oedema

Procedure for recording fluid intake and output measurement

Any patient who has signs and symptoms of fluid imbalance should have their fluid intake and output monitored. Fluid balance should be calculated more frequently if acutely ill. Other indications include: infusions; enteral feeding; nasogastric tubes in place or urinary catherisation.

1   Explain what you will do and gain patient consent.
2   Wash your hands and adhere to standard infection control.
3   Emphasise to the patient and family the importance of measuring all intake and output accurately. Show them the fluid balance chart and demonstrate how to record fluid intake and output on it. If possible, they can participate in this aspect of care.
4   If they wish, provide a measuring jug for fluid intake. Ask the patient to keep a notebook of their fluid intakes (time and volume).
5   Observe for a measure any enteral or parenteral intake and add these to get a cumulative total for intake. The following should also be included: fluid taken with medication; foods that are liquid at room temperature, e.g. ice cream; intravenous medications prepared with solutions; catheter irrigations; and blood transfusions.
6   Fluid output ought to also be recorded as accurately as possible:
  ▪ Urine ought to be measured or weighed
  ▪ Estimate the amount if the patient is incontinent
  ▪ Weigh nappies for infants
  ▪ Measure/weigh liquid faeces, vomit, tube and wound drainage
  ▪ In addition, a urinary output of an adult less than 0.5 mL/kg/hr less than 2 mL/kg/hr for an infant and 1 mL/kg/hr for a child must be reported immediately.

Insensible losses such as sweat or breathing vapour cannot be recorded; however, a daily loss of approximately 800–1000 ml is normal. Patients with burns and fever will have much higher insensible losses and the appreciation of this will rely on clinical judgement. If in doubt, do weigh the patient (at the same time per day). Significant gains or losses in weight will indicate the fluid gained or lost.

Fluid balance is the difference between the total fluid intake and the total fluid output. This should be calculated at the same time every day and needs to be monitored throughout the day. Figure 18.5 shows an incomplete fluid balance chart. What problems can you see in the fluid balance chart?

INACCURATE FLUID BALANCE CHART ⊗

08.00	Oral output	IVI input	Cumulative input	Urine output	Bowels output	Vomit output	Cumulative output
08.00	Tea	100ml??		PU+++	Diarrhoea		?
09.00							
10.00	H20	50ml					
11.00		Tissued				+++	
12.00				Urine output	Soiled bed linen		
13.00		Venflon sited					
14.00							
15.00	Tea	200ml?? Pump not working			80+++		
16.00							
17.00	Juice						

Figure 18.5 Incomplete fluid balance chart

Watch out

Accurate recording of fluid balance is important and patient-specific parameters, including minimum/maximum intake, acceptable urine output, and target fluid balance are needed. Monitoring a patient's fluid balance is a relatively simple task, but recording is often inadequately or inaccurately completed (Bennett, 2010). A study by Perren *et al.* (2011) suggested cumulative fluid balance charts are not accurate and their use should be questioned particularly for critical care patients.

Restoring fluid balance

In mild dehydration, patients are encouraged and assisted to drink more fluids. If unable to do this independently, assistance is provided, e.g. handing cups. Patients must be informed of the target fluid intake and a variety of fluids provided, allowing for the preferences of the patient. Some fluids have a diuretic effect and this is taken into consideration, e.g. tea. Fluids need to be accessible, and made available at regular intervals and between meals. Box 18.2 describes a kidney campaign focusing on hydration.

Box 18.2 Hydration Matters

NHS Kidney Care launched the Hydration Matters campaign in June 2012 to increase awareness of the importance of correct hydration for patients. Its aim was to encourage healthcare staff to monitor fluid balance and take steps to prevent acute kidney injury and other avoidable health complications. Findings included:

- 20–30 per cent of acute kidney injury cases could be avoided or prevented;
- Identification of the patients particularly at risk – are you actively monitoring their fluid balance?
- Fluids are as important as any medication on the prescription chart
- Don't just observe and record any deterioration – act immediately to remedy it.

Parenteral fluid and electrolyte replacement

For some patients, the administration of fluid and electrolytes must be via the parenteral route. Commonly this is intravenously (IV) administered and solutions enter the extracellular compartment directly, which enables efficient and effective delivery. IV fluids are generally prescribed by a doctor but the management of IV therapy is a common nursing responsibility. An infusion is an amount of fluid more than 100 mls for parenteral infusion and administered over a period of time. Continuous infusion is the IV delivery of a fluid at a constant rate over a prescribed period of time. Intermittent infusion is the administration of a small volume infusion, i.e. 50–250 ml over a period of between 20 minutes and 2 hours.

Route of administration

IV fluids may be administered via a variety of lines/catheters:

- Adult peripheral venous catheter or cannula (PVC)
- Central venous catheters (CVCs)
- Skin tunnelled catheters (STC) incorporating implantable ports/Portacaths
- Peripherally inserted central lines (PICC).

Clinical significance

IV solutions can be classified as isotonic, hypotonic or hypertonic. Isotonic solutions are similar in composition (or osmolality) to serum or other body fluids, e.g., 0.9% sodium chloride (normal saline) or 5% glucose is isotonic.

Don't forget!

When monitoring an IV infusion, observe the following:

- Appearance of the PVC infusion site and patency
- Type of fluid infused and rate of flow/rate of electronic infusion
- Response of patient, it can be dramatic in the young or the elderly so close monitoring is needed.

Major complications of IV therapy

IV fluids are given for a variety of reasons but due consideration needs to be given to their use as it can be associated with complications.

- Cannula occlusion/damage
- Infiltration – leakage of non-irritant fluid into tissues surrounding the vein
- Extravastation – infiltration of irritant fluid that cause tissue damage
- Thrombophlebitis
- Pulmonary/air embolism
- Bleeding/haematoma
- Drug error
- Pain
- Shock/fluid overload
- Physical or chemical incompatibility/interaction.

Infection prevention in IV line management

EPIC3 guidelines (Loveday *et al.*, 2014) provide comprehensive recommendations for preventing healthcare-acquired infections in hospital and other acute care settings, based on the best currently available evidence.

- Replace all tubing when the vascular device is changed
- All IV-giving sets for peripheral and central use should be changed every 72 hours unless more frequently is indicated clinically
- Replace blood and blood products IV-giving sets every 12 hours and after every second unit of blood
- Discard intermittent infusions sets immediately after use.

Fluid administration sets

An administration set is used to administer fluids via an infusion bag into the vascular access device. The set contains a number of components as detailed in Figure 18.6. The rationale for preparing and monitoring infusion sets and devices is to ensure patients are given the appropriate treatment, over the appropriate period and in a safe manner. There are a variety of sets dependent on the solution to be administered, e.g. crystalloids, blood. As equipment varies according to the manufacturer, the nurse must be familiar with the equipment used in the hospital/care environment. The 'drips' of fluid will vary in size (i.e. volume) and this will affect the rate at which they can be infused. In normal administration sets for clear fluids, each mL of fluid is determined as 20 drops. Do check the packaging as it will clearly indicate how many drops are in a mL and this knowledge is necessary when calculating flow rates.

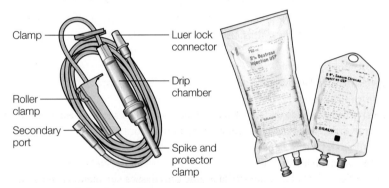

Figure 18.6 (a) and (b) **Fluid administration sets**

Infusion devices

An infusion device is designed to accurately deliver measured amounts of fluid over a period of time. With a gravity device, the roller clamp is used to control the flow which is measured by counting the drops. With a gravity drip rate controller, the desired flow rate is set in drops per minute and controlled by battery or valves.

Infusion pumps use pressure to overcome resistance along the fluid pathway, and pump fluid from the infusion bag via an administration set and calculate the volume delivered. Syringe pumps are low-volume, high-accuracy devices designed to infuse at low flow rates. When choosing an appropriate device, the nurse needs to understand the risk factors to the patient (under-/over-infusion, uneven flow); delivery parameters (accuracy required, infusion rate and volume required) and environmental features (ease of operation, type of patient, child, and neonate).

Watch out

As a point of added safety and best practice, children and young people are connected to electronic pump intravenous infusions and do not have gravity flow infusions.

Procedure for the administration of IV fluids

1 Prepare the work surface and assemble all the necessary equipment.
2 Wash hands and dry hands as per local policy and put on appropriate protective clothing.
3 Maintain hand hygiene.
4 Check the identity of the patient using positive patient identification, the name band and the prescription chart. Two checkers are generally required for IV therapy and one must be a qualified member of staff.
5 Explain the need for IV therapy and the effect of the infusion, using simple, clear language appropriate to their age and understanding.
6 Evaluate the patient's understanding and knowledge of the infusion to be given.
7 Obtain verbal consent. If the patient is a child or someone who cannot give consent, ensure you obtain the parent's/carer's consent.
8 Check that the prescription is complete, correct and legible and indicates the rate of flow or time over which infusion is to be completed.
9 Check name, strength, volume and expiry date of intravenous infusion fluid against the prescription chart.
10 Check that packaging of infusion fluid is intact and inspect the contents for any signs of discoloration, cloudiness or particulate matter.
11 Ensure that you have the correct administration set for the fluid to be administered, do note different administration sets are required for blood, blood products and for electronic devices. Check their expiry date too.
12 Open the packaging and uncoil the tubing: do not let the ends of the tubing become contaminated. Close the clamp by rolling the wheel away from the spiked end.
13 Remove the protective covering from the port of the fluid bag and the protective covering from the spike of the administration set. Do not touch this part – maintain asepsis.
14 Insert the spike of the administration set into the port of the fluid bag, ensuring it is inserted fully.
15 Hang the solution bag on an IV hanger or stand so that it is suspended at the height of approximately 1 metre above the patient's head. Squeeze the drip chamber gently until it is half full of solution. If the chamber is overfilled, lower the bag below the level of the drip chamber and squeeze some fluid back into the fluid bag.
16 Open the roller clamp and allow the fluid to slowly fill the giving set. Loosen or remove the cap at the end of the tubing to get the fluid to flow to the end of the tubing.
17 Tap the tubing to help move the bubbles.
18 When all the air is expelled, close the roller clamp.
19 Maintain sterility of connection and tip of the administration set at all times.
20 The primed administration set can be connected to an electronic device, or the rate can be determined by gravity flow together with the flow clamp.
21 Take the infusion to the bedside on a clinically clean receptacle, i.e. trolley.
22 Check the identity of the patient using the name band, prescription chart and the infusion container.
23 Explain and outline the procedure with the patient.

24 Inspect the PVC infusion site for signs of infection or blockage.

25 Wash hands. The PVC must be cleaned before the administration set line end is attached, to minimise infection risk.

26 Flush venous access to ensure line is patent – do check this step in the local policy.

27 Connect the infusion to the patient using a non-touch technique and lock into position.

28 Secure the tubing with tape to prevent pulling.

29 Commence the new infusion and adjust the rate of flow as prescribed (see calculations below).

30 Ask the patient if they are experiencing any abnormal sensations or reactions.

31 Document the process and all equipment and initiate a fluid chart document.

32 Explain the procedure for maintaining a fluid balance chart to the patient.

33 Dispose of all equipment safely, making sure that it is placed in correct containers, e.g. needles into 'sharps' box, clinical waste in clinical waste bags.

34 Wash and dry hands.

Calculating flow rate in drops per minute (Adult IV infusions)

The prescription for IV infusions can take several forms, e.g. 3000 mls over 24 hours. The nurse calculates the correct flow rate, regulates the infusion and monitors the patient's response. If it is a simple gravity infusion, calculation of the rate in drops per minute is necessary.

$$\frac{\text{Volume of infusion in mL} \times \text{number of drops per mL}}{\text{Time in minutes}} = \text{flow rate in drops per minute}$$

The number of drops per ml will be determined by the administration set being used and is indicated on the packaging. This is the drop factor and is commonly 10, 12, 15 or 20 drops/ml.

Example

A patient is prescribed 600 mLs of 0.9% sodium chloride over 6 hours using a standard administration set with a drop factor of 20 drops per mL.

$$\frac{600 \text{ (volume of infusion)} \times 20 \text{ number of drops per mL}}{360 \text{ (6 hours} \times 60 \text{ minutes)}} = 33.33 \text{ drops/min}$$
$$\text{(round down to 33)}$$

Calculating flow rate in millilitres per hour

Hourly rates of infusion can be calculated by dividing the total infusion volume by the total infusion time in hours.

Example

A patient is prescribed 2000 mLs to be administered over 8 hours.

$$\frac{2000 \text{ (total infusion volume)}}{8 \text{ (total infusion time)}} = 250 \text{ mLs/hour}$$

Activity 18.5

- An adult patient is receiving IV therapy (1 litre of sodium chloride 0.9%) for rehydration. The bag of fluid is prescribed to be administered over 8 hours. What is the drip rate per minute?
- It is observed that the patient has had 600 mL of the bag after just 4 hours. What is the revised drip rate to get this therapy back on track?
- What actions would you take?

Answers:

1   Example 1: 41.66 (round up to 47 drops/min).
2   Example 2: 50 drops/min.
3   Example 3: This is urgent. Record how much had been completed on the medication chart and patient notes, monitor patient for signs of over- or under-hydration state or distress. Observe for signs of the cannula being erratic, i.e. flow varies. Ask the patient is anyone has interfered with the administration set. Calculate the revised drop rate and report to the nurse in charge and doctor, ensuring the infusion is running now to time and the senior staff are aware of your observations and actions.

Complications of PVC and IV therapy

- Catheter-related bloodstream infection: where micro-organisms are introduced into the bloodstream via the PVC and cause bacteraemia
- Extravasation: this is where a vesicant (vein damaging) solution is administered into surrounding tissue
- Haemorrhage: bleeding occurs at puncture site
- Infiltration: non-vesicant solution is administered into surrounding tissue
- Phlebitis: The tunica intima is inflamed.

Care of a PVC site

When a person, either an adult or a child, has an IV infusion, it is recommended that the PVC is sited in the non-dominant arm and not at the position of the antecubital fossa (elbow) or anywhere it can be easily dislodged. The gauge of the cannula must be appropriate for the fluid being administered (i.e. the diameter of the bore). As this is an invasive device, it needs to be monitored and changed if necessary to avoid infection or penetrating and damaging tissues.

The PVC dressing protects the puncture site and minimises the risk of infection between the peripheral cannula surface and the skin. The PVC insertion site is an open wound so the dressing must be sterile and applied using non-touch aseptic technique to prevent contamination. PVC dressings must be replaced when they become; damp, loosened, no longer occlusive or adherent, visibly soiled, or if there is excessive accumulation of fluid under the dressing.

PVC sites ought to be observed whenever:

1   A bolus injection is given.
2   An administration set is changed.
3   Flow rates are checked or altered.

Jackson (1998) developed an assessment scale to indicate the onset of phlebitis termed the Visual Infusion of Phlebitis Score (VIP score) and this gives a practical numerical score to determine when the PVC needs changing. An adapted version can be found at: www.vipscore.net/wp-content/uploads/2012/04/002-IV3000-A4-score-and-vein-card. pdf.

Procedure for removal of peripheral IV cannulae (PVC)

The PVC must be removed in less than 72 hours or when clinically indicated. Removal must be carried out under aseptic conditions as the risks of potential infection remain. The following principles must be applied:

1   Wash and dry hands in accordance with local policy and put on appropriate protective clothing.
2   Maintain hand hygiene.
3   Wear non-sterile gloves and a disposable apron.
4   Remove the dressing by lifting and stretching the dressing towards the nurse to break the dressing integrity and loosen it.
5   Gently remove the PVC.
6   Immediately following the removal of the PVC, apply firm pressure with sterile gauze for 2–3 minutes or until the bleeding has stopped.
7   Cover the puncture site with a sterile, adhesive dressing.
8   Discuss any signs of phlebitis with medical staff and document in the patient's nursing records in conjunction with any treatment/actions taken.
9   Record removal date on Peripheral Cannula Insertion and On-going Care Record sheet or patient notes.
10 Where venous access is limited, the PVC can remain in place for longer than 72 hours, providing there are no signs of infection, and a risk assessment is undertaken regularly and documented.

Blood transfusion

Blood transfusion is one of the clinical skills student nurses can take part in, but it is an advanced practice which may only be undertaken by registered practitioners who have undergone the specified training and assessment, who accept accountability for their actions and who feel competent to undertake the aspect of care. In many areas a senior student nurse can be the second checker with a registered nurse or midwife, provided the registered nurse/midwife is satisfied they are competent to do so. In paediatric areas, blood transfusions and products are usually checked by two qualified staff. It is always advisable to check what the local policy is for the area you work in. Blood transfusion involves the administration of prepared, compatible blood or blood components directly into the recipient's bloodstream via an IV route.

Blood group

A person's blood group is identified by antigens and antibodies present in the blood. Antigens and antibodies are the blood's natural defences against foreign substances. Blood types are inherited and represent contributions from both parents. The International Society of Blood Transfusion states there are four main ones; O, A, B, and AB. The most important blood group system in blood transfusions is the Rhesus system. Each group can be either RhD positive or RhD negative, which means that the blood group can be one of eight types. If this antigen is not present, the blood group is negative, but if the antigen is present, the blood group is known as positive. Figure 18.7 shows blood type compatibility.

Blood types

Blood type	Antigen on red blood cells	Antibodies in plasma	Blood types	Blood types
A	A	anti-B	O and A	A and AB
B	B	anti-A	O and B	B and AB
AB	A and B	neither	O, A, B, and AB	AB only
O	neither	anti-A and anti-B	O only	O, A, B, and AB

Figure 18.7 **Blood group compatibility**

Blood products

Transfusions of blood, blood components and blood products must be requested from the Blood Transfusion laboratory on an individual named patient basis. The use of blood components rather than whole blood has many advantages and is a more efficient use of the blood supply. The patient receives only a specific component which is indicated by their condition, e.g., and a patient with anaemia will only receive red blood cells. Whole blood is indicated if a patient has had significant blood loss and blood volume needs to be restored. Drugs are *never* added to a bag of blood (Figure 18.8).

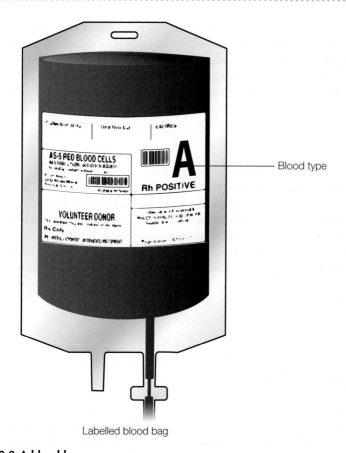

Blood type

Labelled blood bag

Figure 18.8 **A blood bag**

Blood prescription

Generally written consent is not required but patients must be fully informed and give verbal consent to a transfusion and this ought to be documented. Some patients have a cultural and religious objection to receiving a blood transfusion. Blood, blood components or blood products may only be transfused on prescription by a registered medical practitioner. Blood products are in the BNF and a non-medical prescriber (nurse, or other practitioner trained in this skill) may prescribe certain blood products if this is in their area of clinical speciality. A blood sample is required from the patient and the practitioner initially needs to perform a 'cross-match' or check with the patient's blood group. The prescription should specify the date, correct product, quantity required, duration of transfusion, special requirements and any special precautions.

Checking and collection procedure

Red blood cells are stored at 2–6° C, as red cells are damaged at low temperature, and at high temperature there is a tendency for bacterial growth. Platelets are stored at 20–24°

C and gently agitated in the laboratory. Fresh frozen plasma is kept at -30° C, is thawed in the laboratory and should be infused immediately once thawed. It is important that local guidelines are followed to ensure safety in relation to withdrawing blood from the blood bank and its transfer to the clinical area.

Pre-transfusion

Check the following:

- The blood is correctly and legibly prescribed
- The patient/child has patent PVC access
- Discuss the reason for the transfusion with the patient/child/parent
- The indication for the transfusion should be written in the patient's notes by the doctor prescribing the blood component.

Blood must be collected by a member of staff trained in the checking procedure using the blood prescription chart.

Pre-administration

- Check the blood unit or bag is intact and the prescription chart for any special requirements, e.g. for any concomitant drugs such as diuretics
- Check and document patient baseline observations
- Check the expiry date of component blood or blood product and check bag for leaks, discoloration or clumping
- Compatibility checking must be performed by two people at the bedside
- Complete compatibility labels which accompany the blood product and each nurse must sign it and add the date and the time. There will also be a label to attach to a 'Record of Transfusion' form or prescription form, which is then included in the clinical notes as part of the contemporary medical/surgical record.

Administration

Blood and blood products are administered via a blood administration set which has a filter. Platelets are administered via specialist sets. Only electronic infusion pumps that are specified as safe with blood components by the manufacturer must be used, as infusion pumps can damage blood cells. When rapid transfusion is necessary, blood may be warmed during administration using a blood warmer which warms the blood as it passes over a heater element.

Watch out

No identification, then no blood!

Procedure for administration of blood transfusion

1 Following consent, prepare the equipment and remind the patient what you are going to do.

2 Record and document the baseline reading of the patient's temperature, pulse, respiration, blood pressure before the start of each unit. (Report any abnormalities to medical staff and only proceed if they consider this to be appropriate.)

3 Check that the blood/blood component has not passed its expiry date and will not expire during the transfusion episode (that is midnight of the expiry date as stated on the bag).

4 Put on apron, wash hands and put on gloves.

5 Blood should be transfused through a sterile administration set designed for the procedure. The set has a double chamber and must contain a 170-micron filter.

6 Prime the blood administration set with prescribed 0.9% sodium chloride.

7 Attach the administration set to the venous access device, or if using a volumetric IV infusion pump, place the administration set in the infusion pump following the manufacturer's guidelines. Set the rate and volume to be infused as stated on the fluid chart.

8 The two staff members carrying out the patient identity checks and administering the blood must sign the fluid chart prescription, adding the date and time of the commencement of each transfusion.

9 The patient must be observed carefully for 15 minutes after each unit has been connected as this is when a reaction is most likely to occur. During this time the blood component should be infused slowly.

10 Vital signs of temperature, pulse and blood pressure must be recorded; 5, 15, 30, and 60 minutes after infusion begins; and then hourly until infusion is complete and then checked at the end of the transfusion (check hospital blood administration policy and procedure for frequency of observations)

11 Patients must be transfused in an area where they can be readily observed and they should have a call button to obtain assistance.

12 The transfusion should be completed in less than 4 hours and the start and completion time should be recorded.

13 The rate of transfusion should be monitored throughout.

14 Observe urine output volume and colour.

15 The patient should be observed carefully for evidence of a reaction: pain at site of transfusion, loin pain, chest pain, breathing difficulties, anxiety, hypotension (more common in adults than children), collapse, rashes, rigors, or rise in temperature.

16 Report a $1°C$ rise in temperature.

17 In any of these events IMMEDIATELY stop the transfusion and inform the medical staff. The following actions may be taken but need to be prescribed:
a Slow the transfusion.
b Loosen bedclothes/clothing.
c If prescribed, offer analgesia.
d If prescribed, offer antihistamines.

18 Accurately record the quantity of blood administered.

19 Dispose of equipment safely and appropriately following the procedure.

20 Empty blood bags should be kept and sent back to the laboratory.

Table 18.8 shows the adverse effects of transfusion.

Table 18.8 Adverse effects of transfusion on adults and children

Adverse effects in adults	Adverse effects in children
■ Febrile	■ Febrile
■ Urticarial Reaction (rash)	■ Urticarial rash (itchy rash)
■ Anaphylaxis	■ Anaphylaxis
■ Acute haemolytic reaction	■ Pruritus/severe itching of the skin
■ Bacterial contamination	■ Nausea and vomiting
■ Hypothermia	■ Diarrhoea and stomach cramps
■ Potassium imbalance	■ Hypotension (less common)
	■ Increased diastolic BP (associated with febrile non-haemolytic transfusion reaction)
	■ Dyspnoea/shortness of breath (less common)

Don't forget!

Visual observation of the patient is often the best way of assessing the patient during the transfusion. Unconscious patients are more difficult to monitor for signs of transfusion reactions. Try not to start infusions late in the evening (after 20.00h) for patient comfort and so they can easily obtain help if they are having a reaction. A decision chart for transfusion reactions can be found at: www.bcshguidelines.com/documents/ATR_final_version_to_pdf.pdf.

Summary

Patients at times need support and advice on hydration which is essential for optimum functioning. Hydration encompasses water and electrolytes and balance needs to be maintained. Replacement of fluids may be required and one means is via intravenous infusion. Furthermore, this route may also be used for replacement of blood and this gives rise to further nursing challenges and skilled care.

References

Bennett, C. (2010) *'At a Glance' Fluid Balance Bar Chart.* London: NHS Institute for Innovation and Improvement.

Campbell, N. (2011) Dehydration: why is it still a problem? *Nursing Times,* 107(22): 12–15.

Care Quality Commission (2011) *Dignity and Nutrition for Older People: Review of Compliance.* London: CQC.

Chow, J. and Douglas, D. (2008) Fluid and electrolyte management in the premature infant. *Neonatal Network,* 6: 379–386.

EFSA (European Food Safety Authority) (2010) Scientific opinion on dietary reference values for water. EFSA Panel on Dietetic Products, Nutrition, and Allergies. *EFSA Journal*, 8(3): 1459.

Jackson, A. (1998) Infection control: a battle in vein infusion phlebitis. *Nursing Times*; 94(4): 68–71.

Loveday, H.P., Wilson, J.A., Pratt, R.J., *et al.* (2014) epic3: National Evidence-Based Guidelines for Preventing Healthcare-Associated Infections in NHS Hospitals in England, *Journal of Hospital Infection*, 86(S1): S1–S70.

NHS Surrey (2010) Available at: www.surreyi.gov.uk/(F(rdrdwvdr0QPY49PblJseROhBfSw-btGEp_oY4o_WWximyL-Zl03qC8OAD7YEc2MR3cx5e47Z_SYYI9w0zOZtPdBLsVk HZOn1mYJC8ST8E1wd3phu7_DRYi3D5K4Q3K3EXOGRJg2))/get/ShowResourceFile. aspx?ResourceID=419 (accessed 1 March 2016).

NICE (National Institute for Clinical Excellence) (2009) *Diarrhoea and Vomiting in Children: Diarrhoea and Vomiting Caused by Gastroenteritis: Diagnosis, Assessment and Management in Children Younger Than 5 Years*. Clinical guideline no. 84. London: NICE.

NICE (National Institute for Clinical Excellence) (2012) *Patient experiences in adult NHS services: Improving the experience of care for people using adult NHS services*. Available at: www.nice.org.uk/guidance/cg138/chapter/quality-statements (accessed 1 March 2016).

NICE (National Institute for Clinical Excellence) (2013) Intravenous Fluid Therapy in Adults in Hospital. Clinical Guideline no. CG174. London: NICE.

NMC (2010) *Standards for Pre-Registration Nursing Education*. London: NMC.

NPSA (National Patient Safety Agency) (2007) *Safer Care for the Acutely Ill Patient: Learning from Serious Incidents*. London: NPSA.

Perren, A., Markman, M., Merlani, G., Marone, C. and Merlani, P.L. (2011) Fluid balance in critically ill patients: should we rely on it? *Minerva Anestesiologica*, 77(8): 802–811.

Royal College of Nursing, National Patient Safety Agency (2007) *Water for Health. Hydration Best Practice Toolkit for Hospitals and Healthcare*. London: RCN/NPSA.

Thibodeau, G.A. and Patton, K.T. (2012) *Structure & Function of the Body*, 14th edn. St. Louis, MO: Mosby.

Waugh, A. (2007) Problems associated with fluid, electrolyte and acid-base balance. In C. Brooker and M. Nicol (eds) *Nursing Adults: The Practice of Caring*. St Louis, MO: Mosby.

Welch, K. (2010) Fluid balance. *Learning Disability Practice*, 13(6): 33–38.

Index

Please note that page numbers relating to Boxes will be in italics followed by the letter 'B; those relating to Figures will be in italics followed by the letter 'f', while numbers indicating Tables will be in the same format but contain the letter 't'.